INTRODUCTION TO EVIDENCE-BASED PRACTICE AND QUALITY IMPROVEMENT FOR PROFESSIONAL NURSING PRACTICE

INTRODUCTION TO EVIDENCE-BASED PRACTICE AND QUALITY IMPROVEMENT FOR PROFESSIONAL NURSING PRACTICE

A COMPETENCY-BASED APPROACH

Jayne Jennings Dunlap
Texas Woman's University
&
Julee Briscoe Waldrop, Editors
Duke University

cognella®
SAN DIEGO

Bassim Hamadeh, CEO and Publisher
Amanda Martin, Executive Publisher
Amy Smith, Senior Project Editor
Casey Hands, Production Editor
Emely Villavicencio, Senior Graphic Designer
Kylie Bartolome, Licensing Specialist
Stephanie Adams, Senior Marketing Program Manager
Natalie Piccotti, Director of Marketing
Kassie Graves, Senior Vice President, Editorial

Printed in the United States of America.

cognella® | ACADEMIC PUBLISHING
320 South Cedros Ave., Ste. 400, Solana Beach, CA 92075

To my grandmother, Violet Timm Angell, a humble nurse's aide who was at her best in uniform. Violet took pride in ensuring every patient entrusted to her care was left in optimal condition at the end of each shift. She would have loved the chance to become a nurse.

To my parents, John and Jolie Jennings, whose unwavering support and hard work provided unlikely opportunities. To my husband and touchstone, Brian, whose unyielding faith and love have shown me not to fear the unknown. To our children, Addison and Weston, my two greatest sources of inspiration and who I am most proud of.

To the reader holding this textbook: You will touch countless lives throughout your career as a nurse. May you be the one to ensure the patient is the most important person during all healthcare encounters. Follow the evidence closely and carry our noble, most-trusted profession forward through fostering your own best practices.

—Jayne Jennings Dunlap

To my family, Tony (posthumously), Mom, Dad, Joe, Jennifer, Cabe, Dallas, Courtney, Cathe, Penny, and Oliver, who love and support me even if they disagree with my choices sometimes.

To my professional mentors in nursing: Linda D'Angelo, the first nurse practitioner leader I met, who encouraged me to keep learning. To Jennifer D'Auria, who gave me the confidence to seek a clinical practice as an attending in a pediatric residency program and later become the medical director of a newborn nursery. To Linda Beeber, who taught me about being a member of a research team and that as an expert clinician I had a place on the team. To Barbara Turner, who is still teaching me how to be a leader, in all ways.

To my partner and inspiration in the birth of this book, Jayne Jennings Dunlap.

—Julee Briscoe Waldrop

BRIEF CONTENTS

DETAILED CONTENTS

CHAPTER 8 Patient Preferences and Values 141

Elizabeth Miller Walters, Francisco Ayala, and Kathleen Ellis

CHAPTER 9 Fundamentals of Quality Improvement for Nurses 153

Staci S. Reynolds and Bradi B. Granger

Foreword

In today's world where there appears to be less trust in science and less importance placed on evidence-based practice, this is the perfect time for *Introduction to Evidence-Based Practice and Quality Improvement for Professional Nursing Practice: A Competency Based Approach* to be published. Almost daily, healthcare is undergoing dramatic changes and challenges. As we embrace new technologies, procedures, and policies, we are also obligated to evaluate their effectiveness on patient outcomes and healthcare costs. Thus, it is necessary to have not only a working knowledge of research basics but also a comprehension of the role evidence-based practice and quality improvement (EBPQI) can play in driving and promoting such outcomes.

The contents of this transformational book are written in a format that encourages and empowers those who may be hesitant to undertake EBPQI projects because of their uneasiness with the fundamentals of basic research and quality improvement methods. It is also written in a fashion that the novice and experienced nurse alike can find useful in their pursuit of quality improvement projects. It uses a step-by-step approach that guides and assists the reader to develop confidence in their ability to undertake EBPQI projects. The unique feature of this book is that it seems as though the authors are holding your hand and having a one-on-one conversation with the reader, guiding and stimulating their analytical curiosity. It challenges readers to be inquisitive nurses when undertaking quality improvement initiatives. Every detail regarding research methodology, evidence-based practice, and quality improvement is explored, explained, and discussed. Other benefits of this book include the intangible way in which it enhances the clinician's ability to see the benefits and rewards of clinical research and quality improvement projects and their ability to make lasting contributions to the nursing profession. A very unique feature of this book is the use of the Wellness in Action boxes at the end of each chapter. These boxes inspire the learner to consider and explore the many facets of social determinants of health, health promotion, and the need for self-care. Afterall, better health outcomes equal lower healthcare costs, a renewed trust in science, and further supports why we need evidence-based practice and quality improvement.

Ernest J. Grant, PhD, RN, FAAN

Editors' Note to Readers

Message From Jayne

Our main purpose in writing this textbook was to introduce foundational evidence-based practice and quality improvement (EBPQI) competencies to undergraduate nursing students. For several decades, entry-level nursing students have been taught basic research methodologies to the exclusion of EBPQI during undergraduate curriculum. I was one of those students, and when I entered nursing practice, I lacked some of the necessary skills to critically appraise evidence and decide how best to provide care to my patients. I committed to harnessing these skills, and as I have continued to refine them, I long for new nursing students to learn these competencies before entering the profession. I am not alone in this timely longing, and as we now make the paradigm shift away from teaching entry-level nurses about research conduction and toward EBPQI competency throughout our discipline, a first edition text focused on these fundamental principles is necessary. This textbook is mapped to the 2021 American Association of Colleges of Nursing's *The Essentials: Core Competencies for Professional Nursing Education* (see Appendix A) and is likely very different from what you have seen throughout the market to date. We hope this material is adopted and used all over the globe with attention to the local context and educational and practice requirements, with a focus on providing high-quality care based on the best currently available evidence.

Julee and I initially set out to complete this work in third-person language; however, once we began writing, we decided to address our important readership (you) in the first person. Our chapter contributors followed this example, and our collective hope is that the change from a more traditional academic writing approach will increase your engagement and interest in learning the critical content presented throughout this book. We have also included our own brief stories to share why we became nurses so you can come to know us on a more personal level and consider this important question for yourself.

We are passionate about nurse wellness, which should start prior to joining the nursing workforce. With the belief that wellness is a state of action rather than a state of being, we want you to be equipped with wellness practices backed by evidence. You will find Wellness in Action boxes at the end of each chapter, which focus on research-based wellness strategies. These approaches will introduce you to several wellness domains and encourage you to establish and maintain a pattern of self-care now so you will be able to provide sustained patient care later. You can also access customizable information focused on personal evidence-based wellness plans (see Appendix B) to target an issue you might be currently facing.

We will be going through the steps of EBPQI in sequential order throughout each chapter and have included completed critical appraisals of different types of evidence using appraisal tools available online at no cost (Appendix C). We hope access to these completed examples will help you put it all together.

In this textbook there are references to the history of nursing, quality and safety, research and evidence-based practice, and quality improvement. Throughout this text we reference Florence Nightingale. We do this because she is known for being the first nurse to collect data and recognize it as evidence (i.e., hygiene principles) for improvement. We recognize that she was a woman of her times and some of her social ideas may not be well received in the present. There have been many other nurse pioneers in EBP and QI since then, and we thank all of them for lighting the way for us. I wish to recognize and thank the individuals below who have supported me through high-impact mentorship. Each one consistently wields their powerful influence toward evidence-based healthcare education and practice improvements.

Dr. Bernadette Melynk, EBP pioneer who has changed the world through her forward thinking, leadership, and steadfast dedication to patients and nurses.

Dr. Tracy Brewer, educator extraordinaire, clinical scholar, and EBP expert, who shared her idea for this work. Tracy's belief that an undergraduate textbook of this kind is needed now was one of its greatest drivers.

Dean Rosalie Mainous, who connected me with Tracy when I asked for external mentorship as a new faculty member. Rosalie is a true visionary who continues to demonstrate what authentic nursing leadership looks like.

Dean Paula Clutter, whose uncompromising ethical standards and commitment to excellence consistently lead nursing faculty and students to new heights.

Dr. Julee Briscoe Waldrop, human dynamo and gifted guide. Julee bravely agreed to mentor me when I found the courage to walk up to her and ask. Learning from Julee's bright mind and unmatched endurance promotes sustained curiosity and joy.

May you become beneficiaries of the generous investments of these individuals who have deeply inspired me as you participate in learning the content of this book. And may we all continue working with patient-centered dedication to move our profession forward together. Imagine the possibilities if we all commit to EBPQI competency throughout our varied practice settings.

Message From Julee

In her 2015 memoir *Year of Yes*, Shonda Rhimes explains how she has evolved into someone who spends all her time working (extremely hard and successfully) and is a single parent to her children. She doesn't have time or the energy to think about her own health or to have any fun. When her sister challenges her to say yes to something fun or exciting for a change, she balks but eventually decides to commit to saying yes to opportunities that are scary, not in a frightening way but in a way that says, "This will be a big challenge for me. Do I believe in myself enough to try?"

When Jayne asked me if I would co-edit this book with her, I had been working more than one job and was the sole caregiver for my terminally ill husband. My only self-care was a 45-minute run with my dog each day. How could I possibly add one more thing to my plate? I had also co-edited a book before and knew how stressful it could be. Why would I want to do that again? But because she is a dear friend and her vision for this textbook was innovative, I didn't just outright say no; I told her I had to think about it.

My best thinking time is when I am on a run. So, the next morning I thought about my answer. I was spending most of my day doing things I didn't love but needed to be done: going to meetings, caring for our home and my husband. Why shouldn't I do something that challenged me and that I believed in? Who better to do this than me? I gave myself a pep talk, and although I knew there would be challenges, I decided to say "yes."

We started work on the first chapter, and when it was partway written we both had the same nagging thought: "I want to write this in first person." So, we did, despite the advice from experts that textbooks are never to be written in first person. We won the experts over, and we hope we win you, our reader, over too. We wrote this from our nurse hearts, with the sincere belief that you will be a better nurse because you read this textbook. Its content is not going to help you start an intravenous line quicker or prevent infection with your sterile technique, but this content is the foundation for understanding all of the things that you do as a nurse and all of the things that you will do to improve health for your patients and yourself (especially if you read and consider and even do some of the things in the Wellness in Action boxes at the end of each chapter).

Saying yes to this textbook was a big commitment of time and energy, so I needed to also prioritize saying no as other requests came my way. Saying no is a self-care skill that I was not good at. My go-to was to always say yes, with the rationale that if I pleased or helped others, they would like me. Saying yes to this textbook really helped me learn to listen to my heart and taught me that if something was not going to serve me in the future and align with my values and goals, then it was ok to say, "Thank you for asking, but I respectfully decline." Over the past year, I have prioritized writing, editing, and revising this textbook over most other "work" because it was fun. Having fun while doing meaningful work with a purpose makes life worth living. Go live your best life, and make nursing a meaningful part of it—but not all of it.

REFERENCES

Rhimes, S. (2015). *Year of yes: How to dance it out, stand in the sun, and be your own person.* Simon & Schuster.

Acknowledgments

We wish to sincerely thank our chapter contributors and book reviewers for their meaningful work toward making our vision a reality.

Special thanks to Donna Lee Frega, PhD, RN, for her support and excitement about this project and her expert editing. Not only did she go through every word in the book, but she also admits to trying each one of the Wellness in Action box practices.

Reviewers

Donna L. Hamby, DNP, RN, ACNP-BCl
University of Texas Arlington, College of Nursing and Health Innovation

Cynthia D. Beckett, PhD, RNC-OB, LCCE, LSS-BB, CHRC, EBP-C
The Ohio State University College of Nursing/Helene Fuld Health Trust National Institute for Evidence-Based Practice in Nursing and Healthcare

Brenda C. Morris, EdD, RN, CNE, Clinical Professor of Nursing
Edson College of Nursing and Health Innovation, Arizona State University

Barb McClaskey, PhD, APRN-BC, RNC
Pittsburg State University, Pittsburg, Kansas

Andrea M. Smith, PhD, RN
School of Nursing, College of Health Sciences, Sam Houston State University

Amanda Lee Fischer, PhD, RN
Waynesburg University, Waynesburg, PA

CHAPTER 1

Setting the Stage for Clear Understanding of Research, Evidence-Based Practice, and Quality Improvement

Jayne Jennings Dunlap and Julee Briscoe Waldrop

KEY CONCEPTS

Research
Evidence-based practice (EBP)
EBP competencies
Inquiry
Quality improvement (QI)
Evidence-based practice quality improvement (EBPQI)

LEARNING OBJECTIVES

1. Explore the evolution of nursing research, EBP, and QI.
2. Differentiate between research, EBP, and QI.
3. Identify the practicing nurse's role as an EBP and QI team member.
4. Consider competency-based educational activities.
5. Discuss future directions for EBP and QI within the nursing discipline.

> Let whoever is in charge keep this simple question in her head (not, how can I always do this right thing myself but), how can I provide for this right thing to be always done.
>
> —Florence Nightingale (1859)

Introduction

"Why do you want to become a nurse?" This is one of the first questions we ask new nursing students. A very small number will reply that they seek job security, stable health insurance, or upward mobility in healthcare, but the vast majority offer patient-centered reasons for their career choice. Almost unanimously, new students recount a memorable experience involving a nurse as the impetus for their decision to enter the nursing field, recalling vividly why certain details of the encounter remain imprinted in their minds. If the experience was positive, the nurse likely served as a professional role model, and the student seeks the privilege of having a similar impact on others. If the experience was negative, the student often states that they have chosen the nursing profession to prevent harm or poor outcomes from happening to others.

Harm occurs in healthcare every single day, although as trained experts, care providers have a professional obligation to prevent and do no harm. Inaccurate or outdated practices cause poor patient outcomes and increased cost burdens (Institute of Medicine, 2000). Nurses are often at the forefront of care provision, where patients, families, and communities are most vulnerable, so we are well-positioned to advocate (support) for consistently delivering holistic healthcare practices to our patients. Our professional workforce has been chosen as the most trusted in healthcare for 20 straight years, eclipsing all others in ethics and honesty (Saad, 2022). We are dedicated to doing the right thing for our patients, yet given a constantly changing and rapidly evolving healthcare system, how can we "keep up" enough to determine the right thing to do? Hundreds of thousands of research papers are produced on a yearly basis; no one can read them all. It is possible to stay current and sustain a high quality of practice only by knowing how to search for quality evidence on which to base one's nursing practice.

For many decades, undergraduate nursing courses focused on teaching research methodologies to the exclusion of evidence-based practice (EBP) and quality improvement (QI). Although hospitals often have research and QI departments, the QI initiatives are not always evidence-based. Sadly, most nurses, including advanced practice nurses, do not feel competent in EBP (Melnyk et al., 2018), the prerequisite for QI. Nurses must be trained to take an EBP/QI approach to care delivery.

Throughout this textbook, in addition to gaining exposure to the basics of research, you will be introduced to evidence-based practice and quality improvement methods. These will be your mainstay mechanisms to change countless lives throughout your career as a registered nurse. We invite you to join us at the cutting edge of a paradigm shift toward nursing education that trains students to demonstrate EBP and QI competency before their entry into the profession. We hope that by providing you with a clear understanding of research, EBP, and QI processes at the outset of this book, we will set the stage for you to make an early and powerful positive impact in the nursing field. Let's begin this valuable learning journey together now with a look at the past that will help you better understand our present and inform your future.

History and Evolution of Nursing Research, EBP, and QI

Florence Nightingale is recognized as the first nurse to observe nursing care, collect data, and use records for the purpose of improving patient care. An ardent social reformist, pioneering statistician, and prolific writer, she is generally credited with being the first nurse to perform research and apply evidence to change practice (Mackey & Bassendowski, 2017).

Research

Nightingale's earliest research took place in an overcrowded, poorly ventilated facility in which she managed and trained nurses during the Crimean War while observing and documenting which interventions decreased morbidity and mortality in wounded soldiers. She wrote extensively on nursing as a profession and healthcare systems (Nightingale, 1859) and continued to perform epidemiological research and recommend data-driven decisions until the end of her life (McDonald, 2017).

Nursing research grew slowly until the mid-20th century when, in 1946, the Division of Nursing was established within the Office of the Surgeon General. In the 1950s and 1960s, academic nursing established more doctoral programs and predoctoral and postdoctoral fellowships to train nurse researchers. Funding from what is now the Health Resources and Services Administration (HRSA) supported this educational expansion. In 1985, the federal government established the National Institute of Nursing Research (NINR; https://www.ninr.nih.gov/) within the National Institutes of Health (https://www.ninr.nih.gov/aboutninr/history). The NINR has been the major funder of nursing research since its inception. In alignment with the National Academies of Sciences, Engineering, and Medicine's (2021) *The Future of Nursing 2020–2030* report, the NINR's research priorities are to support research that improves health equity.

Today, nursing **research** (i.e., the scientific study of new phenomena) includes clinical research, health systems research, outcomes research, and nursing education research (American Association of Colleges of Nursing [AACN], 2006). New knowledge on these topics provides evidence that practicing nurses need to enhance the quality of care they provide to patients, improve healthcare systems, and advocate for policies that impact populations.

Nurse researchers seek to answer questions about solutions that are not yet known. To find answers to their questions, nurse researchers develop and test hypotheses. *Hypotheses* are simply statements about what the researcher expects the outcome of their study will be. Hypothesis testing includes statistical analysis. The goal of statistical analysis is to allow a determination that the research results are not due to chance.

Research methodologies can be divided broadly into two categories—quantitative and qualitative—based on the type of results they produce. *Quantitative research* generally produces numerical results, and *qualitative research* produces narrative (or word-based) results. All research includes variables. *Variables* are characteristics that can be measured (e.g., age, income, or even a more complex construct like the quality of life). In a specific research study, researchers will label the variables as dependent or independent according to their hypothesis (i.e., what they expect will happen in answer to their research question). A variable is labeled as independent if the researcher expects it to influence another variable. The variable that is expected to be influenced is labeled the dependent variable. Here is a trick to remember:

A baby's weight is "dependent" on (influenced by) its milk intake. How much milk a mother can produce is "independent" of the infant's weight.

Quantitative research designs are further categorized as experimental or observational. *Experimental research* involves the researcher's manipulation of independent variables with the objective of finding out what effect they have on the dependent variable. Because there are often additional variables (that may or may not be considered) that could impact the dependent variable, experimental studies include a control group. In the control group, the researcher does not manipulate the independent variable. At the end of the experiment, the dependent variable is measured in both groups, and results from both groups are compared using statistical analysis to determine whether there is any statistically significant difference in outcomes. On the other hand, in *observational research* the researcher only observes the variables but does not manipulate any variable.

When a research study uses human subjects, the researcher must choose criteria to determine which types of subjects will be included or excluded from the study. A thoughtful choice of criteria allows the researcher to determine whether the study's results can be considered applicable (be generalized) to a broader population of people beyond those in the study. If the sample of participants in the study is random, meaning that everyone who participates in the study has a random chance of being placed in either the experimental group or the control group, then the experiment is classified as a *randomized controlled trial* (*RCT*). A common theme in research evaluation is that an RCT always produces the highest quality of evidence. Results from RCTs are thought to have the least bias and therefore to reveal the answer to the research question closest to the truth. Accordingly, the results are accepted as generalizable and can be applied to everyone. This consideration is problematic, however, in that generalizability to the wider population can be compromised by a biased choice of inclusion criteria. In fact, many current drug-based therapies are based on past RCTs and subsequent systematic reviews comprised almost entirely of subjects who were White men. Although these RCTs included few women and even fewer Black, Indigenous, and people of color (BIPOC), their results were unwisely considered applicable across diverse populations. Furthermore, due to advances in genetics and genomics, we now know that individualized care may be better than care that works for most people, as previously thought. It is important to note that Indigenous healers and ancient therapeutic systems such as Ayurveda and Traditional Chinese Medicine have understood the importance of individualized care for thousands of years. As researchers, we must always be aware of the ways in which our personal values and social context might influence our research perspectives and choices.

Common observational study designs include cross-sectional, cohort, and case-control studies. *Cross-sectional studies* examine a phenomenon of interest at one point in time. Surveys or questionnaires are frequently used in cross-sectional studies to collect information on a specific topic. *Cohort studies* follow a group of people over time and collect data from them at various points over time. Cohort studies can be retrospective (looking at a person's history) or prospective (following people in the cohort into the future). Often, participants in a cohort study have something in common, such as where they live or a certain diagnosis. *Case-control studies* compare people with a specific exposure or condition (case) to a control group of people who are without the exposure or condition but are similar in as many other aspects as possible.

QUANTITATIVE RESEARCH EXAMPLE

Anxiety in pregnancy is associated with poorer pregnancy outcomes. Pregnant women with gestational diabetes mellitus (GDM) experience higher levels of anxiety. Medications for anxiety are not recommended in pregnancy, so other effective treatments are needed. Acupressure, a treatment method in Traditional Chinese Medicine, has been shown to decrease anxiety in other patient populations and has no known risks to the unborn infant. To test whether acupressure is an effective method to decrease anxiety in women with GDM, Bastani (2016) randomly assigned 60 women to two equal groups. A nurse provided one group with acupressure at the true pressure point, and the other received a sham or placebo pressure at a false point on the forearm. The groups were compared afterward using two valid and reliable tools, the Maternal Anxiety Questionnaire and a visual analog scale for severity. The data was analyzed using statistical tests for differences between groups. Results demonstrated a significant difference in the reduction of anxiety in the group who received acupressure at the true point. Therefore, acupressure can be delivered by trained nurses as a safe, effective clinical intervention to decrease anxiety in women with GDM during pregnancy (Bastani, 2016).

Qualitative research differs from quantitative research in that it seeks to describe and understand a phenomenon in depth, adding to what is already known. Qualitative research aims to present more fully what a specific phenomenon means to the people it affects (e.g., how it feels to live with a chronic condition such as diabetes or to lose a loved one to cancer).

Qualitative studies are often the precursor to quantitative studies. When little is known about a phenomenon, a full description of it can provide the knowledge needed to develop more specific quantitative studies to fill in the knowledge gaps.

There are many variations and methods in nursing research besides these basics. You will learn more about evaluating their quality and the strength of their results in Chapters 6 and 7.

QUALITATIVE RESEARCH EXAMPLE

Suicide loss survivors refers to the people who are left behind after someone commits suicide. These people often suffer emotional distress, and their lives are significantly impacted by their loss. To develop effective interventions to help survivors manage their grief, McDaniel et al. (2022) interviewed 28 people who had experienced suicide loss within 6 months after the loss. Each person was asked a similar set of open-ended questions that focused on their life after the loss (e.g., "Can you share something about your life after your loss by suicide?"). The interviews were audio recorded and transcribed. Content analysis revealed three categories: (a) life before suicide where they "saw it coming but couldn't help"; (b) negative emotions; and (c) finding a purpose to move on. These results revealed the need for suicide loss survivors to have community-based access to social and emotional support. Nurses can increase awareness and advocate for services to meet survivors' needs (McDaniel et al., 2022).

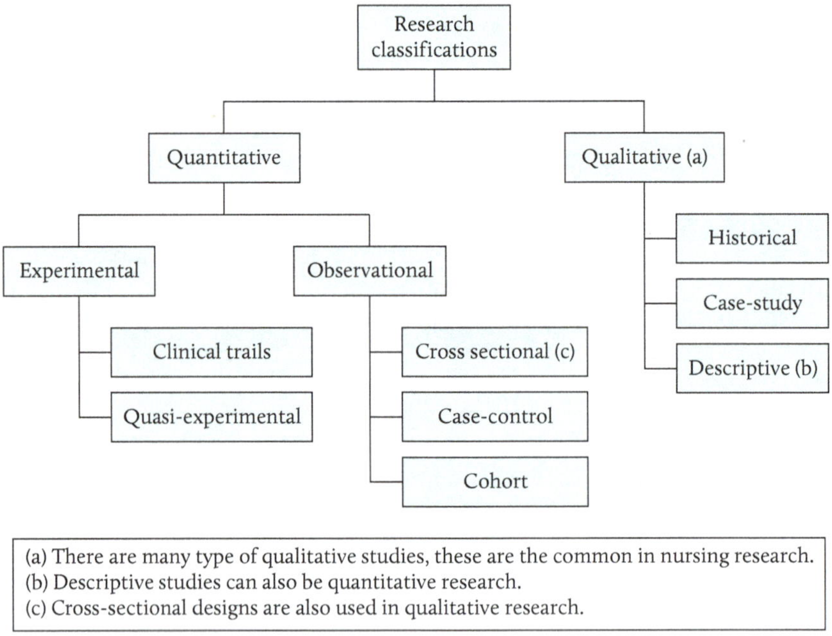

FIGURE 1.1 Classification of Research

Evidence-Based Practice

Evidence-based practice (EBP) is defined as a "three-legged stool" because it includes (a) the best evidence available (research), (b) clinical expertise of the provider, and (c) patient/family preferences/values (see Figure 1.2).

David Sackett is credited with beginning the evidence-based medicine (EBM) movement, and his book *How to Practice and Teach Evidence-Based Medicine* (Sackett et al., 2000) helped to disseminate the concept. In the United Kingdom, Archie Cochrane had a similar vision of evidence-based medicine. His passion was research studies performed using the RCT design. He believed that this type of study design could come closest to answering questions of cause and effect (Thoma & Eaves, 2015). Later, Ian Chalmers and a group of colleagues founded the nonprofit Cochrane collaboration as a repository for systematic reviews of RCTs (https://cochranelibrary.com).

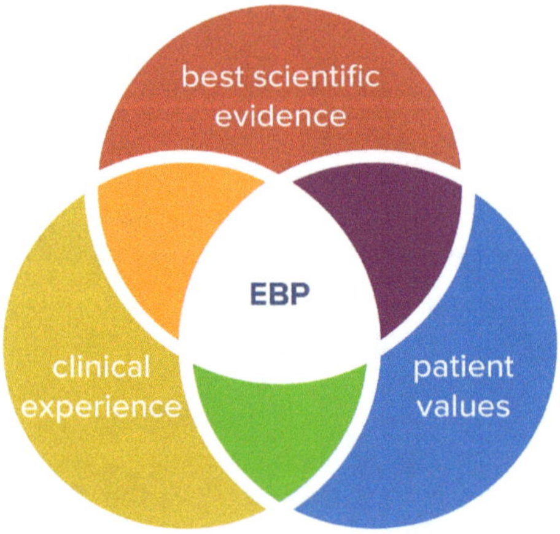

FIGURE 1.2 Evidence-Based Practice Components

As noted above, there are many different types of research. The significance of research studies is based on the quality, quantity, and consistency of their results. Gordan Guyett led the development of a system for rating levels of evidence called Grading of Recommendations Assessment, Development, and Evaluation (GRADE; Guyatt et al., 2008). Clinicians use GRADE to help identify the level of a body of evidence (more than one research study). You will learn more about the levels of evidence in Chapter 6.

The nursing profession has adapted the EBM model slightly. Evidence-based practice (EBP) in nursing, described as a problem-solving approach best accomplished within a context of care, was first popularized by Bernadette Melnyk and Ellen Fineout-Overholt (Fineout-Overholt et al., 2005). Models that support the process of putting evidence into practice have been developed and are being used routinely in many healthcare settings (see Table 1.2). All models broadly include the steps in the EBP process (see Table 1.1).

TABLE 1.1 Steps in the EBP Process

Step in the EBP process	Description	More information
0	Cultivate a spirit of inquiry.	Chapters 1 and 2
1	Identify the problem/ask the question.	Chapters 2 and 3
2	Search for the best evidence.	Chapters 4
3	Critically appraise the evidence.	Chapters 5, 6, and 7
4	Integrate the evidence with your clinical expertise and patient preferences to ensure the best clinical decision.	Chapters 8, 9, and 10
5	Evaluate the outcome(s) of the practice change.	Chapter 11
6	Disseminate the outcome(s).	Chapter 12

MELNYK, ET AL. (2010).

TABLE 1.2 Popular EBP Models

Model	Links and resources
IOWA model	https://uihc.org/evidence-based-practice (Iowa Model Collaborative, 2017)
Model of EBP change	A model for change to evidence-based practice (Rosswurm & Larrabee, 1999)
Johns Hopkins nursing evidence-based practice model	Dang & Dearholt (2017)
Advancing research and clinical practice through close collaboration (ARCC) model	Melnyk et al. (2017)
ACE Star model of EBP	www.acestar.uthscsa.edu (Stevens, 2004).

In 2014, basic-level **EBP competencies** (possession of adequate knowledge and skill) for practicing registered nurses were developed (Melnyk et al., 2014) and are used today (see Table 1.3). In 2003, a national survey of nurses demonstrated a lack of knowledge, beliefs, and skills related to EBP. Although nurses believed EBP improved clinical care, they reported that only 40%–50% of the care they provided was evidence-based (Melnyk et al., 2004). This situation led to campaigns to train nurses in EBP during their formal education and to support that training through continuing development education. Although a follow-up study demonstrated some improvement in nurses' confidence in their ability to implement EBP in the clinical setting, one of its most significant findings was a lack of mentors available to guide and support nurses' EBP education (Melnyk et al., 2012). Melnyk et al.'s 2018 study on nurses' achievement of the 13 EBP competencies revealed that much progress is still to be made. Results revealed that no competency averages reached the competent to very competent range, with most falling in the needs improvement category (Melnyk et al., 2018). The goal is for all nurses to achieve these competencies. You have your work cut out for you!

After learning about the competencies and steps, you can begin your journey as a nurse right now by cultivating a spirit of **inquiry** (i.e., asking for information). In the clinical setting and every other environment in which you observe, learn, or practice as a nurse, ask questions! Ask why things are being done as they are. If you wonder whether there might be a better way to accomplish things, then you are on the path to becoming part of a team to solve the problem and are ready to move on to Step 2. You will learn much more about developing the clinical question in Chapter 4.

TABLE 1.3 Evidence-Based Nursing Competencies

1.	Questions clinical practice
2.	Describes clinical problems using internal evidence
3.	Participates in forming questions
4.	Searches external evidence
5.	Critically appraises pre-appraised evidence
6.	Critically appraises research studies for practice
7.	Participates in the synthesis of evidence
8.	Collects practice data
9.	Integrates evidence into EBP changes
10.	Implements practice change based on three components of EBP
11.	Evaluates practice changes
12.	Disseminates best practices
13.	Participates in strategies to sustain EBP culture

(Melnyk & Fineout-Overholt, 2014)

Quality Improvement

In addition to EBP, the history of **quality improvement (QI**; i.e., systematic care improvement) can be traced back to Florence Nightingale. Ignaz Semmelweis was another early pioneer of QI during the 1800s and is known as the father of infection control. In a teaching hospital in Vienna, Semmelweis observed that there were far fewer infections and deaths among patients of midwives than patients of physicians. Initially, he resisted the notion that the routine handwashing performed by midwives contributed to preventing infection or the transfer of infection from patient to patient; he performed studies to determine whether anything else could account for his observations. Finally, after performing what might be considered the first controlled trial, he was forced to admit that the results demonstrated handwashing to be an effective intervention in limiting the spread of infection. Unfortunately, his ideas were extremely unpopular, and his work was largely ignored. Over 20 years later, researchers whose names you may find more familiar—Pasteur, Koch, and Lister—were given credit for exploring and promoting antiseptic techniques (Best & Neuhauser, 2004).

In 2000, the Institute of Medicine (now the National Academies of Science) published a report entitled *To Err Is Human: Building a Safer Health System*, which highlighted the significant problem of safety in the healthcare system and the harm to patients and care workers caused by errors. In a follow-up report titled *Crossing the Quality Chasm: A New Health System for the 21st Century* (Institute of Medicine, 2001), goals were formulated to improve the quality of care provided by the U.S. healthcare system along with specific principles to guide improvement, including a recommendation for the Six Aims for Improvement: care that is safe, timely, effective, efficient, equitable, and patient-centered (STEEEP).

A model for improvement introduced and developed by Edwards Deming, a celebrated engineer and manufacturing statistician of the 20th century, included plan-do-study-act (PDSA) cycles as an integral part of problem-solving (see Figure 1.3; Langley et al., 2009). Process improvement methodologies like lean and Six Sigma use similar principles. All improvement methods are based on these fundamental questions:

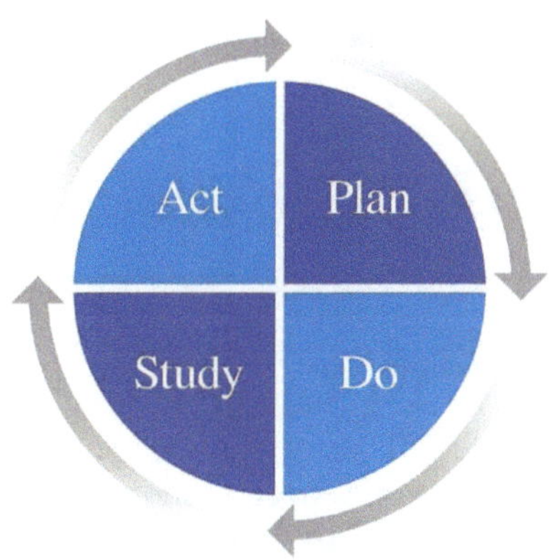

FIGURE 1.3 PDSA Cycle

- What are we trying to accomplish?
- How will we know whether a change is an improvement?
- What change can we make that will result in an improvement?

You will learn more about quality and safety, the model for improvement, why you need data to know whether a change has occurred, and statistical process control (how to measure something to know whether there is an improvement) in Chapters 2 and 11.

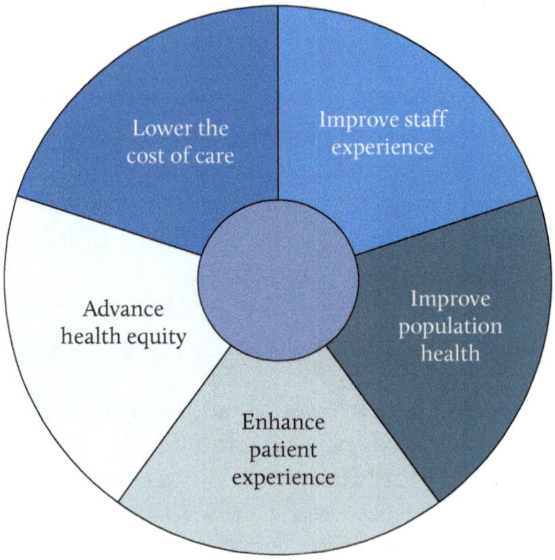

FIGURE 1.4 IHI Quintuple Aim

As adopted by the Institute for Healthcare Improvement (IHI) in 1991, the model for improvement has propelled the quality improvement process and the use of data for improvement. The IHI Quintuple Aims align with EBP to improve the quality of the patient experience, population health, costs of care, provider work–life balance, and health equity (Langley et al., 2009; Itchhaporia, 2021).

Getting Started: Differentiation of Research, EBP, and QI

There is a lethal gap between what is known about achieving improvement and the actual use of knowledge for this purpose. Despite a wealth of papers detailing scientific research evidence for QI, far too often important work ends up on a shelf or within digital databases untouched rather than being broadly and consistently applied to healthcare practice—a sobering symbol of lost opportunity. However, more than 2 decades of EBP-focused research has led to decreased care gaps in some areas. For example, cancer care evidence-to-practice gaps have narrowed from 17 to 15 years (Khan et al., 2021). Unfortunately, at this slow rate, it will take well over the next 100 years to close these costly healthcare gaps. Meanwhile, EBP and QI are needed for every healthcare encounter to help nurses use the best evidence from research to ensure sustained quality care.

As a future nurse, you must understand how research, EBP, and QI are defined so that you can learn how these paradigms differ and connect (see Figure 1.5 and Table 1.4). Although some definition variability exists, consistent use of research, EBP, and QI language and terminology across academic and clinical settings is

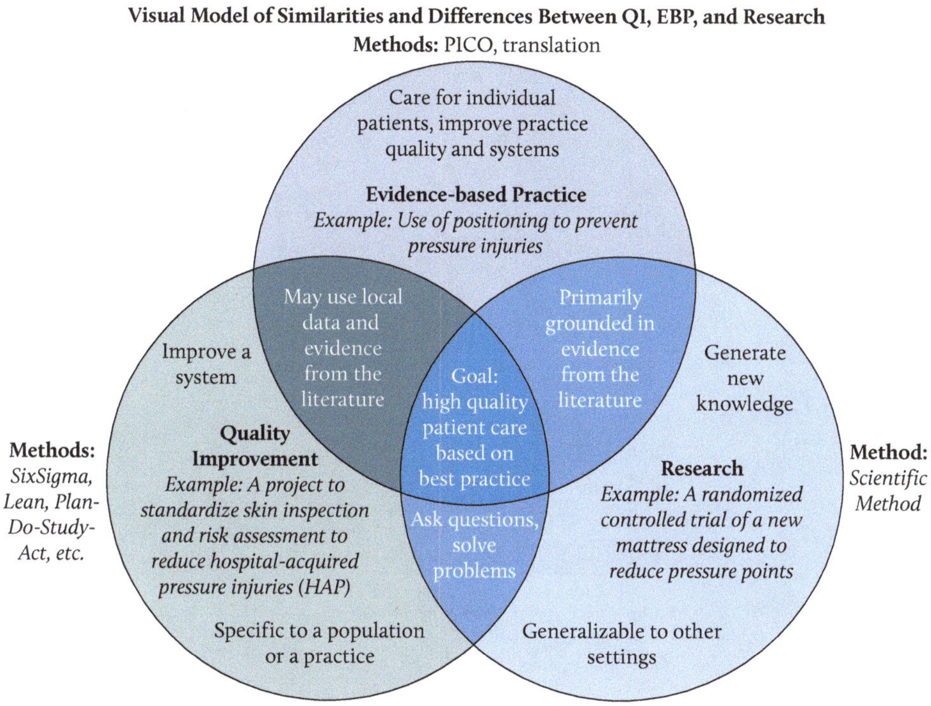

Note: This diagram uses examples related to the prevention of pressure injuries.

FIGURE 1.5 QI, EBP, and Research Visual model

essential. Research is a systematic scientific process used to establish facts and generate new knowledge or theory. EBP is a process used to review, critically appraise, and translate the latest external evidence (data generated from scientific research studies) into practice recommendations. EBP combines (a) the best available research (external evidence), (b) clinical experience, and (C) patient preferences/values to inform clinical decision-making. QI uses rapid cycles of change to improve processes or outcomes following problem identification within a population(s). QI relies on internal evidence (data generated from your own clinical setting or organization) and typically does not involve a systematic search and critical appraisal of evidence. Evidence-based QI (also known as EBP-I) blends the EBP and QI processes by integrating internal and external evidence into the decision-making process about practice change (Hempel et al., 2022; Levin et al., 2010). These projects are becoming more common due to the urgent need to sustain EBP improvements. For more information on internal and external evidence, see Chapter 4. The mountain model is the first framework to integrate EBP and QI as EBPQI (Figure 1.6; Waldrop & Jennings, 2024). As you continue reading this textbook, all the components of this model will be described.

Research aspires to produce generalizable results (findings that can be generalized to a population beyond the participants in the study). Less understood but equally important is the transferability of research results. When research results determine that an intervention is effective, these results should be implemented

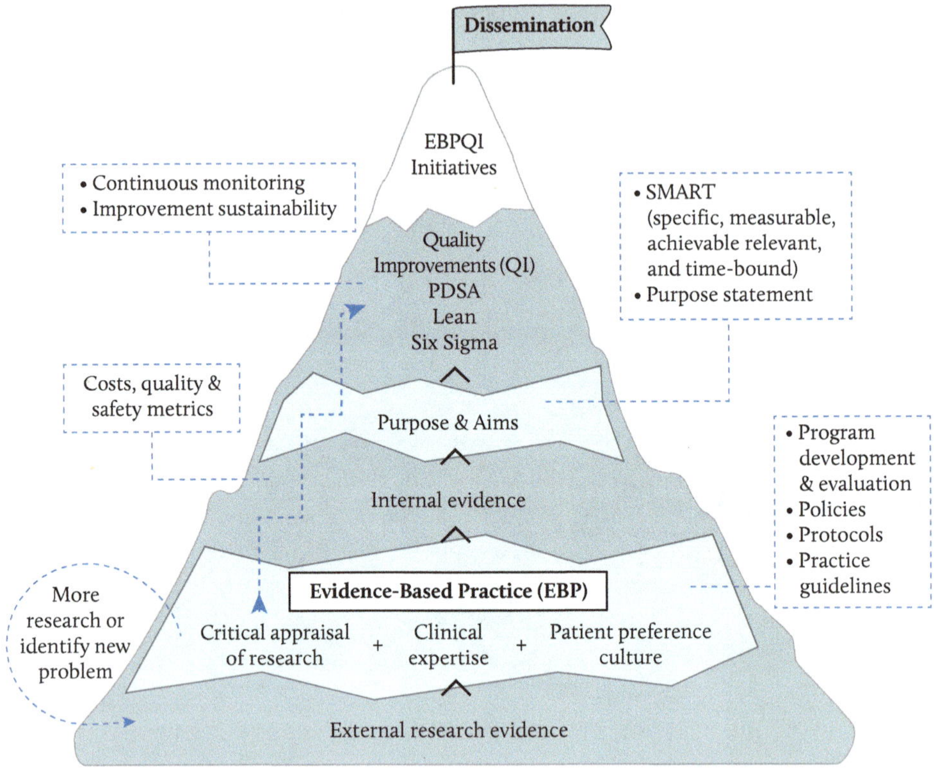

FIGURE 1.6 Mountain Model

into general practice. This is often where the gap between knowledge and the application of knowledge occurs. It can take 15 years or more for research findings to be adapted into general practice (Morris et al., 2011). Granted, research conducted in a controlled setting with participants chosen because they meet specific criteria is not quite an accurate reflection of everyday nursing practice. Nonetheless, nurses are challenged to become a force that shortens this timeline, and putting evidence into practice in your own workplace is one way to do it! Be prepared for some resistance: As nurses put research results into practice in their own settings, the results of their quality improvement efforts may be criticized for not being generalizable because the participants (all the patients affected by the practice change) are not representative of the broader population. This criticism is unjust. An evidence-based QI initiative that has worked in one organization can be transferred and adapted to another so long as the core of the intervention remains the same. For example, following best-practice recommendations, a newborn infant should receive their first hepatitis B vaccine (core intervention) prior to discharge home from the hospital (Committee on Infectious Diseases & Committee on Fetus and Newborn, 2017); however, various aspects of the intervention can differ, such as the use of standing orders, who obtains informed consent, or specific schedule of vaccine administration after birth (Damschroder et al., 2009). Although not always generalizable, EBP and QI work is highly transferable, with clinical and practical significance. This will be discussed further in Chapter 12.

TABLE 1.4 Comparative Representation of Research, EBP, and QI Paradigms for Competency-Based Education

	Research	Evidence-based practice	Quality improvement
Function	Generates new knowledge; replicates evidence; tests or generates theory; improves methods or instrumentation	Translates evidence to recommend best practice	Identifies a problem and incorporates local evidence to improve process and/or outcomes
Methods	Qualitative/quantitative designs; mixed methods	Evidence search	Identify measurements, enact changes, and analyze results to improve systems
Questions	May be directional or nondirectional; can be a research question and/or a hypothesis	PICO (population, intervention, comparison, outcome); PPCO (problem, population/person, change, outcome)	SMART aims (specific, measurable, actionable, relevant, timely)
Focus	New knowledge; replication of former findings; revelations in big data; generation or testing of theory; lived experience	Critical appraisal of current evidence with synthesis	Continuous process improvement; element of time
Process	Uses a variety of research methods and designs to dictate procedure	Produces outcomes through implementation of a practice change in a narrow population through integration of best external evidence, patient/family values, and clinician expertise	Produces internal evidence to evaluate the performance of systems and processes and improve outcomes in the (local) setting
Reliability	May yield highly reliable measures with consistent approach; related concept is validity, which is the accuracy of the measure.	Reliable if considered trustworthy and credible and applicable to the problem	Attempts to increase reliability; greater reliability means less error
Generalizability/ transferability	May be generalizable in quantitative methodologies; seeks transferability if using qualitative methods	Not generalizable but may have transferability	Not generalizable but may have transferability
Significance	Focus on statistical significance or a better understanding of phenomena	Clinical/practical significance	Clinical/practical significance, displayed visually in run or statistical control charts over time

Subsets of research often confused with EBP or QI include:

- Implementation science: scientific study of methods and strategies that facilitate the uptake of EBP and research into regular use.
- Improvement science: research focused on healthcare improvement.
- Translational science: research focused on understanding the scientific and operational principles underlying each step of the translational process.

Important points to remember:

- The term "study" should be used synonymously with "research."
- The terms "project" and "initiative" are used to describe EBP and QI work.
- "Project" may be used in describing research, but "study" should not be used to describe other project types.

Why Do Nurses Need to Understand Research, EBP and QI for Professional Nursing Practice?

If you can't find the answer to a question in the current literature, you should work with research colleagues to help produce the scientific knowledge needed to advance practice. We want to give you the knowledge you need to enter professional practice ready to be a contributing research or EBP and QI team member and team asset!

Who is qualified to carry out research, EBP, and QI? Research is typically conducted by a nurse who has earned a doctor of philosophy (PhD) degree or persons with an advanced science degree as well as additional education and training in research methodology. These individuals are prepared to lead research teams and work with other professionals from various disciplines to complete studies that will provide nurses with new scientific information to translate into clinical practice. The nurses best qualified to lead the translation of research within the nursing discipline are those who have earned a doctor of nursing practice (DNP) degree (think DNP equals EBP). Although all nurses should have a clear EBP understanding and engagement, the DNP degree prepares experts in critical appraisal and evidence synthesis. These nurses are systems thinkers who accelerate practice change. QI projects are carried out by a variety of nurses with QI skills and training, sometimes as members of an interdisciplinary team. The best teams are generally those that incorporate diversity in background and experience. The most pressing problems in healthcare need to be addressed by teams assembled to ensure different paradigm expertise and a multidisciplinary approach. An important point to remember is that EBP and QI are team initiatives. Like team sports, these processes simply cannot be successful without full team engagement.

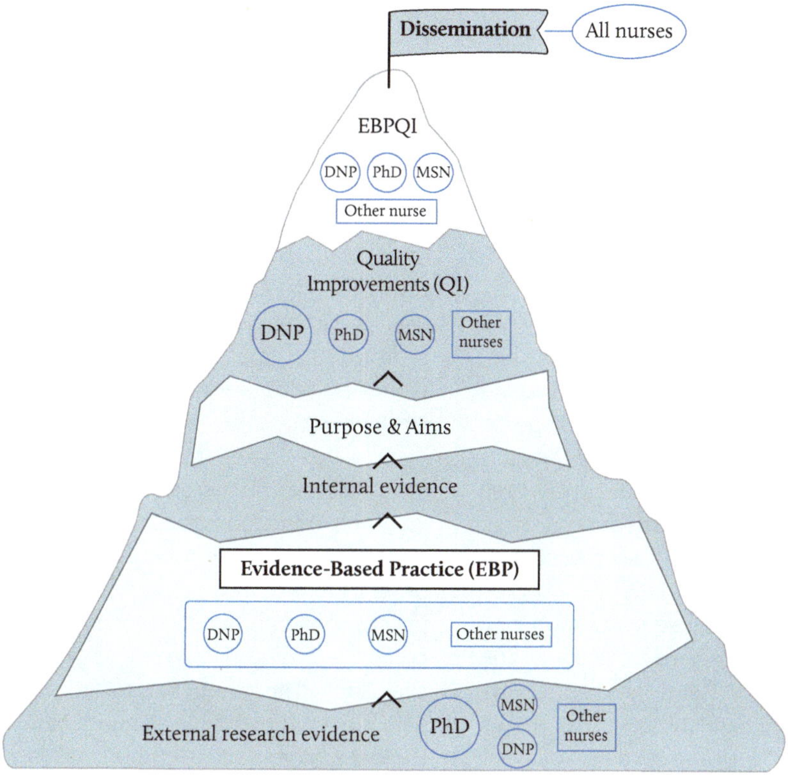

Larger circle represents a leadership role.

FIGURE 1.7 Nurses' Roles in EBPQI

A PERSONAL CASE STUDY

Science is in continual change, and we must try and keep abreast of it.

—C.S. Lewis, 1945

I (Jayne) recently received a call from the spouse of a family member who was experiencing severe abdominal pain. After gathering information, I advised that my relative be taken to the nearest emergency department (ED), where he was admitted following abdominal imaging that revealed kidney stones, gallstones, and a small bowel obstruction. With the patient's permission, his spouse sent me screenshots of the imaging. The clinical picture seemed to fit a very rare condition known as *gallbladder ileus*, which occurs when a gallstone passes through a fistula and obstructs an adhered portion of the gastrointestinal tract.

My husband, a registered dietitian with years of hospital experience, has seen many bowel obstructions in clinical practice, so I asked him to accompany me to the hospital to provide **support**. When we arrived, we were alarmed to find the patient unattended, in extreme pain, and without a nasogastric tube (standard care for initial treatment of a small bowel obstruction, used to decompress the blocked bowel). He was discharged 2 days later without receiving a clinically indicated surgical intervention.

Within 48 hours of discharge, his extreme abdominal pain returned. On my recommendation, he returned to the ED. Repeat imaging revealed that the small bowel obstruction remained. Rather than surgery, however, the medical and surgical team recommended further bowel rest and continued imaging.

I knew that an exploratory laparotomy was likely needed to visibly assess the bowel and perform a surgical intervention, so my husband and I decided to initiate a crucial conversation. I quickly accessed the current literature on small bowel obstruction and reviewed the latest clinical practice recommendations, then merged a call between my husband, myself, the patient, and his spouse. We spoke with the bedside nurse, who provided a thorough status update, but when she was invited to share her thoughts on the patient's care plan, she offered instead to connect us with the surgical team.

During the conference call, the surgical team provider explained why the medical and surgical teams believed that bowel rest, serial labs, and imaging were the best options. I briefly presented the current research evidence and recommendations as well as our concerns that further surgical delay following previous nonsurgical treatment failure would likely lead to complications, increased morbidity, and small bowel obstruction recurrence.

This information was received well, so I requested exploratory surgery, as previous treatments had proved ineffective. I reminded the team that according to evidence-based practice, three pillars must determine care decisions: (a) current research, (b) patient and family values, and (c) clinician preference. I asked whether, following a review of current research and with awareness of our family values, the surgical team would consider weighing those two pillars against clinician preference. The provider agreed that this was a reasonable request and asked the patient whether he would consent to surgery. Now seriously compromised and ill, he chose to trust the medical team's preferred approach and declined surgery. I was heartbroken for my relative and his spouse. They both expressed anger with us for recommending a surgery they hoped to avoid.

My relative was abruptly discharged 2 days later, and within 48 hours I received another frantic call concerning his condition. For the third time, I advised his spouse to seek immediate emergency evaluation. Surgery was performed at last, and a golf ball–sized gallstone was finally removed from the patient's small bowel.

One week later, following the patient's third hospital discharge, the patient's anxious and depleted spouse asked again for my advice as a nurse practitioner. Given her observations of my relative's condition, I suspected postoperative infection and other complications and advised an emergency evaluation. The patient was taken to the hospital for the fourth time and back to surgery. He lost a large portion of his small intestine and will likely have nutritional absorption issues for the duration of his life. At the time of this writing, he has new onset pneumonia, a drain, wound vacuum, and pain pump. His outcome could be lethal, but it might also have been preventable. I am left to wonder whether he could have been spared the cost, complications, and stress he has endured if current EBPs had been followed.

Critical Consideration Checkpoint

1. Throughout the situation described in this personal case study, at what points could a nurse have intervened?
2. As first-line patient care experts, how can nurses be empowered during healthcare encounters to respectfully question a provider's plan of care to ensure that EBP is realized?

As a nurse, you will be called upon to serve in the vital role of research, EBP, and QI team member. The fundamental knowledge you are learning at this very moment will enable you to meet important challenges. As you gain experience and advance in your educational pursuits, you will likely transition from serving as a team member to being the team leader of critically needed EBP and QI efforts. For now, focus on learning the fundamentals of the different paradigms so that you can serve as an active participant in changing healthcare outcomes at the bedside, chairside, and tableside.

Future Responsibilities of the Nursing Profession

In 2021, the National Academies of Sciences, Engineering, and Math published its third report in a series to guide nursing as a profession for the next 10 years. *The Future of Nursing 2020–2030: Charting a Path to Achieve Health Equity* challenges nurses to accept responsibility for addressing the huge inequities in our healthcare system, particularly those related to social determinants of health.

Social determinants of health (*SDoH*) are "conditions in the environments in which people are born, live, learn, work, play, worship, and age [that] affect a wide range of health, functioning, and quality-of-life outcomes and risks). Only 20% of health is determined by the provision of healthcare in a hospital setting or through interactions with healthcare personnel in a clinic or community. A broader 80% of health is determined by conditions in and features of the social environment, including economic stability, the physical environment, education, nutrition, support systems, and accessibility of health services (Office of Disease Prevention and Health Promotion, n.d. (see Figure 1.8).

Health disparities (e.g., average life span) are outcomes of SDoH (such as access to health services) and can be used to measure health equity. Health equity and health

Economic Stability	**Neighborhood and Physical Environment**	**Education**	**Food**	**Community and Social Context**	**Health Care System**
Employment Income Expenses Debt Medical bills Support	Housing Transportation Safety Parks Playgrounds Walkability Zip code/ geography	Literacy Language Early childhood education Vocational training Higher education	Hunger Access to healthy options	Social integration Support systems Community engagement Discrimination Stress	Health coverage Provider availability Provider linguistic and cultural competency Quality of care

Health Outcomes
Mortality, Morbidity, Life expectancy, Health care expenditures, Health status, Functional limitations

FIGURE 1.8 Social Determinants of Health and Related Health Outcomes

disparities are closely related. *Health disparities* are differences in health or key determinants of health (e.g., education, safe housing, and freedom from discrimination) that adversely affect marginalized or excluded groups. According to the Centers for Disease Control and Prevention (2022), *health equity* "is the state in which everyone has a fair and just opportunity to achieve their highest level of health" (para. 1).

Nurses are well positioned to address SDoH because so much of what affects a person's health is unrelated to the clinic or hospital setting (Hood et al., 2016). Improving health does not always require the ability to write a prescription or order a test. The most effective drivers of change are simply nurses—nurses who care; are problem solvers; can reach people where they live, work, or play; and are culturally aware and always learning. Nurses who know how to use evidence in a systematic way to improve problems can do so in many different spaces.

EBPQI

While EBP and QI will continue to be discussed throughout this book, you now know the fundamental differences between research, EBP and QI and we are ready to introduce you to the first model to fully merge EBP and QI to guide practice changes across levels of nursing (see Figure 1.6). This model and the term **evidence-based practice quality improvement** (**EBPQI**) will be used throughout this textbook to inform practice change initiatives.

QI lacks the external, research evidence foundation, and EBP lacks the sustainability offered by QI. Some current blended models and verbiage present in the current literature base merge EP-QI or EBPI, but the full scope of both paradigms is not fully integrated. In the mountain model, nurses can mobilize and use the three pillars of EBP to achieve true QI across the care continuum. The process focus of QI comes from industry, but in healthcare EBP involves practice that is constantly evolving. We are continually engaging in research that is changing, which informs current practice. In nursing at every level, all process changes will be practice changes with the goal of elevating health outcomes.

As a new nurse, you will likely be a member of an EBPQI or a research study team, and different levels of nursing will lead the teams you participate in depending on their education and training. For a research study, the lead nurse would likely have a PhD; for an EBPQI initiative, the lead nurse may have a DNP. We need to work together to optimally impact outcomes at the research or EBPQI or outcome level. Nurses with master's degrees have special skills in certain areas and may contribute in other ways to teams. For example, they may be experts in patient education or a particular disease process.

Where Will You Impact Practice Change?

Areas of professional nursing in which you can affect vital change to address health and healthcare disparities include not only nursing practice but also policymaking, public health, and emergency preparedness and response. All entry-level nurses require knowledge and proficiency to practice as a generalist across the lifespan within a wide variety of care settings. Care spheres for entry-level professional nursing education include wellness, health promotion/disease prevention, chronic disease care management, regenerative/restorative care, and hospice/palliative care (see Figure 1.9). You should be equipped to work with a diverse patient population in all settings.

Today's nursing students, diverse in age, background, and experience, are taking increased responsibility for their active learning and respond well to active learning strategies (AACN, 2021). *Active learning* (creating an action in response to knowledge and clear information regarding needed competencies) is critical to your success as a nursing student as you are trained as a generalist across four spheres of care (see Figure 1.9). We encourage you to engage in active learning approaches to maximize your personal competency levels. Active learning extends beyond the classroom and simulation lab to clinical practice. In a recent study, undergraduate nursing students encountered poor care in clinical settings, and despite feeling an obligation to take action to improve care, the majority said nothing and remained passive spectators (Bickhoff et al., 2017). Cultivating a spirit of inquiry (the primary step in the EBP process) is a step not only toward formulating clinical questions but toward questioning any perceived wrong in real-world settings. If you have doubts, speak up respectfully and ask!

It is especially important that you recognize and question practices or situations that could endanger you as well as your patients. Anyone who has traveled by airplane has heard instructions regarding the first steps to take in the rare event of a change in cabin pressure: "Put on your own oxygen mask first, then assist the person seated next to you." The reason for this clear warning is that individuals cannot help others if they are unable to breathe themselves. Similarly, changes can occur rapidly in a healthcare setting, and it is essential that you remain vigilant and guard your own health and well-being. Think about the image of an oxygen mask and let this remind you of your need to engage in EBP wellness activities so that you are always able to assist others.

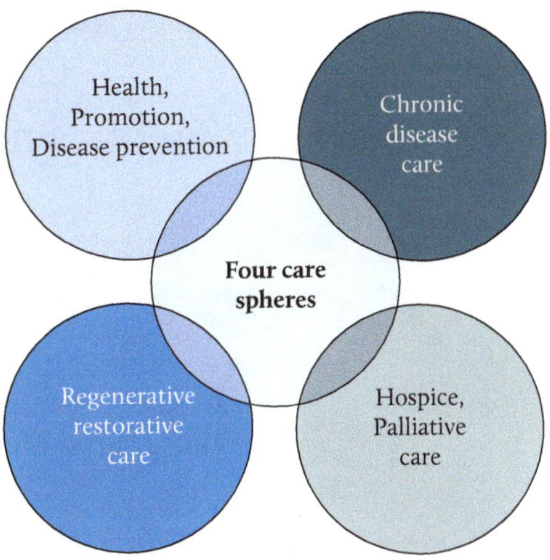

FIGURE 1.9 Four Spheres of Care (AACN, 2021)

WELLNESS IN ACTION: POWER POSE

Power pose: Have you considered engaging in an upright, powerful posture? A recent meta-analysis found that this type of posturing has been linked with feelings of self-confidence and task persistence (Körner et al., 2022). We recommend taking 1 minute right now to try a power pose as you think about your own health as a future nurse, ready to make a positive impact on many people.

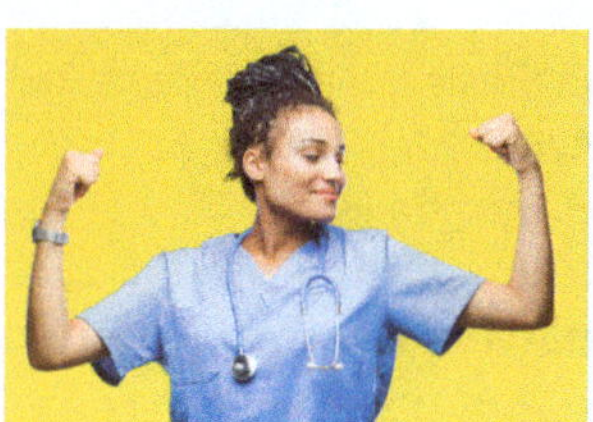

Image 1.1

WRAPPING UP

In summary, nursing requires all three approaches—research, evidence-based practice, and quality improvement—to support the highest quality care for patients. Research must validate that an intervention works for most people or systems. Applying research results (evidence) to practice using an EBP model and QI methods with robust evaluation can lead to sustainable changes in practice. As nurses become more knowledgeable about all three processes and how they work together synergistically, changes in practice will add up to amazing improvements for patients, communities, and even global health efforts.

EBP and QI are the methods nurses employ to help narrow the gaps between knowledge and practice. There is no QI without EBP first, and EBP is not sustainable without QI. Without research, the three-legged EBP stool could not stand. Every nurse must understand the critical connection between research, EBP, and QI. As a nursing student, you are central to your learning experience (AACN, 2021). Make certain to engage in active learning opportunities throughout your professional and personal EBP journey. Prioritize your own wellness to maximize your ability to help others. Begin by deeply considering your wellness now so that you will be prepared to face the future excitement and challenges of the nursing field in optimal condition.

REFLECTION QUESTIONS

1. Nurses are patient care experts. As you work collectively to advance nursing as a professional practice, how can you ensure that patients as individuals are kept at the center of care?
2. Once you complete nursing school, do you desire to advance your own education and training? If so, how does a basic understanding of research, EBP, and QI processes influence which direction you may pursue?

REFERENCES

American Association of Colleges of Nursing. (2021). *Essentials*. Retrieved October 28, 2022, from https://www.aacnnursing.org/Essentials

American Association of Colleges of Nursing. (2006). *Position statement: Nursing research*. https://www.aacnnursing.org/News-Information/Position-Statements-White-Papers/Nursing-Research

Bastani, F. (2016). Effect of acupressure on maternal anxiety in women with gestational diabetes mellitus. *Clinical Nursing Research, 25*(3), 325–341. https://doi.org/10.1177/1054773815579344

Best, M., & Neuhauser, D. (2004). Ignaz Semmelweis and the birth of infection control. *Quality & Safety in Health Care, 13*(3), 233–234. https://doi.org/10.1136/qshc.2004.010918

Bickhoff, L., Sinclair, P. M., & Levett-Jones, T. (2017). Moral courage in undergraduate nursing students: A literature review. *Collegian, 24*(1), 71–83. https://doi.org/10.1016/j.colegn.2015.08.002

Centers for Disease Control and Prevention. (2022, December 16). *Health equity*. https://www.cdc.gov/nchhstp/healthequity/index.html

Committee on Infectious Diseases & Committee on Fetus and Newborn. (2017). Elimination of perinatal hepatitis B: Providing the first vaccine dose within 24 hours of birth. *Pediatrics*, *140*(3), Article e20171870. https://doi.org/10.1542/peds.2017-1870

Damschroder, L. J., Aron, D. C., Keith, R. E., Kirsh, S. R., Alexander, J. A., & Lowery, J. C. (2009). Fostering implementation of health services research findings into practice: A consolidated framework for advancing implementation science. *Implementation Science*, *4*, Article 50. https://doi.org/10.1186/1748-5908-4-50

Dang, D., & Dearholt, S. (2017). *Johns Hopkins nursing evidence-based practice model and guidelines* (3rd ed.). Sigma Theta Tau International.

Fineout-Overholt, E., Melnyk, B. M., & Schultz, A. (2005). Transforming health care from the inside out: Advancing evidence-based practice in the 21st century. *Journal of Professional Nursing: Official Journal of the American Association of Colleges of Nursing*, *21*(6), 335–344. https://doi.org/10.1016/j.profnurs.2005.10.005

Guyatt, G. H., Oxman, A. D., Kunz, R., Vist, G. E., Falck-Ytter, Y., & Schünemann, H. J. (2008). What is "quality of evidence" and why is it important to clinicians? *British Medical Journal*, *336*(7651), 995–998. https://doi.org/10.1136/bmj.39490.551019.BE

Hempel, S., Bolshakova, M., Turner, B. J., Dinalo, J., Rose, D., Motala, A., Fu, N., Clemesha, C. G., Rubenstein, L., & Stockdale, S. (2022). Evidence-based quality improvement: A scoping review of the literature. *Journal of General Internal Medicine*, *37*(16), 4257–4267. https://doi.org/10.1007/s11606-022-07602-5

Hood, C. M., Gennuso, K. P., Swain, G. R., & Catlin, B. B. (2016). County health rankings: Relationships between determinant factors and health outcomes. *American Journal of Preventive Medicine*, *50*(2), 129–135. https://doi.org/10.1016/j.amepre.2015.08.024

Institute of Medicine. (2000). *To err is human: Building a safer health system*. National Academies Press. http://www.ncbi.nlm.nih.gov/books/NBK225182/

Institute of Medicine. (2001). *Crossing the quality chasm: A new health system for the 21st century*. National Academies Press. https://doi.org/10.17226/10027

Iowa Model Collaborative. (2017). Iowa model of evidence-based practice: Revisions and validation. *Worldviews on Evidence-Based Nursing*, *14*(3), 175–182. https://doi.org/10.1111/wvn.12223

Itchhaporia, D. (2021). The evolution of the Quintuple Aim. *Journal of the American College of Cardiology*, *78*(22), 2262–2264. https://doi.org/10.1016/j.jacc.2021.10.018

Khan, S., Chambers, D., & Neta, G. (2021). Revisiting time to translation: Implementation of evidence-based practices (EBPs) in cancer control. *Cancer Causes & Control*, *32*(3), 221–230. https://doi.org/10.1007/s10552-020-01376-z

Körner, R., Röseler, L., Schütz, A., & Bushman, B. J. (2022). Dominance and prestige: Meta-analytic review of experimentally induced body position effects on behavioral, self-report, and physiological dependent variables. *Psychological Bulletin*, *148*, 67–85. https://doi.org/10.1037/bul0000356

Langley, G. J., Moen, R. D., Nolan, K. M., Nolan, T. W., Norman, C. L., & Provost, L. P. (2009). *The improvement guide: A practical approach to enhancing organizational performance* (2nd ed.). Jossey-Bass.

Levin, R. F., Keefer, J. M., Marren, J., Vetter, M., Lauder, B., & Sobolewski, S. (2010). Evidence-based practice improvement: merging 2 paradigms. *Journal of Nursing Care Quality*, *25*(2), 117–126. https://doi.org/10.1097/NCQ.0b013e3181b5f19f

Mackey, A., & Bassendowski, S. (2017). The History of Evidence-Based Practice in Nursing Education and Practice. *Journal of Professional Nursing : Official Journal of the American Association of Colleges of Nursing*, *33*(1), 51–55. https://doi.org/10.1016/j.profnurs.2016.05.009

McDaniel, B. M., Daly, P., Pacheco, C. L., & Crist, J. D. (2022). Experiences with suicide loss: A qualitative study. *Clinical Nursing Research*. Advance online publication. https://doi.org/10.1177/10547738221119344

McDonald, L. (2017). *Florence Nightingale, nursing, and health care today.* Springer. https://doi.org/10.1891/9780826155597

Melnyk, B. M., Fineout-Overholt, E., Fischbeck Feinstein, N., Li, H., Small, L., Wilcox, L., & Kraus, R. (2004). Nurses' perceived knowledge, beliefs, skills, and needs regarding evidence-based practice: Implications for accelerating the paradigm shift. *Worldviews on Evidence-Based Nursing, 1*(3), 185–193. https://doi.org/10.1111/j.1524-475X.2004.04024.x

Melnyk, B. M., Fineout-Overholt, E., Gallagher-Ford, L., & Kaplan, L. (2012). The state of evidence-based practice in US nurses: Critical implications for nurse leaders and educators. *Journal of Nursing Administration, 42*(9), 410–417. https://doi.org/10.1097/NNA.0b013e3182664e0a

Melnyk, B. M., Fineout-Overholt, E., Stillwell, S. B., & Williamson, K. M. (2010). Evidence-based practice: step by step: the seven steps of evidence-based practice. *The American Journal of Nursing, 110*(1), 51–53. https://doi.org/10.1097/01.NAJ.0000366056.06605.d2

Melnyk, B. M., Fineout-Overholt, E., Giggleman, M., & Choy, K. (2017). A test of the ARCC© model improves implementation of evidence-based practice, healthcare culture, and patient outcomes. *Worldviews on Evidence-Based Nursing, 14*(1), 5–9. https://doi.org/10.1111/wvn.12188

Melnyk, B. M., Gallagher-Ford, L., Long, L. E., & Fineout-Overholt, E. (2014). The establishment of evidence-based practice competencies for practicing registered nurses and advanced practice nurses in real-world clinical settings: Proficiencies to improve healthcare quality, reliability, patient outcomes, and costs. *Worldviews on Evidence-Based Nursing, 11*(1), 5–15. https://doi.org/10.1111/wvn.12021

Melnyk, B. M., Gallagher-Ford, L., Zellefrow, C., Tucker, S., Thomas, B., Sinnott, L. T., & Tan, A. (2018). The first U.S. study on nurses' evidence-based practice competencies indicates major deficits that threaten healthcare quality, safety, and patient outcomes. *Worldviews on Evidence-Based Nursing, 15*(1), 16–25. https://doi.org/10.1111/wvn.12269

Morris, Z. S., Wooding, S., & Grant, J. (2011). The answer is 17 years, what is the question: Understanding time lags in translational research. *Journal of the Royal Society of Medicine, 104*(12), 510–520. https://doi.org/10.1258/jrsm.2011.110180

National Academies of Sciences, Engineering, and Medicine. (2021). *The future of nursing 2020–2030: Charting a path to achieve health equity.* National Academies Press. https://www.nationalacademies.org/our-work/the-future-of-nursing-2020-2030

Nightingale, F. (1859). *Notes on nursing: What it is, and what it is not.* Harrison of Pall Mall.

Office of Disease Prevention and Health Promotion. (n.d.). *Social determinants of health.* U.S. Department of Health and Human Services. Retrieved October 31, 2022, from https://health.gov/healthypeople/priority-areas/social-determinants-health

Rosswurm, M. A., & Larrabee, J. H. (1999). A model for change to evidence-based practice. *Journal of Nursing Scholarship, 31*(4), 317–322. https://doi.org/10.1111/j.1547-5069.1999.tb00510.x

Saad, L. (2022, January 12). *Military brass, judges among professions at new image lows.* Gallup. https://news.gallup.com/poll/388649/military-brass-judges-among-professions-new-image-lows.aspx

Sackett, D. L., Straus S. E., Richardson, W. S., Rosenberg, W., & Haynes, R. B. (2000). *Evidence-based medicine: How to practice and teach EBM* (2nd ed.). Churchill Livingstone.

Stevens, K. R. (2004). *ACE Star model of EBP: Knowledge transformation.* Academic Center for Evidence-Based Practice, The University of Texas Health Science Center at San Antonio. www.acestar.uthscsa.edu

Thoma, A., & Eaves, F. F., III. (2015). A brief history of evidence-based medicine (EBM) and the contributions of Dr. David Sackett. *Aesthetic Surgery Journal, 35*(8), NP261–NP263. https://doi.org/10.1093/asj/sjv130

Waldrop, J. B., & Jennings Dunlap, J. (2024). The Mountain Model for evidence-based practice quality improvement. *The American Journal of Nursing,* May.

IMAGE CREDITS

Fig. 1.2: Source: https://health.ucdavis.edu/cnr/evidence_based_practice.html.
Fig. 1.3: Source: https://deming.org/explore/pdsa/.
Fig. 1.4: Source: https://www.oracle.com/ca-en/health/quintuple-aim/.
Fig. 1.5: Crystal A. Grys, "Evidence-Based Practice, Quality Improvement, and Research: A Visual Model," Nursing, vol. 52, no. 11. Copyright © 2022 by Wolters Kluwer.
Fig. 1.8: Source: https://www.kff.org/report-section/beyond-health-care-the-role-of-social-determinants-in-promoting-health-and-health-equity-issue-brief/.
IMG 1.1: Copyright © 2019 Depositphotos/Krakenimages.com.

CHAPTER 2

Quality and Safety as Nursing Practice Mainstays

Bradi B. Granger, Staci S. Reynolds, and Julee Briscoe Waldrop

KEY CONCEPTS

Micro, meso, and macro levels of quality context

Institute of Medicine (IOM)

Quadruple Aim

Quintuple Aim

Six domains of healthcare quality (STEEEP)

National Patient Safety Goals (NPSGs)

Just culture

LEARNING OBJECTIVES

1. Explore the background of healthcare quality and safety.
2. Identify the practicing nurse's role in quality and safety.
3. Discuss impacts of just culture and event reporting.

> Mistakes are a fact of life. It is the response to error that counts.
>
> —Nikki Giovanni

Introduction

What is quality in healthcare, and how do we recognize it? The purpose of this chapter is to introduce the background and underlying principles of healthcare quality, one aspect of which is safety. There are three levels at which the quality and safety of care combine to impact the success and sustainability of quality improvement in healthcare. The first is the **micro level**, which includes the immediate clinical team. As a nurse, this is the level at which you will likely work most often. The **meso level** includes the organization (e.g., the entire hospital), and the **macro level** includes the entire healthcare system. It is important that you understand how your practice and various contextual factors can impact the quality and safety of patient care at each level. For example, in your clinical unit, the staff culture and readiness to implement evidence-based practices may affect practice improvements on the unit (i.e., at the micro level). Similarly, at the meso level, hospital-based policies, the size of the organization, and the range of services provided can impact the ability to improve care. Finally, at the macro level of the larger health system (which may include many hospitals across locations), the quality of care can be impacted by such factors as environmental pressures, demography of the populations served, or locations of affiliated hospitals and clinics (e.g., in urban or rural areas; Fulop & Robert, 2015). Healthcare quality is not only located in hospital settings. Outpatient settings like clinics and community health centers and public health departments are also included.

Let's look at an example of how a nurse improves the quality and safety of care in a busy clinic setting.

MEDICATION RECONCILIATION

Nurse Rogers knows that medication errors, such as wrong prescriptions, incorrect doses, or drug interactions, are common causes of preventable harm. She has noticed an increasing number of patients who reported side effects or interactions from their medications. These issues often arose due to incomplete medication histories, patients seeing multiple providers, or lack of clarity about medication changes. Nurse Rogers discussed this with her colleagues, and together they developed and initiated a protocol where all patients, upon their visit, were required to provide a complete list of their current medications, including over-the-counter drugs, herbal supplements, and vitamins. They developed online patient education materials that highlighted the importance of maintaining an updated list of medications and the potential risks of drug interaction that were accessed by QR code. This included an easily modifiable place to list all medications. This could be reviewed with patients at each visit. In monthly medication reconciliation meetings with the clinic's care providers, physicians, nurse practitioners, and pharmacists, they discussed common drug interactions, recent changes in medication guidelines, and shared experiences and insights. In addition, they worked with the clinic's IT team, and Nurse Rogers designed a more user-friendly interface for medication management within the Electronic Health Record system. This included alerts for potential drug interactions and duplicate therapies. The last initiative was a follow-up phone call to patients from a nurse after any significant medication change to ensure the patient understood the change, check for any early side effects, and answer questions. Through this comprehensive approach, Nurse Rogers was able to lead an EBPQI initiative to reduce medication errors and foster a culture of safety and collaboration within the clinic.

It is important that you as a nurse understand the measurement of quality and understand the foundational evidence that supports contemporary quality measures in the United States and abroad. Not surprisingly, the goals for healthcare quality are universal and have been established or adopted by the National Academy of Medicine (formerly the Institute of Medicine) as well as the World Health Organization. If you are knowledgeable about the standards for care quality and how they are measured, you will be able to identify practices that are substandard and need improvement. Later in this textbook, we will explore measurement methodologies (Chapter 9) and step-by-step strategies for creating an evaluation plan to determine the impact of EBPQI initiatives in clinical practice (Chapter 11).

Background of Healthcare Quality

In recent decades, researchers and providers have focused on improving quality and safety in the U.S. healthcare arena. Their efforts have resulted in a host of related organizations, government agencies, and private foundations and contributed to the evolution of the national quality agenda. These efforts have also introduced numerous new terms, guidelines, and quality metrics that may seem unclear or confusing, but a bit of background should help to clarify when and why these innovations came about.

The roots of healthcare quality and safety can be traced back to the 1800s (see Figure 2.1), when Florence Nightingale collected and reported data that identified an association between poor hospital conditions and high mortality among soldiers in the Crimean War (Nightingale, 1863). Nightingale's findings helped improve the quality of care provision through implementing what we now know as evidence-based practices: frequent handwashing, exposure to natural light, clean drinking water, and other basic sanitation measures (Nightingale, 1859). In the early 1900s, Ernest Codman, a surgeon at Massachusetts General Hospital, initiated the end-results system (Altan et al., 2022), a precursor to outcomes management, by tracking surgical patients and documenting their outcomes to determine the cause of complications, including associations with their surgeon's proficiency and the hospital's efficiency. Codman's advocacy for tracing poor surgical outcomes to their source was not always popular with his fellow practitioners or hospital administrators, but his work to improve healthcare quality assurance and control

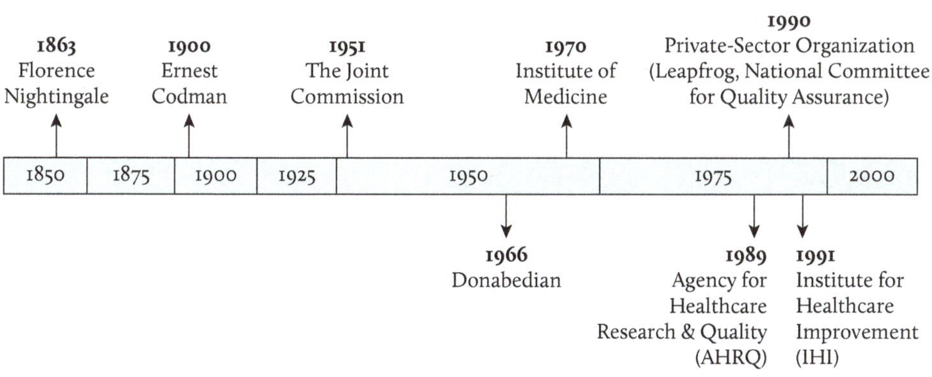

FIGURE 2.1 Timeline of Seminal Events in the History of Healthcare Quality

across levels is now credited for the standardization of surgical practices and the eventual development of The Joint Commission in 1951 (Chun & Bafford, 2014).

In 1966, Avedis Donabedian published "Evaluating the Quality of Medical Care," which added elements of structure, process, and outcomes to the evaluation of quality of care (Donabedian, 1966). Shortly thereafter, the Institute of Medicine (IOM) launched seminal work focused on quality and safety. In 1989, the Agency for Healthcare Research and Quality (AHRQ) was created in response to reports of misuse and overuse of treatments and to data that revealed variations in practice. In 1991, Dr. Don Berwick founded the Institute for Healthcare Improvement, or IHI (Berwick, 1991a), a repository of resources that provide guidance to clinicians who conduct quality improvement initiatives (Berwick, 1991b). A nonprofit organization called The Leapfrog Group was founded in 1998 by a group of independent business leaders in response to the increasing cost and poor quality of healthcare; the aim of this organization is to give consumers a stronger voice to support positive change within the U.S. healthcare system, champion transparency in healthcare, and collect evidence to promote informed consumer choices (The Leapfrog Group, n.d.). You will learn more about these tools and resources in Chapter 9.

Two landmark reports highlighted serious issues in U.S. healthcare and provided a profound continued impetus for change. **The Institute of Medicine (IOM)**, now the National Academy of Medicine (NAM), published the transformative report *To Err Is Human* in 2000, followed by *Crossing the Quality Chasm* in 2001. These reports noted that medical errors caused up to 98,000 deaths annually (Institute of Medicine, 2000, 2001). As the need for improved healthcare quality gained a spotlight, healthcare institutions, organizations, and the government joined in efforts to improve the quality of patient care, including through reimbursement and payment models based on high-quality care delivery (Porter, 2009).

The Quintuple Aim

The transparency of open, public reporting became the backdrop for a quality assessment framework developed by the Institute of Medicine. In 2008, Dr. Donald Berwick and colleagues defined a framework for high-quality care known as the Triple Aim: (a) improving the individual experience of healthcare, (b) improving the health of the populations, and (c) reducing the per capita costs of healthcare. A fourth aim, achieving meaning in work, was eventually included, so the framework became known as the **Quadruple Aim** (Bodenheimer & Sinsky, 2014). In 2021, achieving health equity was added as a fifth aim (Nunday et al., 2022). The **Quintuple Aim** requires all healthcare team members to be highly effective and engaged, provide equitable care, and have a sense of meaning and accomplishment in their contributions (see Chapter 1, Figure 1.4).

Affordable Care Act

In 2010, President Barack Obama signed the Affordable Care Act (ACA) with the intent to modernize the U.S. healthcare system, and in 2011, the Centers for Medicare and Medicaid Services (CMS) released the final rules for Accountable Care Organizations (ACOs), which were established to guide healthcare providers and hospitals toward more coordinated, higher quality, patient-centered care. Healthcare quality and safety issues continue to be researched and addressed as the need for improvement in various areas, or domains, of care are recognized.

The Healthcare Quality Framework (STEEEEP)

The **Six Domains of Healthcare Quality** (**STEEEEP**) is a framework that was first published in 2001 and continues to drive the national quality agenda across all public and private sectors (Institute of Medicine, 2001). The six original domains included safety, timeliness, effectiveness, efficiency, equity, and patient-centeredness. A seventh domain, eco-friendly, has now been added. There is no established hierarchy among the six, nor is their importance linear; in fact, the volume of evidence, metrics, measures, and indicators for each domain is highly variable. Since their origin in 2001, the domains of safety and effectiveness have dominated the landscape, both in terms of funding, political priority, and public awareness. As a result, the bulk of focused academic work and scientific development has targeted the quality domains of safety and effectiveness, resulting in a plethora of related measures, tools, and reimbursement incentives. However, with the birth of the Patient Protection and Affordable Care Act in 2010, the U.S. Congress voted to establish the Patient-Centered Outcomes Research Institute (PCORI). The funding for and national focus on patient-centeredness as a key component of high-quality healthcare has resulted in an increase in tools, care delivery process indicators, and outcome measures associated with patient-centered care.

In 2022, the model for the six quality domains was revised to depict person-centeredness as a ring encompassing all healthcare quality (see Figure 2.2). Also in 2022, the impact of the environment on health was added to the model, creating a

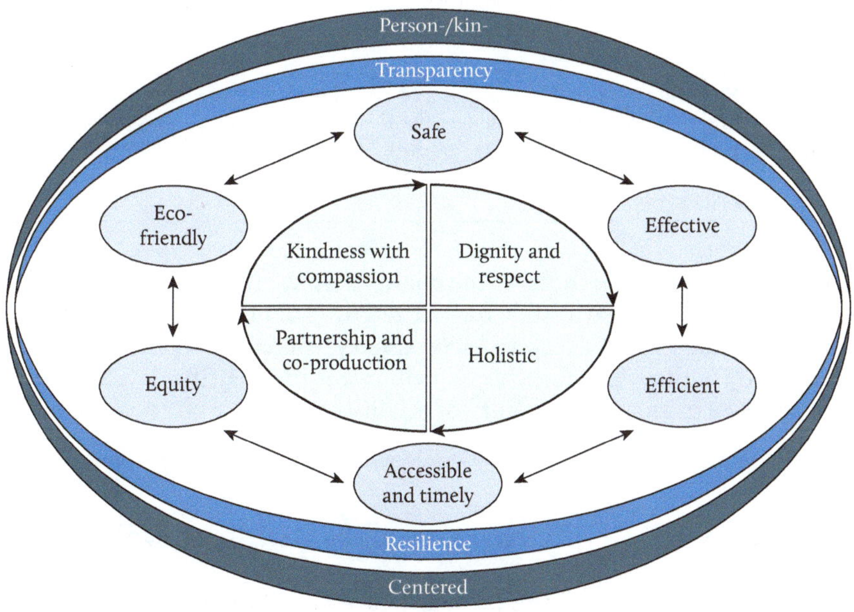

FIGURE 2.2 Seven Domains of Healthcare Quality

TABLE 2.1 Healthcare Quality Domains (STEEEEP) Definitions and Examples for Patients With Heart Failure

Domain	Definition	Example of measure in heart failure
Safe	Avoiding harm to patients from the care that is intended to help them	Healthcare-associated pressure injuries are reduced by routinely checking that nasal cannulas are positioned accurately.
Timely	Reducing wait times and possibly harmful delays for persons who are receiving or providing care	Patients receive a 48-hour follow-up call, and barriers to follow-up care are identified and documented.
Effective	Providing appropriate services based on scientific knowledge only to patients who may benefit from them (avoiding underuse and misuse)	Medications for heart failure to be administered at home are prescribed at time of discharge.
Efficient	Avoiding waste, including waste of equipment, supplies, ideas, and energy	Discharge readiness is documented before 11:00 a.m., and an electronically generated after-visit summary is provided to patients before discharge.
Equitable	Providing care that does not vary in quality because of personal characteristics such as gender, ethnicity, geographic location, or socioeconomic status	Barriers to care are assessed, and social determinants of health are documented and appropriately addressed by the multidisciplinary team (e.g., social work, behavioral health, language translation services).
Eco-friendly	Maintaining a hospital environment that minimizes risks to patients and local communities (e.g., addressing energy use and waste disposal management)	At-home air quality index is assessed, and the at-home area deprivation index is documented.
Patient-centered	Providing care that is respectful of and responsive to individual patient preferences, needs, and values and ensuring that patient values guide all clinical decisions	The patient's preferred language is documented, and a translator is provided as needed.

seventh domain and a fourth "E" in the quality acronym (STEEEEP; see Table 2.1). Most recently, the national agenda has shifted toward identifying and addressing inequities in healthcare delivery and accessibility; this shift will likely also impact priorities and funding, and (one hopes) will result in scientific development and clinical practice to ensure the equity of quality care.

National Organizations for Quality Oversight

Many organizations contribute to healthcare quality oversight. These organizations each play a significant role in setting standards for quality in their particular areas. To meet goals and standards, whether mandated or voluntary requires monitoring and reporting and accountability.

The Department of Health and Human Services

Contemporary oversight of quality in healthcare is organized by the federal executive branch of government under the DHHS (Figure 2.3), which oversees the functions, roles, responsibilities, and reporting relationships of 12 federal operating divisions, six of which are directly responsible for various aspects of healthcare quality, education, regulation, and funding. These six divisions (listed alphabetically) are the Agency for Healthcare Research and Quality (AHRQ), the

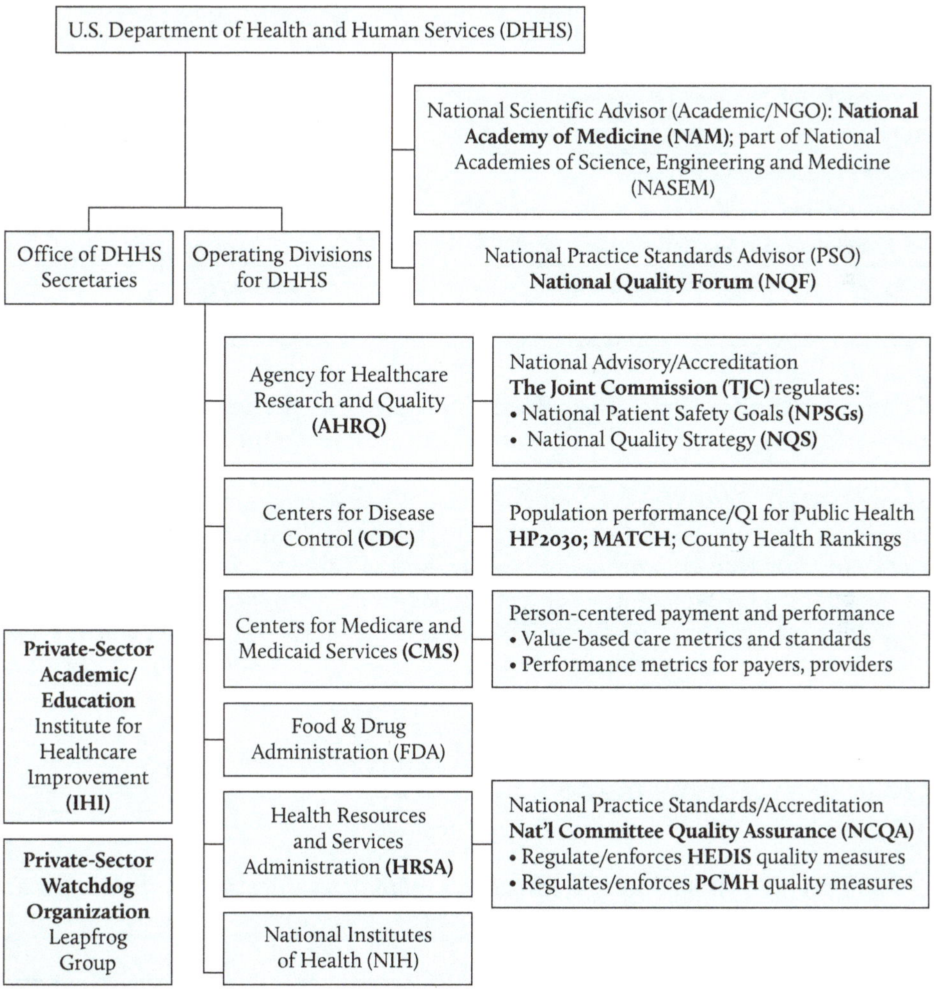

Key:
NPSG - National Patient Safety Goals
HEDIS - Healthcare Effectiveness Data and Information Set
PCMH - Patient-Centered Medical Home

FIGURE 2.3 Organizational Hierarchy for Creation, Regulation, and Enforcement of Quality

TABLE 2.2 Department of Health and Human Services Quality Oversight Agencies and Organizations

Agency or organization	Acronym	Website
Department of Health and Human Services	DHHS	https://www.hhs.gov/
National Academy of Medicine	NAM	https://nam.edu/
National Quality Forum	NQF	https://www.qualityforum.org/
Agency for Healthcare Research and Quality	AHRQ	https://www.ahrq.gov/
The Joint Commission	TJC	https://www.jointcommission.org
Centers for Disease Control and Prevention	CDC	https://www.cdc.gov/
Centers for Medicare and Medicaid Services	CMS	https://www.cms.gov/
Health Resources and Services Administration	HRSA	https://www.hrsa.gov/
National Committee Quality Assurance	NCQA	https://www.ncqa.org/
Institute for Healthcare Improvement	IHI	https://www.ihi.org/
Leapfrog Group	Leapfrog	https://www.leapfroggroup.org/

Centers for Disease Control and Prevention (CDC), the Centers for Medicare and Medicaid Services (CMS), the Food and Drug Administration (FDA), the Health Resources and Services Administration (HRSA), and the National Institutes of Health (NIH). Of these, the first three are directly responsible for regulatory, accreditation, and educational activities for hospitals, health systems, payers, and clinicians, and thus they are described in detail in Table 2.2. The overarching goal of the DHHS and each of its operating divisions is to provide the highest quality of care to patients and their families across all settings (e.g., home, clinic, acute care, specialty services, skilled nursing, hospice). Information about individual agencies can be found at their websites.

National Academy of Medicine (NAM)

The National Academy of Medicine (NAM), known as the Institute of Medicine (IOM) until 2015, is a nonprofit, nongovernmental organization. Operating as an honorary, elected membership body, NAM provides unbiased, evidence-based, and authoritative information on health, health policy, biomedical science, and technology to policymakers, professionals, leaders across both government and nongovernmental sectors of society, and the public at large. The National Academy of Medicine is a part of the National Academies of Sciences, Engineering, and Medicine.

The role of NAM is to generate evidence-based recommendations and reports on key issues impacting health. Most of these studies are requested and funded by the federal government. Other sponsors include private industry, foundations, and local governments, as well as the academy itself. All reports are available online free of charge by the National Academies Press (https://nam.edu).

The Future of Nursing reports have been developed by the IOM/NAM since 1990 and provide direction for the nursing workforce and profession in the coming decade. The most recent report, *The Future of Nursing 2020–2030: Charting a Path to Health Equity*, was published in 2021 (National Academies of Sciences, Engineering, and Medicine, 2021). The report envisions nurses as leaders in addressing health inequities based on our fundamental views of optimizing health instead of curing disease. Nurses are also integrated into diverse settings both in practice and personally where we can have an impact on the health and well-being of the nation. Because improving health is dependent on correcting social determinants of health and systemic racism, these underlying issues are a priority for nurses to address. However, in order for nurses to optimize their expertise, nursing organizations, state and federal governmental agencies, and nursing educational institutions will have to come together. Nurses can better use their knowledge and skills when restrictions on their practice are lifted and reimbursement is provided for their efforts. Lastly, nurses must also recognize that we need to care for ourselves in order to care for others. This is one reason why we have added wellness information and activity suggestions to each chapter in this book!

The National Quality Forum (NQF)

The NQF is a nonprofit, nonpartisan, membership-based organization under contract to the DHHS. The NQF works to catalyze improvements in healthcare through NQF-selected measures and standards that enhance value, safety, and patient outcomes. Selection of these measures by the NQF membership is done through consensus; however, experts who represent diverse interests from every healthcare sector make recommendations on measures based on evidence, discussion, debate, and input from end users and key stakeholders at every level.

The NQF measures are focused on five basic areas of healthcare quality: immunization, Alzheimer's and dementia, care coordination, the healthcare workforce, and person-centered care. Standards within these five areas are selected through the NQF process of stakeholder consensus, and they are set as standards for quality within their respective domains of the healthcare quality framework. Not all domains of the framework are addressed by NQF standards, but some are (effectiveness and person-centeredness primarily).

The Agency for Healthcare Research and Quality (AHRQ)

The Agency for Healthcare Research and Quality (AHRQ) is the lead federal agency charged with improving the safety and quality of healthcare for all Americans. From 2011–2017, on behalf of the DHHS, it led the National Quality Strategy (NQS), a national (not federal) initiative established to serve as a catalyst and compass for a nationwide focus on quality improvement efforts. The NQS was the first-ever national effort backed by legislation to align public- and private-sector stakeholders to achieve one goal: better health and healthcare for all Americans.

Core competencies associated with AHRQ include (a) health systems research, (b) practice improvement, and (c) data and analytics. Practicing nurses can utilize AHRQ's resources to help improve the quality of care provided to patients. For example, an interprofessional team at Morgan Stanley Children's Hospital used one resource, the Comprehensive Unit-Based Safety Program method (AHRQ, n.d.), to improve operating room efficiency. A priority aim was to improve *first case on-time start* (*FCOTS*; i.e., avoid a delayed start time of the first surgery of the day). The team's strategy involved switching staff responsibilities to task night shift nurses with beginning preparations for the day's surgeries before the arrival of the day shift. As a result of this change, FCOTS percentages improved each year over the 5 years reported compared to before the practice changes were implemented (Raman et al., 2022). TeamSTEPPS® is another tool provided by AHRQ and is a curriculum that helps optimize patient outcomes by improving communication and teamwork among all healthcare members (https://www.ahrq.gov/teamstepps-program/index.html) .

The Joint Commission (TJC)

The Joint Commission (TJC) was founded in 1951 as an independent, nonprofit organization. As the nation's oldest and largest standards-setting and accrediting body in healthcare, TJC aims to improve healthcare quality through the accreditation of healthcare settings (hospitals, home care, skilled nursing facilities, nursing care centers, behavioral healthcare centers, ambulatory care centers, and laboratories). TJC's central office provides a hub for interaction with federal government leaders on regulatory and policy issues to improve healthcare quality for the public. TJC activities focus on establishing quality standards, evaluating the performance of individual healthcare organizations, and providing education to organizations to support continuous quality improvement. TJC certification is recognized nationally as a gold seal of quality approval and an acknowledgment of competency and skill in providing safe and effective care. TJC accreditation is a DHHS requirement for financial reimbursement of CMS funding; any setting receiving federal Medicare and Medicaid funding for care delivery must meet the standards for accreditation established by TJC and be periodically reevaluated and reaccredited. Internationally, hospitals may be accredited by DNV (https://www.dnv.com/services/hospital-accreditation-7516). Their standards are approved by CMS and can be applied by any hospital to support the development of continual improvement of healthcare quality and safety.

In 2003, TJC adopted and implemented the **National Patient Safety Goals (NPSGs)** to promote quality improvement and ensure that patient safety meets set standards in all accredited organizations. The NPSGs apply across the three chapters of the TJC: Hospital Chapter, Ambulatory Health Chapter, and Nursing Care Center Chapter. The following are among the highest priority goals:

- Identify patients correctly.
- Prevent infection.
- Improve staff communication.

- Identify patient safety risks.
- Prevent mistakes in surgery.
- Use medicines safely.
- Use alarms safely.

Major focus areas include promoting surgical safety and preventing hospital-acquired infections, medication errors, inpatient suicide, and specific clinical harms such as falls and pressure ulcers. In 2023, a health equity safety goal (NPSG #16) was added; this goal represents a landmark step toward establishing standards and measures to ensure equitable care because although "equity" has been a key quality domain since the original definition and establishment of healthcare quality by the IOM in 2001, recognition of standards and measures for equity have not been detailed (TJC, 2023).

Centers for Disease Control and Prevention (CDC)

The Centers for Disease Control and Prevention (CDC) is the nation's leading science-based organization dedicated to protecting the public's health. During the COVID-19 pandemic, the CDC provided necessary guidance on how to keep patients and healthcare workers safe, including guidelines for COVID-19 testing, use of personal protective equipment, and treatment of the virus. Practicing nurses can find many useful resources through the CDC, such as guidance on maintaining urinary catheters and central venous access devices to help prevent healthcare-associated infections (CDC, 2022).

Health Resources and Services Administration (HRSA)

HRSA programs provide equitable healthcare to people who are geographically isolated and economically or medically vulnerable. Quality measures for HRSA are established by the National Committee on Quality Assurance and implemented across programs that deliver care to people with low incomes, residents of rural areas, American Indians and Alaska Natives, people with HIV, pregnant people, mothers and their families, and those otherwise unable to access high-quality healthcare. HRSA oversees quality and accreditation for programs that serve the underserved (e.g., by providing discounts on prescription drugs to safety net providers or facilitating organ, bone marrow, and cord blood transplantation for those unable to access these types of specialty care).

The National Committee on Quality Assurance (NCQA)

The National Committee on Quality Assurance (NCQA) was established in 1991 to develop and enforce quality standards such as the Healthcare Effectiveness Data and Information Set (HEDIS).

HEDIS is a comprehensive set of standardized performance measures designed to provide purchasers and consumers with information needed for reliable comparison of health plan performance. HEDIS measures relate to a variety of significant public health issues, such as cancer, heart disease, smoking, asthma, and diabetes. Healthcare organizations can use HEDIS performance data to identify performance gaps and opportunities for improvement, establish realistic targets for improvement, track improvement or monitor the success of quality improvement initiatives, and provide a set of measurement standards that allow comparison with other plans (see Table 2.3).

TABLE 2.3 Healthcare Effectiveness Data and Information Set (HEDIS) for Hospital and Outpatient Care Settings

Measures by quality domain	Hospital setting (TJC standards and NPSGs)	Outpatient setting (HEDIS)
Safe falls risk example	Proportion of patients assessed for falls risk on admission Proportion of patients for whom falls prevention measures were documented Proportion of actual falls and falls with injury of those at risk per 1,000 patient days	*Discussing Fall Risk.* The percentage of Medicare members 65 years of age and older who were seen by a practitioner in the past 12 months and who discussed falls or problems with balance or walking with their current practitioner. *Managing Fall Risk.* The percentage of Medicare members 65 years of age and older who had a fall or had problems with balance or walking in the past 12 months, who were seen by a practitioner in the past 12 months, and who received a recommendation for how to prevent falls or treat problems with balance or walking from their current practitioner.
Timely transitions of care and planning for all-cause readmission examples	Follow-up after acute admission: Provide a 48-hour follow-up call. Identify and document barriers to follow-up care. Review the after-visit summary with patient at discharge and transmit to primary care provider.	Patients discharged from the hospital should be seen by their primary care provider within 30 days of discharge to prevent the patient from being readmitted. The percentage of discharges for members 18 years of age and older who had each of the following. Four rates are reported: 1. Notification of inpatient admission: documentation of receipt of notification of inpatient admission on the day of admission through 2 days after the admission (3 total days). 2. Receipt of discharge information: documentation of receipt of discharge information on the day of discharge through 2 days after the discharge (3 total days). 3. Patient engagement after inpatient discharge: documentation of patient engagement (e.g., office visits, visits to the home, telehealth) provided within 30 days after discharge. 4. Medication reconciliation post-discharge: documentation of medication reconciliation on the date of discharge through 30 days after discharge (31 total days).

Measures by quality domain	Hospital setting (TJC standards and NPSGs)	Outpatient setting (HEDIS)
Effective cardiac care example	Provide guideline-directed medications at the time of discharge. Provide at least 60 minutes of education for medications and post-discharge planning needs.	Patients 18–85 years of age who had a diagnosis of hypertension and whose blood pressure was adequately controlled (<140/90mmHg) during the measurement year. The percentage of members 18 years of age and older during the measurement year who were hospitalized with a diagnosis of acute myocardial infarction and who received persistent beta-blocker treatment for 6 months after discharge.
Efficient avoidance of acute care utilization	Reduce readmission rates; report proportion of planned versus unplanned (occurring within 30 days of an acute care admission).	For members 18 years of age and older, the risk-adjusted ratio of observed-to-expected acute inpatient and observation stay discharges during the measurement year. Also, the risk-adjusted ratio of observed-to-expected emergency department visits during the measurement year.
Equitable social needs screening example	Providing care that does not vary in quality because of personal characteristics such as gender, ethnicity, geographic location, and socioeconomic status (NPSG #16)	The percentage of members who were screened, using prespecified instruments, at least once during the measurement period for unmet food, housing, and transportation needs and received a corresponding intervention if they screened positive.
Person-centered experience of care example	Hospital Consumer Assessment of Healthcare Providers and Systems [HCAHPS]*	Consumer Assessment of Healthcare Providers and Systems [CAHPS]*: This measure provides information on the experiences of commercial and Medicaid members with the organization and gives a general indication of how well the organization meets members' expectations. Results summarize member experiences through ratings, composites, and question summary rates. Four global rating questions reflect overall satisfaction: 1. Rating of all healthcare 2. Rating of health plan 3. Rating of personal doctor 4. Rating of specialist seen most often Five composite scores summarize responses in key areas: 1. Claims processing (commercial only) 2. Customer service 3. Getting care quickly 4. Getting needed care 5. How well doctors communicate Item-specific question summary rates are reported for the rating questions and each composite question. Question summary rates are also reported individually for one item summarizing the following concept: 1. Coordination of care

**The eco-friendly quality domain is not yet addressed in the HEDIS.*

Nursing Organizations and Nurse-Led Initiatives

Professional nursing organizations and nurse-led initiatives are engaged in improving the quality and safety of healthcare. In 2014, the American Academy of Nursing was the first nursing organization to partner with other medical and healthcare organizations, such as the American Board of Internal Medicine, to encourage conversations in healthcare about which evidence-based practices should be considered of current value. Here are five practices that have been deemed potentially unsafe:

- Automatically initiating continuous electronic fetal heart rate monitoring during labor for women without risk factors
- Allowing older adults to remain in bed or get up only to sit in a chair during their hospital stay
- Using physical restraints with an older hospitalized patient
- Waking the patient for routine care when their condition or care does not specifically require it
- Placing or maintaining a urinary catheter in a patient when there is no specific indication to do so

Have you seen any of these practices being used while on your clinical rotations? As you learned in Chapter 1, it can take approximately 15 years for a change in practice to become the new normal, so there is likely still room for you to consider improvements in these areas. See Table 2.4 for more examples of nurse-led endeavors.

TABLE 2.4 Nursing Organizations and Initiatives Focused on Improving Quality in Healthcare

Organization	Initiative	Description	For more information
American Academy of Nursing	Choosing Wisely Campaign	Encourages patients and nurses to question healthcare practices and identify the evidence behind them	https://www.aannet.org/americanacademyofnursing/initiatives/choosing-wisely
American Nurses Association	National Alliance for Quality Care (NAQC); Quality and Safety Education for Nurses (QSEN)	NAQC works in tandem with QSEN to advance high-quality, patient-centered healthcare	https://www.nursingworld.org/practice-policy/naqc/

Organization	Initiative	Description	For more information
Registered Nurses Association of Ontario	Best Practice Guidelines (BPG)	Systematically developed evidence-based recommendations for nursing practice comprising 10 categories: children and youth, clinical, equity, diversity and inclusion, foundational, health system, healthy work environment, mental health and substance use, older adults, and population health	https://rnao.ca/bpg/guidelines
American Organization of Nursing Leadership (AONL)/ American Association of Critical Care Nurses (AACN)	Healthy Work Environment	Has developed nine elements of a healthy work environment contributing to high-quality and safe patient care (e.g., adequate numbers of qualified nurses present, shared decision making at all levels)	https://www.aonl.org/elements-healthy-practice-environment

Identifying Specific Clinical Problems and Population Health Issues

You now have a sense of the big picture of quality metrics and regulation, but how can you, as a nurse, identify healthcare problems? There are practice-focused ways to identify healthcare problems. Your observations or personal experiences—what you see and hear in your daily practice—will often provide your first insight into a problem that can be addressed. A coworker may come to you with a concern. A patient may alert you to an issue that is worrisome from their perspective. You may realize that you or others lack the knowledge to attend to a specific patient care need. Perhaps the standard of care has recently been changed and your unit has not made corresponding updates in practice to meet the new standard. Perhaps you have attended a conference or professional organization meeting and heard about a new practice that has improved care elsewhere. The problem you identify may be broad and chronic or small and specific to your organization or unit. When you think you have found a problem, ask yourself, "What evidence do I have to support that this is a problem?"

Your workplace will provide a variety of locations in which to search for evidence. Many problems in healthcare organizations, especially hospitals, are tracked by the national/international safety and quality organizations described previously in this chapter. Data on how well an organization meets their standards is often available to the public. Such benchmarking allows potential patients and other

TABLE 2.5 Example Quality Care Indicators Dashboard

Healthcare-associated infection (HAI) rates	United Acres Hospital	State average	National average	Areas for improvement
CLASBI	1.22	2.0	1.0	X
CAUTI	0.5	1.5	1.0	
Surgical site infection (SSI)	1.8	2.0	1.0	X
MRSA bacteremia	2.0	1.5	1.0	X
Clostridioides difficile (C. diff)	0.4	1.0	1.0	

CLABSI = central line-associated bloodstream infection; CAUTI = catheter-associated urinary tract infection; MRSA = Methicillin-resistant Staphylococcus aureus

interested groups to compare certain aspects of quality (between hospitals or healthcare organizations) and thus make an informed choice about where they wish to receive (and pay) for their care (see Table 2.5).

Adverse Events

Despite advances and improvements in quality over the past few decades, the prevalence of adverse events and patient harm continues to present hospitals with opportunities for improvement. A study by Bates and colleagues (2023) found evidence of patient harm in nearly 1 in 4 hospital admissions, and 25% of this harm was preventable; such findings highlight the need for an ongoing focus on quality and safety in healthcare. Decades ago, the main takeaway from the IOM (2000) report *To Err Is Human* was that errors responsible for harm were primarily due to systems problems rather than human errors. Human errors occur when the conduct of an individual or group unintentionally causes (or could have caused) an undesirable outcome (IOM, 2000). Human errors are inevitable, even among the most conscientious nurses who consistently practice the highest care standards, and typically result from a system(s) failure or process breakdown (Marx, 2001). Although humans do commit errors, a focus on making healthcare systems safer continues to be of paramount importance.

The Joint Commission (n.d.) conducts evaluations of healthcare organizations with the purpose of inspiring them to hold the highest standards of quality and safety and pursue continuous quality improvement. To identify opportunities for improvement, hospitals accredited by TJC keep track of sentinel events. A *sentinel event* is a patient safety event that results in death, permanent harm, or severe temporary harm (TJC, 2021). These events are often high on an organization's list of problems needing a solution. The most common sentinel event reported to TJC in 2021 were falls. As you will see in future chapters, nurses can play a leadership role in preventing falls and other events that pose harm.

Healthcare organizations try to prevent sentinel events by collecting data on adverse events and near misses. Reports that generate this information are commonly referred to as *incident reports*. An *adverse event* is any event that resulted in an undesirable outcome (e.g., longer hospital stay, harm to the patient, death) not caused by the underlying disease process. Of particular importance, but often overlooked and underreported, are near misses and close calls. A *near miss* or *close call* is an event that could have resulted in a patient injury but did not due to mere chance (AHRQ, 2019). TJC describes a near miss as a patient safety event that didn't make it to the patient (Marks et al., 2013). As a nurse, you will likely experience or witness multiple near misses throughout your nursing career. It is important to pay attention to these close calls. You should view them as symptoms of areas that require attention rather than as proof that healthcare system safeguards are effective. Ignoring a near miss only increases the chance that a patient will be harmed next time (Ulrich, 2015).

A care omission, or care left undone, is harder to measure than an error but can be equally harmful. Most studies on care omissions are cross-sectional surveys that ask nurses to self-report how often they do not complete specific aspects of care. In one study, only 15% of nurses surveyed said that they always reported care left undone (Ulrich & Kear, 2014). Similarly, a retrospective review of 100 patient charts found that between 8% and 84% of 32 identified care tasks had been partly or fully omitted during each patient's stay (Saar et al., 2021). Care omissions are harder to track and less likely to be reported than close calls, but when data on omissions is collected and used to identify trends and find systematic errors, it can be very valuable.

Incident reports should trigger a nonpunitive (i.e., not aimed at punishment) investigation of the situation with a focus on improving the system to prevent recurrence (rather than on finding someone to blame). Healthcare workers are often reluctant to report incidents or near misses because they fear retaliation. One way in which systems can address such reluctance is to establish a "just culture."

The concept of "just culture" was an underlying principle of the landmark report *To Err Is Human* by the Institute of Medicine (2000). **Just culture** is an industry-related concept based on systems thinking, which assumes that mistakes are not solely the fault of individuals but rather are a product of the organizational culture; therefore, organizational mistakes affecting workplace safety are investigated through a lens of justice and problem solving versus blame and punishment (Boysen, 2013).

A just culture supports the reporting of all types of errors (adverse events, near misses, omissions in care) because the organization understands and emphasizes that mistakes are generally the result of a faulty culture or systems failure rather than individual misconduct. Reports are encouraged because they help the organization to improve processes and systems to prevent or decrease the occurrence of errors. Healthcare leaders have a duty to (a) recognize the inevitability of errors, (b) design systems that decrease the risk or frequency of errors, and (c) avoid punitive reactions to honest mistakes (Pelletier, 2023). Awareness of your professional and site-specific responsibilities related to the quality of care, including the prevention and reporting of events, is central to your work as a nurse and patient advocate. In a just culture, the question asked following a problematic event should be "What went wrong?" rather than "Who is to blame?" Let's consider some sample cases of how errors can be addressed using communication and reporting.

REAL-WORLD EXAMPLE: MEDICATION ERROR

A 5-year-old boy with no known allergies receives a Bicillin (penicillin antibiotic) injection at an outpatient clinic to treat strep throat. Per clinic routine, his parents are asked to stay with him in the waiting room for 20 minutes while the staff monitored his reaction. A few minutes later, the nurse who administered the injection (Nurse 1) checks on the patient and thinks that he seems flushed and lethargic. She checks his vital signs and notes that the patient's pulse is rapid and weak and his systolic blood pressure has decreased considerably compared to before the injection. Suddenly, the child slides off his chair onto the floor and is difficult to rouse. The nurse promptly activates the clinic's rapid response team and moves the patient onto a table in an exam room with assistance from his parents. Another nurse (Nurse 2) and a physician soon arrive in the room. The physician gathers a brief history, quickly examines the patient, delivers a diagnosis of anaphylaxis (severe, life-threatening allergic reaction), and verbally states, "He needs epi now!" Nurse 2 retrieves a syringe and a vial of epinephrine from a drawer, and the physician orders, "Give it now." While Nurse 1 notifies emergency services and continues to recheck the patient, Nurse 2 administers the full contents of the 1 mg vial of epinephrine, approximately 10 times the recommended dose, into the child's upper arm. The child instantly vomits due to a rapid blood pressure increase, screams that his head hurts, and begins to sob.

Outcome: Following this incident, the clinic response team communicated with one another and quickly realized the medication error. When emergency services arrived, the team reported the patient's status and reaction to the medication injection; however, the physician refused to chart that she had given a verbal order for epinephrine with no specified dosage for fear of repercussions as a senior staff member. Nurses 1 and 2 understood that this was vital information, and unless it was entered into the electronic medical record, the providers to whom they had just verbally handed off care would not have access to accurate, timely information on which to base appropriate care for the patient. Nurse 1 encouraged the team to engage in an immediate debriefing, after which the physician completed accurate electronic charting of the event and reported the error in real time to ensure that the child would receive informed inpatient care and that the event would be investigated. The harm to the patient and potential for a dangerous outcome were serious but temporary, and the child experienced complete recovery, likely due to urgent care coordination, subsequent interventions, and continued monitoring.

Within 1 week, following a review, a second debriefing with clinic administrators occurred, during which evidence was presented to the entire team involved in the event. They learned that epinephrine dosage errors are common (Kanwar et al., 2010) and system-level practice changes were needed. Later that month, in all clinics within the large healthcare system, epinephrine vials were replaced with age-appropriate epi pens to reduce the opportunity for dosing errors. There have been no known cases of medication errors related to epinephrine across clinic sites since this improvement was made, years ago.

Real-World Reflection

What comes to your mind when you consider the unintentional occurrences along the healthcare continuum outlined in this example? The case involved an honest medication error and broken system processes. As we learned in Chapter 1, nursing is not a solo profession; we work as part of a system. The scenario involved team nursing, with more than one nurse providing direct patient care. Reflecting on this case may help you to think critically about the safety and quality of care you will provide as a nurse.

In this case the error was reported in a timely fashion, and ultimately, future harm was likely prevented due to local and system-level changes resulting from adherence to proper reporting mechanisms. Remember that adopting a systems mindset as a nurse requires thinking beyond blame and which person should be held responsible for errors. Individual behavior can indeed result in errors, yet viewing healthcare delivery from a systems perspective enables nurses to identify and respond to threats to safety within healthcare and find effective, comprehensive, and long-lasting solutions (Pelletier, 2023).

1. What do you think were the process breakdowns during this emergency?
2. How could a few moments of clarification during the emergency communication have prevented harm?
3. What type of events (sentinel, near miss, care omission) are outlined in this case?
4. What would have been the risks to the patient, team, organization, or future patients had the nurse(s) decided not to report this event?

The case above involves communication. Nurses can take charge of communication issues and use evidence to support improvements and reduce errors. In a systematic review of 18 studies, communication (nurse to nurse, nurse to patient, nurse to provider) issues were found to be the most common reasons for care being left undone (He et al., 2022). The TeamSTEPPS® initiative from IHI is one method used to improve quality metrics that hinge on clear communication (https://www.ahrq.gov/teamstepps-program/index.html).

The daily safety huddle is a TeamSTEPPS tool for (a) improving communication equitably among all healthcare workers involved in a patient's care and (b) facilitating trust when there is a patient safety concern so that immediate action can be undertaken. *Huddles* are brief meetings (10 minutes or less) that typically occur at the start of the workday or shift. As an example, Aldawood et al. (2020) report that one pediatric intensive care multidisciplinary team (e.g., physicians, nurses, dieticians, physiotherapists) increased their use of the daily huddle on their unit from 73% to 97% over 9 months. By increasing the systematic use of huddles, over 340 safety issues were addressed, with the majority related to infection control and medication errors. A bonus was that members of each of the different disciplines involved developed a more complete understanding of the roles and responsibilities of the others, especially of nursing!

Healthcare Employee and Patient Satisfaction

As you search for evidence that a problem exists, you should consider the perspectives of staff and employees. Evidence has demonstrated that satisfied employees are more likely to stay at their current place of employment (Pressley & Garside, 2023). Successful employee retention can save an organization the expense of hiring and training new staff. To determine how employees feel about their employment, organizations often request that they complete "climate surveys." Climate surveys can include questions about issues such as safety, diversity, equity, inclusion, and belonging. The results from these surveys can be used to identify areas for improvement.

If you have ever been a patient, you have likely been asked to respond to a survey about your experience at the healthcare organization. Organizations use various surveys to assess patient satisfaction. The Hospital Consumer Assessment of Healthcare Providers and Systems (HCAHPS) instrument was developed by the U.S. Centers for Medicare & Medicaid Service (CMS; 2023) to assess the quality of care during patient experiences. An organization's reimbursement by CMS is tied to how well its scores reflect high patient satisfaction. Another patient satisfaction survey, referred to as the "Press Ganey" after the company that developed it (https://www.pressganey.com/), is used by many hospitals and healthcare organizations to identify areas for improvement. Because nurses are involved in patient encounters in most settings, there are generally questions specific to nursing on patient satisfaction surveys; therefore, nurses can and should become involved in identifying issues that may be leading to lower scores (see Table 2.6 for examples).

Social Determinants of Health

In Chapter 1, you were introduced to social determinants of health (SDOH) that lead to health disparities (a major, chronic problem in healthcare). If you are observant, you will probably note the impact of SDOH on your patients. It is important to reflect on how SDOH impact the patients or populations for whom you care because when a presenting health problem is strongly associated with SDOH, simply treating its symptoms will not address (and may perpetuate) root causes of the problem.

TABLE 2.6 Examples of Questions Patients Answer About Their Nursing Care Experience

During this hospital stay or patient encounter:	Never	Sometimes	Usually	Always
How often did nurses treat you with courtesy and respect?				
How often did nurses listen carefully to you?				
How often did nurses explain things in a way you could understand?				

As an individual nurse, you may feel powerless to address complex social problems on a broad scale, but you can use evidence-based strategies to make a difference in the quality of care you provide to your patients and to make leadership changes on your unit. Your attitudes, beliefs, and behaviors impact everyone for whom and with whom you provide care. Let's look at a sample case and consider evidence-based strategies.

CASE STUDY: PREMATURE BIRTH

Carlos was born prematurely at 28 weeks gestation, weighing just 1.2 kg, to a 19-year-old single mother who lives in a low-income area of the city. The mother had limited prenatal care during her pregnancy due to a lack of transportation, inadequate financial resources, and a history of substance use during this pregnancy. After Carlos was born, he was immediately admitted to the neonatal intensive care unit due to his prematurity, low birth weight, and respiratory distress syndrome.

What SDOH can you identify in this case (refer to Chapter 1, Figure 1.7)? How are they related to an increased risk of poorer health for Carlos and his mother? We are confident you identified many SDOH issues, but let's discuss an obvious one: limited access to healthcare. Carlos's mother had limited access to prenatal care due to a lack of transportation and financial resources. Lack of adequate prenatal care has long been known to be associated with adverse birth outcomes, such as prematurity and low birth weight (Harrison & Goldenberg, 2015), which may contribute to subsequent health issues for Carlos.

Limited access to healthcare is certainly a sweeping problem, but you can be on your way to addressing this problem for your patient(s) by seeking out evidence related to the problem as well as potential solutions. Chapter 3 will show you how to begin. As a nurse caring for Carlos and his family, you can demonstrate equity in your care as well as work to improve the overall equity of care provided in your unit or your organization. Remember, equitable care is one of the STEEEEP domains of healthcare quality!

Climate Change and Health Issues

Social determinants of health intersect with the environment. The negative effects of climate change often have the greatest impact on populations who have contributed the least to the problem. For example, you have probably heard news reports about older persons dying in heat waves. Over the past 20 years, temperature change has led to a 53.7% increase in health-related deaths in people over 65 years of age (Watts et al., 2021). What can be done about this problem? How can systems be changed to help prevent these deaths?

As you might guess, nurses were early advocates for improving the environment to improve health. Florence Nightingale published work on the topic of ventilation and light in 1859, and the International Council of Nurses position statement on nurses, climate change and health urges nurses to actively address environmental issues (2018). The mission of the Alliance of Nurses for Health Environments (n.d.) is to promote an "understanding that optimal health requires good nutrition, adequate mobility, a healthy environment, and social support. Nurse members are committed to taking evidence-based action to improve the health of themselves and others while also healing the planet" (Our Mission section). By engaging in responsible personal practice (see Wellness in Action box below), you can inspire others. Working together, nurses can improve the problems of climate change, but it will take all of us to make a difference.

WRAPPING UP

As a nurse, you are part of a group that interacts the most with patients across healthcare settings and throughout the care continuum, with significant responsibility for identifying quality and safety issues as well as problem-solving evidence-based ways to improve. This chapter provides foundational knowledge about (a) how healthcare quality and safety are organized within the United States and (b) how to identify problems and evidence/data to drive improvement.

REFLECTION QUESTIONS

1. What is the leading cause of errors in healthcare?
2. How can you work toward maximizing effective team communication in your nursing practice setting?
3. Suppose your unit plans to initiate weekly team "huddles." What is the purpose of regular engagement in this activity?
4. As a new nurse, you are involved in a near-miss event. Your supervisor asks you not to fill out a digital event report form because no harm has reached the patient. Mandatory completion of written reports for such events is outlined in your institutional policy. What action will you take, and why?

WELLNESS IN ACTION: DECREASING ENERGY USE (CARBON FOOTPRINT)

All of us are being impacted by climate change. Have you heard the slogan "Reduce, Reuse, and Recycle"? This is the guiding principle for reducing your individual carbon footprint. Greenhouse gas emissions, the major cause of climate change, are measured *per person*! In 2020, the average emissions per person in the United States were 14.6 tons of CO_2 equivalent, which is more than double the average for the rest of the world (https://www.un.org/en/actnow/ten-actions). The United Nations ACT NOW campaign recommends 10 actions—things each individual can do right now—to limit climate change:

1. Save energy at home by switching to LED bulbs: These bulbs serve a dual purpose, as they save energy and don't need to be changed as often.

2. Walking, biking, or taking public transport = fewer cars on the roads: During the COVID-19 pandemic, the air quality in many major cities improved significantly because people were staying home and not driving their cars.
3. Eat more vegetables: Growing vegetables rather than raising animals for meat results in fewer greenhouse gasses (think of how much waste cows and pigs produce).
4. Consider your travel destinations: Airplanes require immense amounts of fossil fuels.
5. Throw away less food: In a landfill, foods produce methane, another greenhouse gas.
6. Reduce, reuse, repair, and recycle: These practices preserve resources and natural space on the planet.
7. Change your home's energy source: If possible, switch to wind or solar power.
8. Switch to an electric vehicle: You will appreciate the big savings as fossil fuel prices continue to increase.
9. Make your money count: Choose to spend it on products from companies that use environmental resources responsibly and limit fuel use and waste production.
10. Speak up: Let others know how you feel about climate change and whether you are embracing any of these recommendations. Role modeling is one of the most effective methods of fostering behavior change in others.

REFERENCES

Agency for Healthcare Research and Quality. (n.d.). *The CUSP method*. https://www.ahrq.gov/hai/cusp/index.html

Agency for Healthcare Research and Quality. (2019, September 7). *Adverse events, near misses, and errors*. Patient Safety Network. https://psnet.ahrq.gov/primer/adverse-events-near-misses-and-errors

Aldawood, F., Kazzaz, Y., AlShehri, A., Alali, H., & Al-Surimi, K. (2020). Enhancing teamwork communication and patient safety responsiveness in a paediatric intensive care unit using the daily safety huddle tool. *BMJ Open Quality*, *9*(1), e000753. https://doi.org/10.1136/bmjoq-2019-000753

Alliance of Nurses for Health Environments. (n.d.). *Home page*. https://www.nursesdrawdown.org

Altan, D., Leya, G. A., & Chang, D. C. (2022). Tracking the "end result" and long-term patient outcomes—Failure to rescue and the shrinking denominator. *JAMA Surgery*, *157*(3), 268. https://doi.org/10.1001/jamasurg.2021.6905

Bates, D. W., Levine, D. M., Salmasian, H., Syrowatka, A., Shahian, D. M., Lipsitz, S., Zebrowski, J. P., Myers, L. C., ... Mort, E. (2023). The safety of inpatient health care. *New England Journal of Medicine*, *388*(2), 142–153. https://doi.org/10.1056/NEJMsa2206117

Berwick, D. M. (1991a). Blazing the trail of quality: The HFHS quality management process. *Frontiers of Health Services Management*, *7*(4), 47–50. https://www.ncbi.nlm.nih.gov/pubmed/10110631

Berwick, D. M. (1991b). Controlling variation in health care: A consultation from Walter Shewhart. *Medical Care, 29*(12), 1212–1225. https://www.ncbi.nlm.nih.gov/pubmed/1745079

Berwick, D. M., Nolan, T. W., & Whittington, J. (2008). The Triple Aim: Care, health, and cost. *Health Affairs, 27*(3), 759–769. https://doi.org/10.1377/hlthaff.27.3.759

Bodenheimer, T., & Sinsky, C. (2014). From Triple to Quadruple Aim: Care of the patient requires care of the provider. *Annals of Family Medicine, 12*(6), 573–576. https://doi.org/10.1370/afm.1713

Boysen, P. G., II. (2013). Just culture: A foundation for balanced accountability and patient safety. *Ochsner Journal, 13*(3), 400–406. https://www.ncbi.nlm.nih.gov/pubmed/24052772

Centers for Disease Control and Prevention. (2022). *CDC 24/7*. https://www.cdc.gov/about/index.html

Chun, J., & Bafford, A. C. (2014). History and background of quality measurement. *Clinics in Colon and Rectal Surgery, 27*(1), 5–9. https://doi.org/10.1055/s-0034-1366912

Donabedian, A. (1966). Evaluating the Quality of Medical Care. *The Milbank Memorial Fund Quarterly, 44*(3), 166–206. https://doi.org/10.2307/3348969

Fulop, N., & Robert, G. (2015). *Context for successful quality improvement*. The Health Foundation. https://www.health.org.uk/sites/default/files/ContextForSuccessfulQualityImprovement.pdf

Harrison, M. S., & Goldenberg, R. L. (2015). Global burden of prematurity. *Seminars in Fetal & Neonatal Medicine, 21*, 74–79. httpa://doi.org/10.1016/j.siny.2015.12.007

He, M., Zhu, X., Dong, Y., Zhang, S., Fang, S., Wang, W., ... & Sun, J. (2022). Exploring the role of communication in missed nursing care: A systematic review. *Journal of Advanced Nursing, 78*(12), 4019–4033.

Institute of Medicine. (2000). *To err is human: Building a safer health system*. National Academies Press. http://www.ncbi.nlm.nih.gov/books/NBK225182/

Institute of Medicine. (2001). *Crossing the quality chasm: A new health system for the 21st century*. National Academies Press. http://www.ncbi.nlm.nih.gov/books/NBK222274/

International Council of Nurses. (2018) *Position statements. Nurses, climate change and health*, https://www.icn.ch/sites/default/files/inline-files/ICN%20PS%20Nurses%252c%20climate%20change%20and%20health%20FINAL%20.pdf

The Joint Commission. (n.d.). *Who we are*. Retrieved January 29, 2023, from https://www.jointcommission.org/who-we-are

The Joint Commission. (2021). *Sentinel event data: General information and 2021 update*. https://www.jointcommission.org/-/media/tjc/documents/resources/patient-safety-topics/sentinel-event/sentinel-event-general-information-and-2021-update.pdf

The Joint Commission. (2023). *R3 Report Issue 38: National Patient Safety Goal to improve health equity*. https://www.jointcommission.org/standards/r3-report/r3-report-issue-38-national-patient-safety-goal-to-improve-health-care-equity/#.Y9eyfezMKjA

The Leapfrog Group. (n.d.). *Home page*. Retrieved January 25, 2023, from https://www.leapfroggroup.org

Kanwar, M., Irvin, C. B., Frank, J. J., Weber, K., & Rosman, H. (2010). Confusion about epinephrine dosing leading to iatrogenic overdose: A life-threatening problem with a potential solution. *Annals of Emergency Medicine, 55*, 341–344. https://doi.org/10.1016/j.annemergmed.2009.11.008

Marks, C. M., Kasda, E., Pain, L., & Wu, A. W. (2013). "That was a close call": Endorsing a broad definition of near misses in health care. *The Joint Commission Journal on Quality and Patient Safety, 39*(10), 475–479. https://doi.org/10.1016/S1553-7250(13)39061-8

Marx, D. (2001). *Patient safety and the just culture: A primer for healthcare executives.* Trustees of Columbia University. https://www.chpso.org/sites/mail/files/file-attachments/marx_primer.pdf

National Academies of Sciences, Engineering, and Medicine. (2021). *The future of nursing 2020–2030: Charting a Path to Achieve Health Equity.* National Academies Press. https://doi.org/10.17226/25982

Nightingale, F. (1859). *Notes on nursing: What it is and what it is not.* Harrison of Pall Mall.

Nightingale, F. (1863). *Notes on hospitals* (3rd ed.). Longman, Roberts, and Green.

Nunday, S., Cooper, L. A., & Mate, K. S. (2022). The Quintuple Aim for health care improvement: A new imperative to advance health equity. *JAMA, 327*(6), 521–522. https://doi.org/10.1001/jama.2021.25181

Pelletier, L., R. (2023). *HQ Solutions: Resource for the healthcare quality professional.* Lippincott Williams and Wilkins.

Porter, M. E. (2009). A strategy for health care reform—Toward a value-based system. *The New England Journal of Medicine, 361*(2), 109–112. https://doi.org/10.1056/NEJMp0904131

Pressley, C., & Garside, J. (2023). Safeguarding the retention of nurses: A systematic review on determinants of nurses intentions to stay. *Nursing Open, 10*(5), 2842–2858 https://doi.org/10.1002/nop2.1588

Raman, D. L., Bixby, E., C., Wang, K., Rossi, D., Arora, S...Vitale, M. G. (2022). A comprehensive unit-based safety program to improve perioperative efficiency in adolescent idiopathic scoliosis. *Journal of Pediatric Orthopedics, 42*(3), 123–130.

Saar, L., Unbeck, M., Bachnick, S., Gehri, B., & Simon, M. (2021). Exploring omissions in nursing care using retrospective chart review: An observational study. *International Journal of Nursing Studies, 122*, 10409. https://doi.org/10.1016/j.ijnurstu.2021.104009

Ulrich, B. (2015). Near misses and close calls: what they are and why you should report them. *Nephrology Nursing Journal, 42*(3), 205. https://link.gale.com/apps/doc/A421624251/AONE?u=anon~7b9c2090&sid=googleScholar&xid=209febob

Ulrich, B., & Kear, T. (2014). Patient Safety and Patient Safety Culture: Foundations of Excellent Health Care Delivery. *Nephrology Nursing Journal : Aournal of the American Nephrology Nurses' Association, 41*(5), 447–456.

U.S. Centers for Medicare and Medicaid Services. (2023, September 6). *HCAHPS: Patients' perspectives of care survey.* https://www.cms.gov/medicare/quality/initiatives/hospital-quality-initiative/hcahps-patients-perspectives-care-survey#:~:text=HCAHPS%20(pronounced%20%22H%2Dcaps,perceptions%20of%20their%20hospital%20experience

Watts, N., Amann, M., Arnell, N., Ayeb-Karlsson, S., Beagley, J., Belesova, K., Boykoff, M., Byass, P., Cai, W., Campbell-Lendrum, D., Capstick, S., Chambers, J., Coleman, S., Dalin, C., Daly, M., Dasandi, N., Dasgupta, S., Davies, M., Di Napoli, C., Dominguez-Salas, P., ... Costello, A. (2021). The 2020 report of The Lancet Countdown on health and climate change: responding to converging crises. *Lancet (London, England), 397*(10269), 129–170. https://doi.org/10.1016/S0140-6736(20)32290-X

IMAGE CREDITS

Fig. 2.2: Peter Irwin Lachman, Paul Batalden, and Kris Vanhaecht, "A Multidimensional Quality Model: An Opportunity for Patients, Their Kin, Healthcare Providers and Professionals in the New Covid-19 Period," F1000Research, vol. 9, no. 1140, p. 6. Copyright © by Peter Irwin Lachman, Paul Batalden, and Kris Vanhaecht (CC by 4.0) at https://f1000research.com/articles/9-1140/v1.

CHAPTER 3

Clinical Questions and Specific Aims

Julee Briscoe Waldrop

KEY CONCEPTS

Population, intervention, comparison, and outcome (PICO) question

Problem, population, change, outcomes (PPCO) question

SMART aims

LEARNING OBJECTIVES

1. Develop questions to guide your search for the evidence using a framework-guided approach.
2. Analyze an aim statement using SMART components.

> Intention without action is just a wish.
>
> —Vex King, *Good Vibes, Good Life*

Introduction

Now that you have learned about identifying a clinical or health systems issue (Chapter 2), you are probably thinking, "Well, yes, that is a problem, but how do you figure out how to address it?" You will need to find the research evidence to address the identified health-related problem, but before you can do that, you need to understand the problem or issue in general. You must thoroughly understand an issue before you try to solve it. In this chapter, you will learn about statement frameworks you can use to build searchable clinical or health issue questions and EBPQI initiative aims. Nurses are highly skilled at identifying what changes need to occur in healthcare from the front lines, but evidence is required to support practice changes. This is why the step you will learn about now is critical for every nurse engaging in the EBPQI process to understand. Let's go ahead and get started with some examples.

Example 1: Sleep in Adolescence

You are a nurse in an adolescent behavioral health clinic. You have noticed that when you ask your patients how much sleep they get each night, they often report much less than the recommended hours per night. You know that poor sleep habits (including too little sleep) can impact mental health, but you are unsure about the impact or if there is a nonpharmacological way to improve sleep that might help your patients. Where do you start to find the evidence you need to support clinical decision-making?

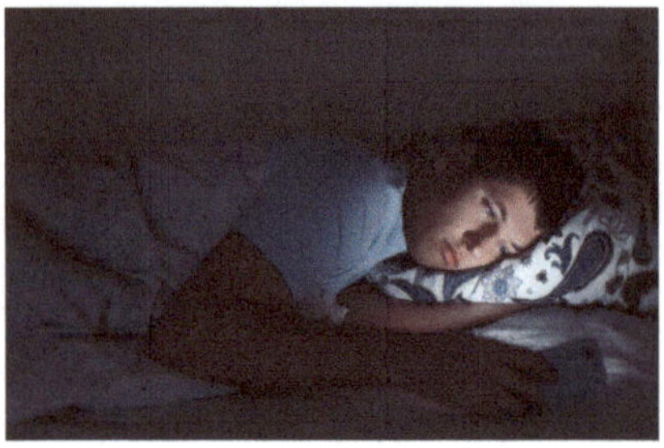
Image 3.1

Example 1: External or Research Evidence on the Problem

In this case, you need more information about the problem. How can you ask a question that will help you find this information systematically (i.e., not using Google)? The information-seeking question on the larger health issues is sometimes called the *background question* (Melnyk & Fineout-Overholt, 2023). Background questions are the foundation for *foreground questions*, or questions about solutions to the problem or how well an intervention, program, or practice change might work.

A way to ask a question about a problem (e.g., high blood pressure) is to think about the outcome of the problem or issue if not treated or if a change in how we do things doesn't occur. In this question, you only have the problem and population (P) and the outcome (O). The problem can be inclusive of many things. It could be a disease or symptom; it could be a behavior; it could be a process or a policy. The problem can be more specific when you add the affected population. The outcome is what you are interested in: what you want to improve. It could be the consequence of a disease. In this case, the problem is "too little sleep" in adolescents, and the outcome is "mental health." The background question you formulate is "In adolescents, how does lack of sleep impact mental health?" In Chapter 4, you will learn how to search for the evidence you need by using this type of question to become more of an expert on the problem. You will search for the evidence from the literature: published research or other professional publications (practice guidelines or recommendations).

Example 2: Patient Falls

During your clinical rotations, you notice that one of the metrics on the unit's dashboard is patient falls. Patient falls are a significant safety concern in the

TABLE 3.1 Background Question Examples

Background question	**To better help you understand an issue or problem**		
Element	Definition	Example 1	Example 2
Problem/ population (P)	Who?	Adolescents who don't sleep enough	Falls in hospitalized patients
Outcome (O)	What about the population and the exposure (issue/problem) do I want to examine?	Mental health	Consequences
Question example		In adolescents, how does lack of sleep impact mental health?	In patients in the hospital who fall, what are the consequences?

hospital and long-term care settings. The national benchmark for falls per 1,000 patient days is 3.2 (Agency for Healthcare Research and Quality, 2019). Your unit's fall rate is hovering around 6 per 1,000 patient days. Reducing and, ideally, preventing patient falls is a nursing responsibility. You wonder, why this is such a big deal?

Example 2: External or Research Evidence on the Problem

In this case, the problem is "falls" in hospitalized patients and the outcome is "consequences." With a broad outcome like this, you can better find information on the entire extent of the problem. You can narrow it to a more specific outcome of interest in your setting later if desired. Finding this type of evidence (from research databases like PubMed and Cinahl) is external evidence. Table 3.1 is an example of how the elements of a question help you write a background question.

Example 1: Internal Evidence on the Problem

But for now, let's move on to the second part of being an expert on the problem: finding evidence that supports your observation that sleep is a problem for your patients at *this* clinic. This is called *internal evidence*, or evidence from your local setting, which is different from evidence about the problem in general. You have observed and noted the problem anecdotally (i.e., based on personal experience) in this case. Is there another way you could find some evidence about the extent of the problem within your patient population? If asking about sleep is a routine question on your history form, then could you do a retrospective chart review of a sample of patients (e.g., all patients on Monday and Tuesday of this past week) and collect data that documents the number of patients who reported less than the recommended hours of sleep? Or you could start a spreadsheet on Monday and prospectively keep track of this new information for 2 days. Either way, be sure to count how many patients you tracked overall so that you can calculate a baseline rate or percentage. Once you have the data to confirm that this is an issue in your clinic, you are ready to find solutions or ways you can consider addressing the problem.

Example 2: Internal Evidence on the Problem

Since your hospital unit is already tracking patient falls, you won't have to collect this data yourself (like you did in the clinic example above), but you will need to find out who (or what department) collects it and how you might be able to gain access to it. Once you do this, you find out that the unit does have more falls than the benchmark (see Chapter 9 for more information on benchmarks and metrics). This is your internal evidence that falls are indeed a problem in this unit, so ideas for solutions will be welcomed.

Next, you want to look for solutions, and this is where the clinical question on solutions comes in.

Clinical Question on Solutions to the Problem or Issue

Did you know there are many different ways to write a clinical question? Most of them are variations on the traditional **population, intervention, comparison, and outcome (PICO) question**. The components of interest should guide the formulation of the question. The PICO question framework was developed by medicine, focusing on treatments or interventions. This framework works best to guide a search for evidence to support the answer to a question seeking the most effective treatment for a specific patient population with a specific health problem (Huang et al., 2006). In general, the comparison (C) component is the one that is the most difficult to include. In the classic PICO, the population (P) can include many adjectives, such as age, gender, disease, symptoms, or current treatment. The intervention (I) and comparison (C) can incorporate all therapies (e.g., drugs, procedures, tests, surgeries, usual care, or placebo), and then the outcome (O) happens as the result of the I and C. Often, an outcome is whether or not there was an improvement in the disease or symptoms. You may want to include a few other elements in your question, such as a specific timeframe (PICO) or setting (PICOS). We will revisit the PICO format in Chapter 5.

The traditional PICO question seeks to find the best available research evidence to support evidence-based practice (EBP) and privileges experimental research and medical interventions. The best evidence is usually defined with a hierarchical approach, often a pyramid (see Figure 3.1). The top of the pyramid reflects the highest level of evidence and includes systematic reviews with meta-analyses composed of randomized control trials (RCTs). As mentioned in Chapter 1, most research studies have excluded minority populations; therefore, depending on your population, the PICO question may reveal significant gaps in evidence for nondominant populations.

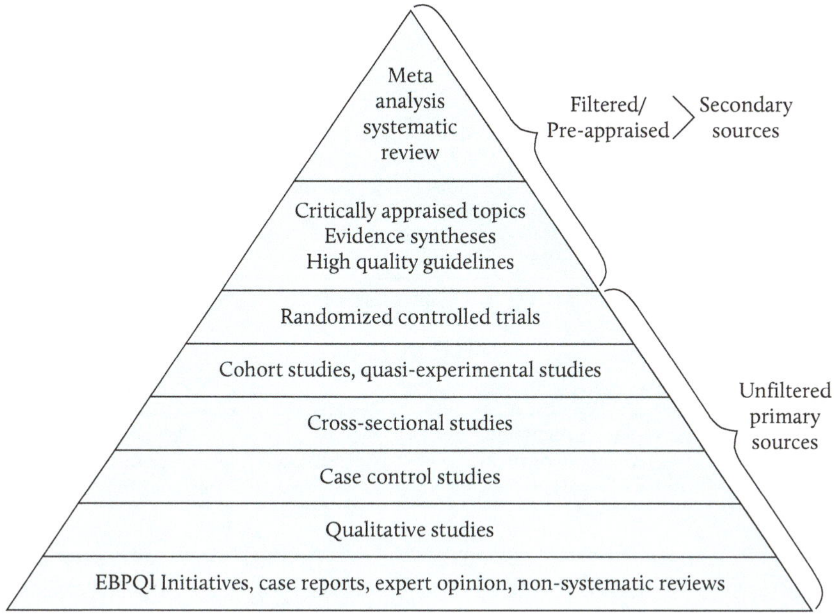

FIGURE 3.1 Evidence Pyramid

Example 1: Clinical Question Development

Using the PICO format, your problem/population is "adolescents who don't get the recommended hours of sleep at night." You do not have a specific solution yet, so to keep an open mind about what might help, you can simply use the term "interventions." Your comparison can be "no intervention" or "usual care," and your outcome or goal of the interventions is "hours of sleep."

Example 2: Clinical Question Development

Again, using the PICO format, your problem/population is "hospitalized patients," and again, you do not know what the best solutions are, so you can repeat the use of "interventions." Your comparison can be "no intervention or care as usual," and your outcome is "numbers or rate of falls." Using a table like Table 4.2 can help you write your clinical question.

Although you have not yet learned how to search for and find the research (evidence), you will need to help your patients with these problems, and you may have some ideas already on what to do. But ideas are only as good as the evidence that supports them, which is why we go through this systematic process every time. Also, this process will reveal if there is enough or a high enough quality of evidence to change practice. What happens if you don't find enough evidence for solutions? If you don't find enough evidence to support a change in practice to address the problem, this indicates that more research needs to be done before

TABLE 3.2 PICO Framework Examples

PICO Element	Definition	Example 1	Example 2
Population/ problem	Who?	Adolescents who don't get enough sleep	Hospitalized patients
Intervention	What is done to improve sleep?	Interventions	Interventions
Comparison	Intervention, or no intervention?	Care as usual	Care as usual
Outcome	What is the desired outcome?	Hours of sleep	Number or rate of falls
Question example	In adolescents, what interventions impact hours of sleep?		In hospitalized patients, what interventions impact falls?

you make a change. If this is the case, you can be part of the research process. Nurse scientists need you to tell them what areas you see in practice should be investigated through research. Your recognition of clinical issues is an important part of the research process. If you are passionate about improving the health of your patients, you can volunteer to be part of a research team too. Remember that the PICO framework can also work well for writing a research question that focuses on an intervention's effectiveness.

A good research question may also include the "how," or method, for investigating the problem and the "what" you want to find out. Because there are many different study designs, there are many different types of questions. We introduced research study designs in Chapter 1. Some studies aim to find out more about a problem and explore and describe it in a way that has not been done before (observational). Some studies are designed to see what happens after an intervention is tested (experimental). You will learn even more about study designs in Chapters 5–7.

The traditional PICO format for a guiding question is less accurate when it concerns an issue or a process instead of a population/problem and how to "treat it." Despite its widespread use, there is limited evidence to support its efficacy, especially in nursing (Eriksen & Frandsen, 2018; Schiavenato & Chu, 2021). So don't feel confined to using this format. There are emerging formats that might suit your situation better. Many problems nurses encounter are not related to treatments. For example, they may be related to management, systems of care, program effectiveness, policies, or public disaster responses. Nurses identify many problems that impact health in every aspect of their lives, not just the workplace.

PPCO Question

Maybe a **problem, population, change, outcomes (PPCO) question** will be needed (Waldrop et al., 2024). This acronym reflects a combination of the background and the foreground questions, with the first "P" representing the problem you wish

TABLE 3.3 PPCO Question

Element	Description	Example 1	Example 2
Problem (P)	What is the problem in general and specifically in your local context?	Social media and sleep	Patient falls
Population (P)	Who does the problem impact?	Adolescents	Hospitalized patients
Change (C)	What has been recommended or done to improve the problem?	Sleep interventions	Fall prevention interventions
Outcomes (O)	How is improvement reported (measured)?	Sleep quantity and quality	Fall rate

to address. This problem "P" reminds you that you need to ask that background question to be sure you are well-informed on the problem in general and in your local context before you start looking for evidence-based solutions. The second "P" is for the population, which should always be specified, as you still need to know who the problem impacts. Next, the "C" is for change. What has been recommended or already done (research evidence) to improve the problem? The "O is for outcome: How will you know the change made a difference? If we redid the above problem using the PCCO statement, it would look like what is presented in Table 3.3.

Another acronym that is overarching and inclusive of additional aspects of an EBPQI initiative is PURPOSE (Cullen et al., 2022). A PURPOSE question includes components that provide more guidance to you for future implementation and evaluation of an EBPQI initiative, such as who the users are and who will be responsible for the outcomes, where the initiative will take place, and how many resources it will require.

TABLE 3.4 PURPOSE Statement

Element	Description	Example 1	Example 2
Patient/ population (P)	Who is being affected by the problem, and who do you want to benefit from the improvement? Always think about who might be most disadvantaged by the problem. (Look at it from your health equity lens or health equity glasses.)	Adolescents	Hospitalized patients
Users (U)	Who will need to change their behavior? Or what process will need to change?	Workflow process to allow for patient education time	Workflow processes to allow for prevention interventions by hospital staff

(Continued)

TABLE 3.4 *(Continued)*

Element	Description	Example 1	Example 2
Responsible team (R)	Who all needs to be involved for the initiative to be successful?	Primarily RN, but all staff and providers will need to be involved.	Primarily RN, but other team/staff members who provide care for patients may be involved.
Problem (P)	(the first P from the PPCO question above). The specific target (issue) for the EBP change	Sleep hours less than recommendations	Fall rate is higher than the desired.
Outcomes (O)	The measurable goal or aim of the initiative	Increased average hours of sleep per night	Decreased fall rate
Setting (S)	Where the EBP/QI initiative will take place (describe it)	Clinic	Hospital unit
Effort (E)	Can be the time frame for completion and/or resources needed	Resource of RN time and changes in the workflow to include patient education time will need to be planned and agreed upon prior to the start of the intervention.	Prevention interventions selected may take time and will need to be planned and policies written and approved prior to the start of practice change.

Any of these elements can be used to help you search the literature for research to support your EBPQI initiative. An added benefit to the PURPOSE statement is that you can easily build on it to write specific and measurable aims for the initiative.

Introduction to GOALS/AIMS

We will talk about AIMS some more in Chapter 9, but remember from Chapter 1 that all good EBPQI initiatives start with three questions:

- What are we trying to accomplish?
- How will we know whether a change is an improvement?
- What change can we make that will result in an improvement?

Writing aims is our guide for how to answer these questions. An acronym developed by George Doran (1981) is **SMART**, which stands for specific, measurable, attainable, realistic, and timely. Ask yourself these questions as you are thinking about your aims.

TABLE 3.5 SMART Aims

Component	Description
Specific	Be specific about the who, what, where, and when. What are you trying to accomplish? What change will be made to result in an improvement? Who is going to be part of the change process? Where will the changes take place? When will the change happen?
Measurable	How will we know there has been an improvement? How will we measure the improvement?
Attainable	Is your aim attainable? Do you have the resources or tools you need? If not, can you find a way to get them?
Realistic	Is your aim realistic given the tools and resources you have? This may include time and effort of personnel as well. Do you have enough people? If not, how can you make a change in your aim or in the resources to achieve your aim?
Timely	What is the timeline you need to achieve your aim? Is there a deadline? If not, how do you create a sense of urgency to motivate team members to make the change happen?

Example 1. Teenagers who sleep less than the recommended hours per night will increase their reported number of hours per night by 10% at their next clinic visit after receiving sleep hygiene education from a nurse at regular clinic visits.

Example 2. The fall rate on Unit X will decrease by 25% in the 6 months after initiation of a falls prevention bundle.

Let's analyze these aims based on the SMART principles (see Table 3.6).

TABLE 3.6 Analysis of SMART Aims Examples

Principle	Description	Example 1	Example 2
Specific	Who?	Adolescents	Hospitalized patients
	What changed?	Will receive sleep hygiene education from RN	Fall prevention bundle
	When and where?	At clinic visit	Begins with each patient's admission assessment and continues for the rest of the hospital stay on Unit X
Measurable	What is being measured?	Number of hours of sleep: increase by 10%. Example: If a teen currently reports sleeping an average of 6 hours per night, a 10% increase would be 6 hours and 36 minutes.	Number of falls per 1,000 hospital days (if the fall rate was 6/1,000 patient days, a 25% decrease would be 4.5/1,000 patient days)

(Continued)

TABLE 3.6 *(Continued)*

Principle	Description	Example 1	Example 2
Attainable	Resources needed?	The biggest resource needed here is RN time to do the education. Before you begin this project, you will need to know how long the education sessions will take and how all responsibilities can still be met.	The biggest resource needed here is RN and other staff time (as fall prevention is everyone's responsibility) to do the bundle of interventions. Before you begin this project, you will need to develop a plan for integrating these practices changes into the unit's workflow. All staff will likely be affected.
Realistic	Can it be achieved?	An aim to increase sleep by half an hour on average is realistic.	An aim to improve fall rates by 25% should be realistic. Research (evidence) has demonstrated improvements with similar bundles of over 40% (Melin, 2018; Spano-Szekely et al., 2019).
Timely	What time period will the change take place and outcomes be assessed?	The timing of the change will be at one clinic visit, and measuring the outcome will be the next clinic visit for the patient.	Each month the unit/hospital collects and reports fall data on each unit and hospital-wide. You will not have to make any changes here or collect any of this information yourself.

These are examples of outcome-based aims. In EBPQI initiatives, there are also process or feasibility aims and measures. These are aims that measure if the intervention or behavior change actually occurred. There are also balancing aims or measures. These aims are intended to keep you aware of potential unintended consequences or processes that might be negatively impacted by the EBPQI initiative.

For example, in our sleeping example, a process measure or aim could be a checklist of how many of the sleep hygiene recommendations were followed each night. A SMART aim statement might be "At least 1 out of 10 sleeping recommendations will be used each night." A balancing measure might be that the teen's grades do not drop in the next reporting period. This aim might be "The adolescent will not receive lower grades in the next reporting period." Since better sleep correlates with increased memory and productivity (see Wellness in Action box), it is predicted that grades may actually improve!

In the fall example, a process measure or aim might be "A fall risk assessment is documented on admission for 90% of patients." If a fall risk assessment is not being performed, then it is unlikely the indicated fall prevention measures are being implemented for the patient. A balancing measure might be related to other responsibilities that nurses have, such as medication administration. If nurses are spending time on fall prevention, another responsibility might suffer. A balancing measure might be "There will be no decrease in the percentage of medications that are given on time to patients."

WELLNESS IN ACTION: SLEEP

It is well known that sleep has many benefits and is one of the cheapest therapies around! As a nursing student, one of the biggest benefits is improved memory (Walker et al., 2003) and increased productivity (Curcio et al., 2006). Longer term benefits are decreased risk of infection and chronic disease by improving your immune system and your mood (Irwin et al., 2016; Palagini et al., 2022). The American Heart Association recently added sleep to make up its eight healthy habits (Lloyd-Jones et al., 2022). So, try to get at least 7 and preferably 8 hours of sleep per night. Follow the sleep hygiene recommendations below.

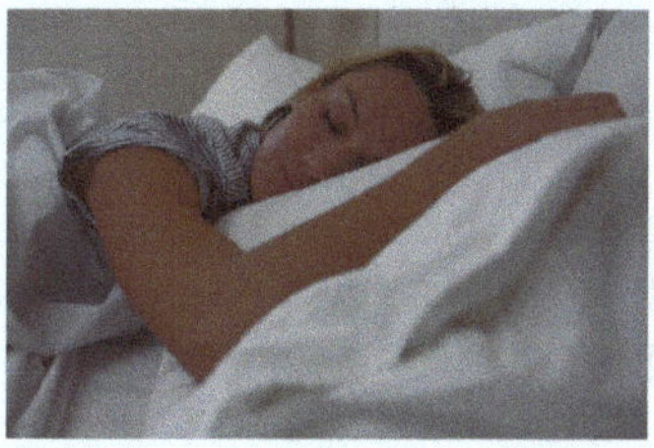

Image 3.2

COMPONENTS OF SLEEP HYGIENE

1. Develop and keep a regular sleep schedule.
2. Avoid caffeine and nicotine in the evening.
3. Avoid alcohol. Although alcohol may help you fall asleep, it can disrupt sleep throughout the night.
4. Exercise regularly; it relieves strees and helps you fall asleep more quickly.
5. Make sure your bedroom is cool. A temperature in the 60s promotes sleep.
6. Keep your bedroom quiet. Use earplugs, or white noise can help if you feel it is too quiet.
7. Sleep on a comfortable surface that is supportive.
8. Avoid screens in the hour before bed and once in bed.
9. Make sure your bedroom is dark to help with your circadian rhythm.
10. Manage stress and practice relaxation techniques because stess can interfere with sleep.
11. Avoid large meals before bed. Try to be finished with your meal at least 2–3 hours before bedtime.

Source: National Sleep Foundation (2024)

WRAPPING UP

Clinical or health system problems and issues are present in every setting. Your ability to find evidence of solutions starts with a solid, well-formulated question for searching the evidence. Whether you use a PICO or a PPCO question, the outcome should be a systematic search for the best quality and most current evidence on which to base your nursing practice. Being able to write SMART aims will guide you as you continue learning to improve care using EBPQI principles.

REFLECTION QUESTIONS

Hand Hygiene Example

Many hospitals struggled with healthcare acquired infection rates during the COVID-19 pandemic, but since 2021 most have been able to return to pre-pandemic levels. However, your unit has had an increase in infections over the last 6 months and is currently at 10 per 10,000 patient days. Your organizations benchmark is set at six per 10,000 patient days. You need to write some questions to help you find the evidence to support an EBPQI initiative to improve your infection rate!

Using any of the models presented above:

1. Write a problem question.
2. Write a PICO solution question.
3. Write a PPCO question.

The CDC website provides best practices to promote hand hygiene and reduce infection rates (https://www.cdc.gov/handhygiene/index.html).

REFERENCES

Agency for Healthcare Research and Quality. (2019, September 7). *Falls*. Patient Safety Network. https://psnet.ahrq.gov/primer/falls

Chaput, J.-P., Dutil, C., Featherstone, R., Ross, R., Giangregorio, L., Saunders, T. J., Janssen, I., Poitras, V. J., Kho, M. E., Ross-White, A., Zankar, S., & Carrier, J. (2020). Sleep timing, sleep consistency, and health in adults: A systematic review. *Applied Physiology, Nutrition, and Metabolism = Physiologie Appliquee, Nutrition Et Metabolisme*, *45*(10 (Suppl. 2)), S232–S247. https://doi.org/10.1139/apnm-2020-0032

Cullen, L., Hanrahan, K., Farrington, M. M., Tucker, S. J., & Edmonds, S. (2022). *Evidence-based practice in action* (2nd ed.). Sigma Theta Tau International.

Curcio, G., Ferrara, M., & De Gennaro, L. (2006). Sleep loss, learning capacity and academic performance. *Sleep Medicine Reviews*, *10*(5), 323–337. https://doi.org/10.1016/j.smrv.2005.11.001

Doran, G. (1981). There's a S.M.A.R.T. way to write management's goals and objectives. *Management Review*, *70*, 35–36.

Eriksen, M. B., & Frandsen, T. F. (2018). The impact of patient, intervention, comparison, outcome (PICO) as a search strategy tool on literature search quality: A systematic review. *Journal of the Medical Library Association*, *106*(4), 420–431. https://doi.org/10.5195/jmla.2018.345

Huang, X., Lin, J., & Demner-Fushman, D. (2006). Evaluation of PICO as a knowledge representation for clinical questions. *AMIA Annual Symposium Proceedings*, *2006*, 359–363.

Irwin, M. R., Olmstead, R., & Carroll, J. E. (2016). Sleep disturbance, sleep duration, and inflammation: A systematic review and meta-analysis of cohort studies and experimental sleep deprivation. *Biological Psychiatry*, *80*(1), 40–52. https://doi.org/10.1016/j.biopsych.2015.05.014

Lloyd-Jones, D. M., Allen, N. B., Anderson, C. A. M., Black, T., Brewer, L. C., Foraker, R. E., Grandner, M. A., Lavretsky, H., Perak, A. M., Sharma, G., & Rosamond, W. (2022). Life's essential 8: Updating and enhancing the American Heart Association's construct of

cardiovascular health: A presidential advisory from the American Heart Association. *Circulation, 146*(5), e18–e43. https://doi.org/10.1161/CIR.0000000000001078
Melin C. M. (2018). Reducing falls in the inpatient hospital setting. *International Journal of Evidence-Based Healthcare, 16*(1), 25–31. https://doi.org/10.1097/XEB.0000000000000115
Melnyk, B., & Fineout-Overholt, E. (2023). *Evidence-based practice in nursing & healthcare: A guide to best practice* (5th ed.). Lippincott Williams & Wilkins.
National Sleep Foundation (2024). 10 tips for a better night's sleep. https://www.thensf.org/sleep-tips/
Palagini, L., Hertenstein, E., Riemann, D., & Nissen, C. (2022). Sleep, insomnia and mental health. *Journal of Sleep Research, 31*(4), Article e13628. https://doi.org/10.1111/jsr.13628
Schiavenato, M., & Chu, F. (2021). PICO: What it is and what it is not. *Nurse Education in Practice, 56*, Article 103194. https://doi.org/10.1016/j.nepr.2021.103194
Spano-Szekely, L., Winkler, A., Waters, C., Dealmeida, S., Brandt, K., Williamson, M., Blum, C., Gasper, L., & Wright, F. (2019). Individualized fall prevention program in an acute care setting: An evidence-based practice improvement. *Journal of Nursing Care Quality, 34*(2), 127–132. https://doi.org/10.1097/NCQ.0000000000000344
Walker, M. P., Brakefield, T., Hobson, J. A., & Stickgold, R. (2003). Dissociable stages of human memory consolidation and reconsolidation. *Nature, 425*(6958), 616–620. https://doi.org/10.1038/nature01930
Waldrop, J. & Jennings-Dunlap. (2024). The Mountain Model for evidence-based practice quality improvement. *The American Journal of Nursing,* May, in press.

IMAGE CREDITS

CHAPTER 4

The Nurse's Role in Searching for Evidence

A Foundation to Explore and Embrace Evidence

Niki Cobb, Erin Whitaker, and Tracy Brewer

KEY CONCEPTS

Inclusion/exclusion criteria
Filters/limiters
Keywords
Articles
Credibility
Journals
Grey literature
Databases
Platforms

LEARNING OBJECTIVES

1. Discuss the value of accessing evidence-based information to inform healthcare decision-making.
2. Develop a strategy for searching for evidence.
3. Search the evidence through a clinical question that addresses a practice issue.
4. Identify various sources of evidence by type.
5. Place evidence within a hierarchy pyramid according to strength.

> To believe without evidence is a demonstration of ignorance and folly.
>
> —Socrates

Introduction

Nurses across healthcare settings, especially those who provide direct patient care, rely on current evidence-based information to inform best practice. As discussed in Chapter 3, nurses play a key role in identifying problems, so they must know how to seek and find reliable evidence to solve problems affecting the patients and populations to whom they provide care. In this chapter, we will focus on how to identify evidence sources by type, strength, and placement within the evidence hierarchy. We will prepare you to apply what you learned in Chapter 3 to search for evidence through a systematic process involving keywords related to an example of a focused clinical question that addresses a specific issue or topic. When you enter the nursing profession, you will be ready to use this important EBP skill as a healthcare team member!

When should nurses search for answers to clinical questions? Nurses and clinicians cultivate numerous questions at the point of care every day. Del Fiol et al. (2014) found that at least one question arises for every two patients seen, yet only 51% of clinicians seek answers to these questions. Unfortunately, there can be barriers to pursuing solutions to clinical questions, such as a care provider's lack of time, skill at seeking information, or access to information. As a nurse, it is your obligation to seek answers to clinical questions, regardless of barriers, to ensure healthcare quality and safety.

When confronted with a clinical issue, you should ask yourself, "What is the best available evidence to answer this question?" You might be tempted to use Google or another search engine for information, which would be a quick and easy way to search but unlikely to produce the most timely, valid, and reliable scientific evidence. Internet search engines often provide less reliable search results because they do not use controlled medical vocabulary terms that have specific, universal meanings in a healthcare/medical context. Additionally, results from a Google search are often overwhelming in quantity, and their accuracy or truthfulness can be difficult to verify due to search flaws, low quality of site content, and numerous other reasons. Nurses need current and highly credible sources to provide evidence-based care (Skeith, 2019). "Would an artificial intelligence (AI) source be more helpful?" you might wonder. An AI source might produce credible information, but you will be required to spend time verifying it. When clinical issues that affect your patients need to be addressed, you will want an efficient method to produce the most credible, high-quality evidence available to promote improvements.

Before we discuss skills for searching and collecting the best evidence, we must describe what we mean by "evidence." *Evidence* is "something presented in support of the truth or accuracy of a claim" (Merriam-Webster, n.d.), but how can you assess the truth (validity) and accuracy (reliability) of evidence to answer your clinical question? You learn to do this by becoming "information literate."

Information literacy involves not just *finding* information but critically appraising, synthesizing, and applying it (the next chapters will address this process further). Information-literate nursing professionals seek knowledge regularly throughout their careers. In 2013, the Association of College & Research Libraries (ACRL) released information literacy competency standards specific to the skills, resources, and language that nurses must have to promote and ensure EBP (ACRL, 2013; Adams, 2014). You are pursuing information literacy as you read this textbook, but don't forget that many types of professionals are information literate and may be available to share their expertise. If your search for evidence feels intimidating, consider taking a team approach! Librarians are experts in information literacy and can provide vital assistance with the search and retrieval of various types of evidence. Consulting a librarian can save you significant time and produce valuable information. If you do not have access to a librarian in your academic or practice setting, you can seek out trusted mentors to help you with this process. We will discuss mentorship in detail in Chapter 13.

Hierarchy of Evidence

As discussed in Chapter 1, all evidence is not of equal quality. Characteristics of research studies are evaluated hierarchically to classify or categorize the quality of evidence. There are many examples of evidence pyramids in the literature, with slight differences among them regarding what is included at each level; however, all are similar in their general categories and the increased rigor of levels from the bottom to the top of the pyramid. Consider the hierarchy of evidence pyramid in Figure 4.1. The design of the research study is the primary characteristic included, and there are various types of evidence at each level of the pyramid. Note that the rigor of study design increases as you move up the pyramid; this is only one aspect of the quality of evidence, however. You will learn more about how to evaluate the quality of your evidence in Chapters 5, 6, and 7.

Note that the evidence hierarchy pyramid is divided into two segments. The top segment or point of the pyramid refers to filtered or preappraised synthesized evidence based on experimental research studies, usually RCTs, known as *systematic reviews*. The tip includes the highest level of a systematic review: a meta-analysis of an outcome from multiple RCTs. Of note, systematic reviews

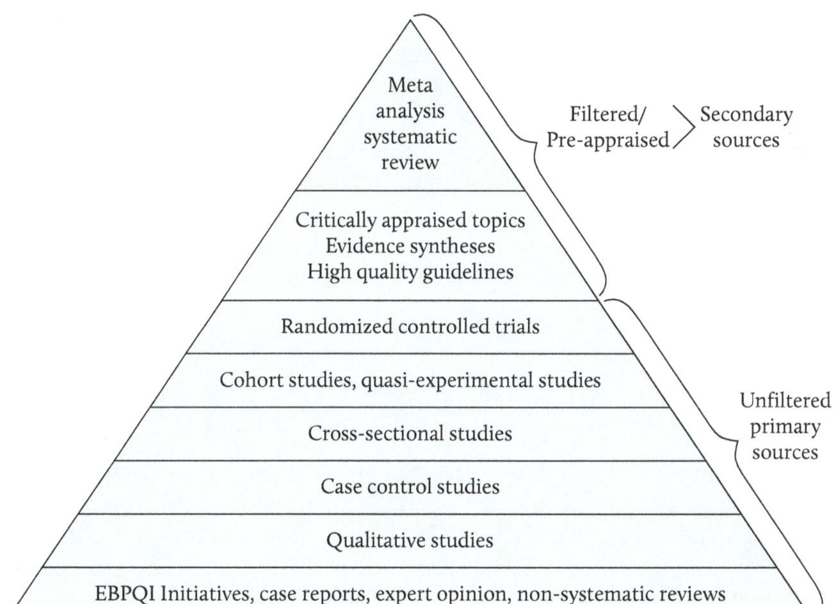

FIGURE 4.1 Hierarchy of Evidence Pyramid

of studies that are not RCTs and of qualitative studies are increasing in the nursing literature. These systematic reviews, while offering a synthesis based on the included studies, would still be describing associations, not cause and effect (e.g., the review includes cohort studies), or describing a phenomenon (e.g., the review includes qualitative studies) and their quality would be at the level of the research studies that they include. Also included at the top of the pyramid are evidence-based guidelines based on systematic reviews. These types of evidence are described as *secondary sources*. Notice that the pyramid tip is small, signifying that less evidence is available at this high level. The lower segment includes individual research studies based on the study design. For example, a randomized control trial (as discussed in Chapter 1) using experimental designs will most likely predict cause and effect between an intervention and outcome; thus, it is higher on the pyramid. A cohort study or a qualitative study intended to describe the characteristics of a phenomenon or individual variable implies associations but not cause and effect; therefore, these are lower on the pyramid. Individual studies are considered primary sources. You will learn more about how to critically appraise systematic reviews and quantitative experimental research studies in Chapter 5 and qualitative research studies in Chapter 6. The bottom tier of the pyramid is considered foundational and includes nonresearch and other types of evidence. Note the broadness at the pyramid's base, signifying how much more of this type of evidence exists. In Chapter 7, we will discuss in depth how to explore and critically appraise various types of nonresearch and other evidence.

Each level of the pyramid can provide evidence that is essential to answering a clinical question. Regardless of the tier or level to which a type of research evidence belongs, you must consider the amount of risk or harm associated with the intervention(s) or practice changes the evidence describes. The level of evidence you are willing to consider for making a practice change will be determined by the potential risk of harm or adverse events associated with the interventions in the evidence (Dang et al., 2022; Melnyk & Fineout-Overhold, 2023). For example, findings based on systematic reviews of RCTs will garner more confidence if the quality of the systematic review is high. Most nursing interventions do not carry a high risk of harm or lend themselves to RCTs, so very few systematic reviews exist on nursing care practices. Although the evidence you find will most likely be from the lower tiers of the pyramid, this evidence will still be valuable to your decision-making as you strive to provide the safest possible patient care.

From Clinical Question to Search

In previous chapters, you learned that the purpose of your formatted question is to aid your search for the best external literature (research). You also learned that it is essential to take time to develop a clear question for your clinical issue because your search strategy will use terms from the question in order to conduct a precise and unbiased search.

Let's consider a hypothetical evidence search based on actual events. We're going to travel back in time to 2020, at the height of the COVID-19 pandemic.

Little was known about the transmissibility of the SARS-CoV-2 virus at that time. In July 2020, the World Health Organization (WHO) published a scientific brief on the modes of transmission of the SARS-CoV-2 virus and associated implications for prevention and precautions within and outside healthcare facilities. The virus transmission was thought to occur through direct, indirect, or close contact with infected people (WHO, 2020), so nurses were asking questions about optimal hand hygiene practices to reduce cross-contamination and the spread of the SARS-CoV-2 virus through direct contact (Hillier, 2020).

Imagine that you are a nurse working in a hospital setting and the world has just shut down. Your general medical-surgical unit has been mandated to care for patients with this new contagious disease (COVID-19), but no one is sure how the infection is transmitted. You are leading a team of nurses, using the steps of the EBP process to develop a clinical question and create a systematic search strategy to look for any available evidence on best practices for preventing cross-contamination of hospital-acquired infections (HAIs). First, you take time to carefully develop your question.

PICO question: In hospitalized patients (P), how does nurses' handwashing (I), compared to glove use (C), affect hospital-acquired infection rates (O)?

Inclusion and Exclusion Criteria

Before beginning a database search, you must specify which types of evidence to include or exclude from your search (because you don't want to consider every report ever published in your field!). **Inclusion criteria**, which you predetermine before the search, are the detailed study characteristics that a research report must include in order for your search to select it as helpful in answering your question. Establishing inclusion criteria will help to ensure consistency in study characteristics that align with your clinical question (Stern & McArthur, 2014). For example, you may determine inclusion criteria based on the following:

- Study design types (e.g., systematic reviews, RCTs, phenomenology)
- Participant or population characteristics (e.g., age, sex, race/ethnicity, diagnosis, location)
- Intervention types or issues of interest (e.g., specific therapy, exposure, risk behavior)
- Outcome measure types (e.g., outcomes expected from the intervention or clinical changes, risk of disease, rate of adverse events, types of measurement)

To balance your inclusion criteria, you must also predetermine exclusion criteria before you begin your search (Stern & McArthur, 2014). **Exclusion criteria** are those characteristics that will result in a study being excluded from your search because it will not help to answer your question. For example, if you are looking for studies on adult patients with COVID-19, you will exclude studies that focus on the pediatric population only.

Filters

Inclusion and exclusion criteria are often confused with database filters, which serve different purposes. **Filters**, also referred to as **limiters**, are applied to narrow down the evidence returned from your search to make it more relevant to answering your question. Filters are applied to the database *before* reviewing individual article results. For example, you can use filtering to narrow a search by study design (RCTs, systematic review), publication type (journal article, book), language (English), publication year, population age, or full text–only options (Hartzell et al., 2023). Be careful not to apply too many filters, however, or you may exclude relevant information (Dang et al., 2022). In your search for best practices in hand hygiene, for example, you could decide to filter the years of publication from 2020 to the current year to capture the most recent evidence since the COVID-19 pandemic.

Using the PICO question developed for identifying optimal hand hygiene practices to reduce cross-contamination of infection, you should now determine the inclusion and exclusion criteria you will apply for your search. We suggest that you keep your initial inclusion/exclusion criteria broad to ensure that you don't miss an important report. There are several ways to define each element of the PICO to establish your inclusion/exclusion criteria. Consider the characteristics and criteria choices presented in Table 4.1.

TABLE 4.1 Inclusion/Exclusion Criteria

	Criteria	Include	Exclude
Population	Characteristics of your hospitalized patients (e.g., age, diagnosis, type of hospital or unit location)	Adults (>18 years of age)	Children (<18 years of age)
Intervention	Time of handwashing (e.g., before entering the room, before touching the patient, after exposure to body fluids, after touching the patient, after touching the surfaces surrounding the patient, before leaving the room) Agents used for handwashing (e.g., soap [type of soap] and water [hot or cold], alcohol-based sanitizers) and how the soap or hand sanitizer is dispensed Duration of handwashing (e.g., in time increments, by surface coverage)	All types of hand hygiene at all points of care	Not applicable
Comparison	Type of gloves (e.g., sterile or nonsterile), when to wear and/or change Use with or without hand hygiene practices	Include all types of gloves and all aspects of glove use.	Not applicable
Outcome	Hospital-acquired infection rates (how measured?), types of infections, compliance in hand hygiene rates or gloving	Hospital-acquired infection rate; iatrogenic infection rate	Preexisting or coexisting infection

To summarize, inclusion and exclusion criteria are used to improve the relevance of the literature you collect. Before deciding on inclusion and exclusion criteria, you must define each element of your PICO or PPCO question specific to your clinical inquiry. These definitions will predetermine the characteristics of studies that you will include or exclude from your search results. Specified study characteristics for inclusion/exclusion are not easily searched with **keywords** (i.e., filters/limits you would apply for database searching). You will need to read, at a minimum, the title and abstract to decide whether to include or exclude an article. If precise interpretation is required, you may need to screen the full-text article.

Fundamentals of Database Searching

Now that you have determined your PICO or PPCO question and identified your inclusion and exclusion criteria, the next step is to build your search strategy. Let's discuss the elements and mechanics of database searching.

A term you will frequently encounter during your search is article. An **article** is a publication that gathers and synthesizes information about a specific topic, study, or subject. On the hierarchy of evidence, articles encompass all the types of evidence you seek. As you gather evidence, it is essential to remember that all works contain inherent biases (effects of factors or assumptions that skew viewpoints, findings, or outcomes). For example, an article will include information that the author *wants* us to understand, but the details of the article (the journal in which it appears, who wrote it, who published it, whether any organization funded it) provide clues as to the article's credibility. **Credibility** is the reliability of a source. To determine a source's credibility, we must ask questions such as "Can and why should this source be trusted?" Both information and disinformation are readily available, and it can be challenging to distinguish credible sources and evidence from suspect ones. Fortunately, we can offer a tip that will help you to choose wisely: Consider whether an article has been vetted through a peer-review process and published in a respected scholarly journal.

Peer review is a process that ensures integrity in publication. After an article is submitted for publication, the publication's editor sends it to experts (peer reviewers) in the discipline who read it and assess its credibility. Peer reviewers provide comments, questions, and suggestions based on their expertise on the subject. This process helps to ensure that the information in an article is factual, well-represented, and adheres to the field's conventions. You will learn more about peer review in Chapter 12.

As you begin searching the literature, you will notice that many articles are published in journals. **Journals** are serial publications comprised of articles and other works by experts in a specific field. There are many nursing-specific journals, such as the *American Journal of Nursing*, as well as specialty-specific journals, such as the *Journal of Pediatric Surgical Nursing*. Each issue of a journal generally includes peer-reviewed articles as well as some non-peer-reviewed material relevant to the discipline, such as editorials, commentaries, and case reports. Unfortunately, there are also journals that do not hold similar high standards, do not provide true peer review or editorial services. Their primary aim is to generate revenue from author processing charges to publish your manuscript. Although not foolproof, using reputable databases decreases your chance of finding this type of journal during your search (Oermann et al., 2022).

Some materials, referred to as **grey literature**, are published to be shared with a specific disciplinary audience but are not formally peer reviewed or published in scholarly channels such as journals, trade publications, or periodicals. Grey literature includes material such as dissertations, preprints, white papers, and conference proceedings; these can be good sources of evidence when you have assessed their credibility.

Selection of Databases

Journals and articles can often be discovered in databases. **Databases** are collections of resources (such as journals, trade publications, and periodicals) that are curated, typically electronic, and frequently updated. Databases will likely yield the most relevant, high-quality evidence to answer your clinical question. Typically, databases are subject-specific. Collections of databases are often housed on platforms. **Platforms** allow users to search a single database or several simultaneously (if they are owned by the same companies). Some databases are free to the public; others require a subscription.

PubMed

PubMed is a publicly available government site (https://pubmed.gov) and a premier biomedical, health, and life sciences literature search system. PubMed was created and is maintained by the National Center for Biotechnology Information (NCBI) at the U.S. National Library of Medicine (NLM), located at the National Institutes of Health, which serves as an agency under the U.S. Department of Health and Human Services. PubMed provides over 35 million citations and is an excellent resource for locating research and other evidence (NLM, n.d.-d). Full-text content for some articles may be available from PubMed Central (a free public database) or publisher websites, but other articles may require subscription access from the publisher or database platform site to view the full content. You can contact your academic, institutional, or public library for assistance with accessing full-text content. A primary component of PubMed is MEDLINE, NLM's premier bibliographic database, which provides nearly 30 million biomedical references indexed using NLM's Medical Subject Headings (MeSH; NLM, n.d.-b). Subject headings aid users in locating materials by using a set of terms or phrases, known as *controlled vocabulary* (EBSCO, n.d.). Some advantages of subject headings are that they reveal specific terms used when classifying articles and provide additional headings or subheadings for your search. MeSH are subject headings developed and cataloged by a team of reviewers to help users identify related resources within the MEDLINE database. As the MEDLINE database serves as a component of PubMed, MeSH terms can be used to search within the PubMed database along with keywords (NLM, n.d.-a). You will learn more about subject headings and see an example for searching with MeSH terms later in this chapter.

PubMed's interface has several beneficial features, such as the visibility of similar resources for full-text records and the creation of an NCBI account for saving, organizing, and receiving updates about saved searches and citations. Your NCBI account can be used across several NLM databases (NLM, n.d.-c). PubMed and other databases have similarities and specific differences related to their use.

CINAHL Complete

CINAHL is an acronym for Cumulative Indexes of Nursing and Allied Health Literature databases. Access is provided through their EBSCOhost platform. CINHAL is a great resource for research and other evidence; it provides an authoritative index of nursing and allied health journals as well as content for over 7,000 journals (EBSCO, n.d.). CINAHL Complete also allows access to use CINHAL subject headings, which use controlled vocabulary with a hierarchical arrangement of terms for indexing articles and are similar to PubMed's MeSH (ESBCO, n.d.). CINAHL is a subscription-based resource (i.e., access to full-text articles requires payment). It can be helpful to consult with your librarian (if you have access to this resource) for assistance in locating articles within this database.

Cochrane Library

The Cochrane Library is an excellent resource for locating systematic reviews and other resources. The Cochrane Library, published by Wiley, consists of multiple databases provided by Cochrane, an international network that provides evidence to support medical and healthcare decision-making. The Cochrane Library databases include the Cochrane Database of Systematic Reviews, Cochrane Central Register of Controlled Trials (CENTRAL), and Cochrane Clinical Answers. The databases provide featured content in special collections on curated topics and allow the user to search for content provided by the McMaster Health Forum's repositories: Health Systems Evidence and Social Systems Evidence (Cochrane Library, n.d.).

See Table 4.2. for links to tutorials for up-to-date training on how to use them.

TABLE 4.2 Electronic Databases

Database	Defining characteristics	Link to training tutorial
PubMed	Multilanguage, international database A free resource supporting the search and retrieval of biomedical and life science literature Contains 35 million citations and abstracts of biomedical literature Provided by the National Library of Medicine, National Center for Biotechnology Information, and the National Institutes of Health	Online training https://learn.nlm.nih.gov/documentation/training-packets/T0042010P/ PubMed YouTube playlist (English) https://www.youtube.com/playlist?list=PL7dF9e2qSW0YkmxDTsUG6p4hJjYOPT0Uj PubMed YouTube playlist (Spanish) https://www.youtube.com/playlist?list=PL7dF9e2qSW0Y8MqgB0rLnrJH-ypnsj0OH
CINAHL Complete	Contains journals in nursing and 17 allied health fields, as well as biomedicine, consumer health Additional topics include exercise science, health administration, nursing education, and public health Contains journal articles, ebooks, evidence-based care sheets, quick lessons, legal cases, clinical trials, gray literature, etc. Audience: nurses, medical personnel, social workers, counselors, occupational therapists, physical therapists, speech therapists, audiologists, etc. Contains literature back to 1937 Provides a search term thesaurus for searching literature in the nursing and allied fields	CINAHL YouTube video training https://www.youtube.com/results?search_query=cinahl+database+ebsco+channel Basic searching—link to PowerPoint and video https://connect.ebsco.com/s/article/CINAHL-Databases-Basic-Searching-Tutorial?language=en_US Advanced search—link to PowerPoint and video https://connect.ebsco.com/s/article/CINAHL-Databases-Advanced-Searching-Tutorial?language=en_US CINAHL and MeSH headings—link to Power Point and video https://connect.ebsco.com/s/article/Using-the-CINAHL-MeSH-Headings-Feature-in-EBSCOhost-Tutorial?language=en_US
Cochrane Library	Cochrane Library is a collection of databases containing the leading resources for high-quality systematic reviews in health care. Cochrane reviews are peer-reviewed. It contains the *Cochrane Handbook for System Reviews of Interventions* and the *Cochrane Handbook for Diagnostic Test Accuracy Reviews*. It contains the Cochrane Central Register of Controlled Trials (CENTRAL) and the Cochrane Clinical Answers for "actionable" point-of-care decision-making.	Cochrane Library Users Guide—PowerPoint https://www.wiley.com/en-us/customer-success/cochrane/cochrane-library-user-guide How to Use Cochrane PICO search—PowerPoint https://www.wiley.com/en-us/customer-success/cochrane/how-to-use-pico-search Cochrane Training: Learning Live https://training.cochrane.org/learning-events/learning-live

Building the Search Strategy

To begin your search, you will use the elements of your clinical question to select keywords and synonyms that align with your search goals. After determining search terms, you will use operators and search strategy enhancers (discussed in this section) to perform your search in a database or platform.

Most databases are configured to run keyword searches. Unlike platforms such as Google, which allow users to phrase searches in the form of questions (natural language to most users), many databases require users to compile searches of essential words or phrases. For example, suppose you wanted to search for sources on the PICO question we considered earlier: "In hospitalized patients, how does nurses' handwashing, compared to glove use, affect hospital-acquired infection rates?" You might pick out "hospital," "handwashing," and "infection" as keywords to form your search. Synonyms for these keywords could also be included.

Some databases allow users to search sets of predefined words and phrases called subject headings. *Subject headings* are control vocabulary used by a database or platform to index articles relevant to a specific term or specialization, substance, or publication type. Not every article may be indexed by subject headings, so we always use them in combination with keywords. A good tip is to think of subject headings as sprinkles! The primary function of sprinkles is to enhance a dessert, such as a cake, cookie, or ice cream (and the list goes on). Although sprinkles alone can be wonderful, their intended purpose is to work in combination with something else—desserts. Similarly, subject headings are intended to work in combination with keywords. Combining your subject headings with your keywords will increase the possibility of capturing articles related to your topic that could be missed by your keyword search strategy alone.

You can connect your search terms using words like AND, OR, and NOT. These terms are called *Boolean operators*, and they indicate the relationship between your search's keywords, phrases, or subject headings (Figure 4.2). Adding the operator "AND" to your search will tell the platform or database that you want to include both terms in your search. For example, you might combine the terms "handwashing" AND "sanitizer" to expand your results. The operator "OR" indicates to the platform that you want your search to include results that cover two or more terms. For example, you could search for "patient" OR "inpatient" to widen your search net. Finally, the operator "NOT" tells the platform or database that you want to exclude results. For example, if you searched "handwashing" NOT "gloves," your results would include items related to handwashing but not those related to gloves.

Using our PICO or PPCO question from the beginning of this chapter, we could perform a simple search for "handwashing," but it is unlikely that this would return relevant results. However, if we combined terms using Boolean operators, the results would be more focused. The more Boolean operators your search contains, the narrower your search becomes.

For example, a search with the keywords "hospital AND patient AND handwashing OR gloves AND infection" would be broader and less focused than one using "hospital AND adult AND patient AND handwashing NOT gloves AND hospital-acquired infection."

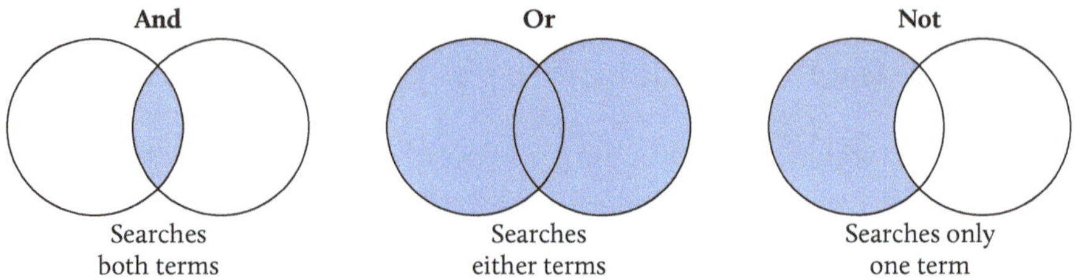

FIGURE 4.2 Boolean Operator Diagrams

TABLE 4.3 TQP Functions

Function	Symbol	Example	Purpose
Truncation	*	Infect* = infect, infects, infection, infected, etc.	Truncating a search term lets a database platform know that you are looking for results that have multiple endings of the key word.
Quotation marks	Be sure you use straight quote marks (") instead of the traditional curly quotes (", ")	"hand hygiene"	Using quotation marks around a search term lets the database platform know that you want to search the term as a phrase rather than each of the words individually.
Parentheses	( )	Hospital* AND (patient* OR inpatient*)	Using parentheses around search terms allows you to keep terms together. The database platform looks for the terms "patient" or "inpatient" along with the first term "hospital."

Finally, truncation, quotation marks, and parentheses (TQP) can be used to refine your search strategy, especially in combination with Boolean operators. These concepts are described in more detail in Table 4.3.

Searching for Evidence

Using your PICO search terms, you can begin to arrange your terms using the Boolean operators AND, OR, and NOT. If we were to break down our PICO question into search terms using the methods described above, it might look something like this:

POPULATION: hospital* AND (patient* OR inpatient*)

INTERVENTION: "hand wash*" OR handwash* OR "hand hygiene" OR "hand sanitation"

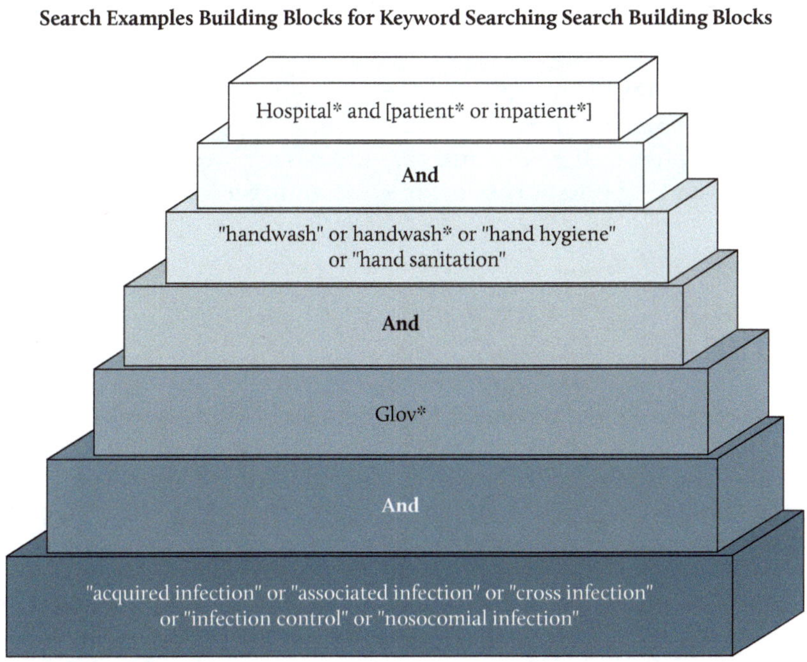

FIGURE 4.3 Search Example's Building Blocks for Keyword Searching

COMPARISON: glove*

OUTCOME: "acquired infection*" OR "associated infection*" OR "cross infection*" OR "infection control" OR "nosocomial infection*"

Figure 4.3 shows an example of how you can arrange your PICO keywords. These building blocks will be the foundation for your search strategy.

Searching a Database Using Your Keywords and Terms

When you perform a search in PubMed or other databases, you will find a search box or boxes in which to insert your keywords. For example, PubMed has a simple search box and an advanced search builder. Usually, you will want to use advanced search builders because they allow more options for your search strategy. Depending on the database, you can apply filters and limiters at the onset.

A simple search in PubMed based only on your PICO question words "hospital AND handwashing AND gloves AND infection" yields 424 results. If you use the building blocks approach and PubMed's advanced search builder, your search will look like this: (hospital* AND (patient* OR inpatient*) AND ("hand wash*" OR handwash* OR "hand hygiene" OR "hand sanitation") AND glov* AND ("acquired infection*" OR "associated infection*" OR "cross infection*" OR "infection control*" OR "nosocomial infection*"). There will be 91 article citations retrieved with this more specific search process. You can also add a limiter; in this case, you will want only articles written after the start of the COVID-19 pandemic. If you add 2019 as a limit, the search will return only articles published since January 1, 2019. Now there are only 9 articles. If you feel that your results are too narrow, you can always broaden them by eliminating one of the terms or changing a Boolean operator (e.g., AND to OR).

Information Access

During your search, you may come across resources behind paywalls. Access to an article behind a paywall requires payment or a subscription. If you have access to a librarian, make sure to consult with them before paying; your institution may have or be able to obtain access to the resource. If not, your librarian can often find an accessible alternative resource.

Conversely, some resources are open access. *Open access* refers to resources that are publicly available at no cost. These resources do not require an institutional affiliation to read or download, and access to them does not depend on whether your university, college, hospital, or organization has a subscription. You should be aware, however, that a payment has been made to keep them open to all. Many governmental organizations that fund research with taxpayer dollars now mandate that researchers publish in open-access journals. The rationale is that if the public (taxpayers) have paid for the research, they deserve to be able to read it and know the results.

As you consider sources with paid and open access, it is essential to remember that one is not inherently more authoritative or credible than the other. Just because an article is behind a paywall does not mean that it will be of better quality or more beneficial for your practice than an open-access article. It is incumbent on you as a future nurse to investigate the reliability and relevance of evidence through critical appraisal (see Chapters 5, 6, and 7).

The Librarian as a Resource

Ultimately, your expert librarian is one of your greatest assets during your search process. Just as you will be an expert in your nursing practice, librarians are experts at searching for evidence. You and your librarian can create sophisticated search strategies together using the combined knowledge of your fields, as illustrated in this chapter. Librarians can provide various resources and related materials to grow your search abilities.

Librarians often curate subject-specific lists of resources called *research guides*. These guides (called *LibGuides* at some institutions) are updated consistently with information about the subjects they cover. Research guides typically also include information about contacting your librarians, tips for research and writing, and database tutorials (many of which are free to access).

Finishing Up the Search Process

Now that you have searched your chosen databases for evidence and have a list of possible articles to review, don't forget about your predetermined inclusion/exclusion criteria. Let's say that the following are two of the articles found in your search. You must read the abstract or summary of the article to determine whether it meets your inclusion criteria or should be excluded.

1. Hillier, M. D. (2020). Using effective hand hygiene practice to prevent and control infection. *Nursing Standard*, *35*(5), 45–50. https://pubmed.ncbi.nlm.nih.gov/32337862/

From reading the abstract, you determine that the article meets the inclusion criteria on the intervention (handwashing), but there is no mention of a patient population, a comparison with glove use, or an outcome related to infection rates. You might decide to exclude it at this point; however, the smarter choice would be to obtain and read the full text of the article to determine whether it provides any useful information or should be excluded.

What about the next one?

2. Prasad, P., Brown, L., Ma, S., McDavid, A., Rudmann, A., Lent, D., Regan-Webster, P., Valcin, E. K., Graman, P., & Apostolakos, M. (2021). "If the glove fits": Hospital-wide universal gloving is associated with improved hand hygiene and may reduce clostridioides difficile infection. *Infection Control & Hospital Epidemiology*, *42*(11), 1351–1355. https://pubmed.ncbi.nlm.nih.gov/33888164/

After reading the abstract of this article, you determine that it is a research study and meets all the inclusion criteria. The population is adult patients, there is a comparison of hand hygiene and glove use interventions, and infection rates are the outcome of interest. You will want to read this one not only for evidence but to integrate important aspects of their project with your EBPQI initiative!

Next Step: Critical Appraisal

Critical appraisal is a vital and fundamental skill that is key to making sound recommendations about evidence obtained through an EBP approach to decision-making. Critically appraising a piece of literature accomplishes several things: It helps you to gain a deeper understanding of the research (particularly of the quality and strength of the evidence), and it helps you to decide whether the evidence provided is needed to answer your question.

Unfortunately, critical appraisal may be skipped or overlooked in real-world settings because nurses often view it as one of the most difficult steps in EBP and feel that they lack the skill or competence to perform it (Melnyk et al., 2014). Omitting critical appraisal from the EBP process creates a dangerous situation in which poorly conducted work (research, literature reviews, quality improvement,

EBP initiatives) or inadequate evidence may be used to inform decisions, thus placing the patients, clinicians, organizations, and communities served at risk for less-than-best outcomes.

Critical appraisal is the process of evaluating a study or piece of literature for its worth. When we critically appraise a piece of evidence, we must ask:

- Is the work able to be duplicated under similar conditions? (reliability)
- Are the results a true reflection of what they are intended to measure? (validity)
- Is this work applicable to the issue I am wondering about? (applicability)

The next three chapters will guide you in critically appraising quantitative research evidence (Chapter 5), qualitative research evidence (Chapter 6), and other types of evidence (Chapter 7).

WELLNESS IN ACTION: PHYSICAL ACTIVITY

You have likely remained seated as you read this chapter, so let's prepare to move our bodies in addition to our minds. Regular physical activity has been strongly and consistently linked to preventing many chronic diseases and ensuring a longer lifespan (Reiner et al., 2013; Ruegsegger & Booth, 2018; Warburton et al., 2006). Can you engage in physical activity right now or, at least, today? Here are some ideas you can implement immediately to support our compelling recommendation to engage in routine physical activity. Choose one or more of the physical activities below, but be sure to adapt your activity to your current health status, ability, accessibility, and comfort level.

- Do 10 jumping jacks, 10 sit-ups, and/or 10 push-ups (or as many as you desire).
- Try taking stairs up/down and back instead of the elevator.
- Bank your steps/movement before periods of time when you know you will be sitting.
- Take a walk (short or long) using a brisk pace (if possible).
- Go to a gym/health center. Explore and try some equipment and/or enroll in a fitness class.
- Choose another type of preferred exercise. Put it on your calendar to remind you to engage in it regularly.
- Track your activity progress.

We have a spectrum of physical movement levels on our authorship team. Some of us enjoy (or commit to) walking, running, cycling, and/or swimming, and some have physical limitations requiring modified activities. What we know for certain is that physical movement is practical and tremendously beneficial. House cleaning or gardening count as movement, and this type of physical activity adds up. As a nursing student, you may be routinely sedentary; you may sit for long periods of time during computer work, and we encourage you to challenge this lifestyle. As a nurse, you may need to be very active because our profession often requires movement, so you will want to get ready! Please join us, as you see fit, in embarking on a lifelong movement journey with short- and long-term benefits to help your brain and body. It is never too late to start.

WRAPPING UP

After reading and participating in this chapter, we encourage you to review and reflect on your newly acquired literature search knowledge and skills as you prepare to learn more in the next chapters about critical appraisal of various types of evidence you have accessed or may access in the future. Remember that although literature searching takes time and some practice, your investment in this valuable EBP step is a gift to your future patients. It will allow you to enter the nursing profession with hands-on practice experience searching literature. The COVID-19 pandemic has reminded us of how quickly the world can change and how rapidly healthcare must evolve in response. Nurses must be ready and able to look at the best current evidence to answer new clinical questions as they arise.

REFLECTION QUESTIONS

1. Why is it important that nurses know when to access literature/evidence to answer clinical questions?
2. How can you continue learning about literature/evidence searching to hone the fundamental skills introduced in this chapter?
3. When a problem arises, how does the nurse know whether exploration of evidence is needed?

REFERENCES

Adams, N. E. (2014). A comparison of evidence-based practice and the ACRL information literacy standards: Implications for information literacy practice. *College & Research Libraries, 75*(2), 232–248. https://doi.org/10.5860/crl12-417

Association of College & Research Libraries. (2013, October). *Information Literacy Competency Standards for Nursing.* American Library Association. https://www.ala.org/acrl/standards/nursing

Cochrane Library. (n.d.). *About the Cochrane Library.* Wiley. Retrieved March 8, 2023, from https://www.cochranelibrary.com/about/about-cochrane-library

Dang, D., Dearholt, S., Bissett, K., Ascenzi, J., & Whalen, M. (2022). *Johns Hopkins evidence-based practice for nurses and healthcare professionals: Models and guidelines* (4th ed.). Sigma Theta Tau International.

Del Fiol, G., Workman, T. E., & Gorman, P. N. (2014). Clinical questions raised by clinicians at the point of care: A systematic review. *JAMA International Medicine, 174*(5), 710–718. https://doi.org/10.1001/jamainternmed.2014.368

EBSCO. (n.d.). *CINAHL Database.* Retrieved March 8, 2023, from https://www.ebsco.com/products/research-databases/cinahl-database#:~:text=CINAHL%20includes%201%2C314%20journals%20with%20searchable%20cited%20references

Hartzell, T. A., Fineout-Overholt, E., & Kelley, C. B. (2023). Finding relevant evidence to answer clinical questions. In B. Melnyk & E. Fineout-Overholt (Eds.), *Evidence-based practice in nursing & healthcare: A guide to best practice* (5th ed., pp. 55–92). Wolters Kluwer.

Hillier, M. D. (2020). Using effective hand hygiene practice to prevent and control infection. *Nursing Standard, 35*(5), 45–50. https://doi.org/10.7748/ns.2020.e11552

Melnyk, B., & Fineout-Overholt, E. (2023). Making the case for evidence-based practice and cultivating a spirit of Inquiry. In B. Melnyk & E. Fineout-Overholt (Eds.), *Evidence-based practice in nursing & healthcare: A guide to best practice* (5th ed., pp. 7–32). Wolters Kluwer.

Melnyk, B. M., Gallagher-Ford, L., Long, L. E., & Fineout-Overholt, E. (2014). The establishment of evidence-based practice competencies for practicing registered nurses and advanced practice nurses in real-world clinical settings: Proficiencies to improve healthcare quality, reliability, patient outcomes, and costs. *Worldviews on Evidence-Based Nursing, 11*(1), 5–15. https://doi.org/10.1111/wvn.12021

Merriam-Webster. (n.d.). *Evidence.* In *Merrian-Webster.com dictionary.* Retrieved March 3, 2023, from https://www.merriam-webster.com/thesaurus/evidence

National Library of Medicine. (n.d.-a). *Medical Subject Headings.* Retrieved March 7, 2023, from https://www.nlm.nih.gov/mesh/meshhome.html

National Library of Medicine. (n.d.-b). *Medline overview.* Retrieved March 7, 2023, from https://www.nlm.nih.gov/medline/medline_overview.html

National Library of Medicine. (n.d.-c). *My NCBI help.* Retrieved March 7, 2023, from https://www.ncbi.nlm.nih.gov/books/NBK3842/#MyNCBI.What_Is_My_NCBI

National Library of Medicine. (n.d.-d). *PubMed overview.* Retrieved March 7, 2023, from https://pubmed.ncbi.nlm.nih.gov/about/

Oermann, M. H., Nicoll, L. H., Carter-Templeton, H., Owens, J. K., Wrigley, J., Ledbetter, L. S., & Chinn, P. L. (2022). How to identify predatory journals in a search: Precautions for nurses. *Nursing, 52*(4), 41–45. https://doi.org/10.1097/01.NURSE.0000823280.93554.1a

Reiner, M., Niermann, C., Jekauc, D., & Woll, A. (2013). Long-term health benefits of physical activity: A systematic review of longitudinal studies. *BMC Public Health, 13,* Article 813. https://doi.org/10.1186/1471-2458-13-813

Ruegsegger, G. N., & Booth, F. W. (2018). Health benefits of exercise. *Cold Spring Harbor Perspectives in Medicine, 8*(7), Article a029694. https://doi.org/10.1101/cshperspect.a029694

Skeith, J. (2019, February 21). *"I'll just Google it": The case against internet searching for clinical evidence.* EBSCO. https://www.ebsco.com/sites/g/files/nabnos191/files/acquiadam-assets/The-Case-Against-Internet-Searching-for-Cinical-Evidence-White-Paper.pdf

Stern, C., & McArthur, A. (2014). Developing the review question and inclusion criteria. *American Journal of Nursing, 114*(4), 53–56.

Warburton, D. E., Nicol, C. W., & Bredin, S. S. (2006). Health benefits of physical activity: The evidence. *Canadian Medical Association Journal, 174*(6), 801–809. https://doi.org/10.1503/cmaj.051351

World Health Organization. (2020, July 9). *Transmission of SARS-CoV-2: Implications for infection prevention precautions.* https://www.who.int/news-room/commentaries/detail/transmission-of-sars-cov-2-implications-for-infection-prevention-precautions

CHAPTER 5

Critically Appraising Quantitative Evidence

Tracy L. Brewer, Melissa Hessock, and Jayne Jennings Dunlap

KEY CONCEPTS

Critique
Critical appraisal
Body of evidence
Bias
Quantitative evidence
Primary sources
Synthesis

LEARNING OBJECTIVES

1. Describe the role of quantitative research evidence in making EBPQI recommendations.
2. List the four steps of the critical appraisal process.
3. Use a hierarchy to determine levels of evidence.
4. Differentiate between different types of quantitative research evidence.
5. Identify resources that nurses and EBPQI teams use to critically appraise research evidence.

> Positivity, confidence, and persistence are key in life, so never give up on yourself.
>
> —Khalid

Introduction

Tracy's story:

> In the early '90s, I was working as a staff nurse in the mother-baby unit in a small rural hospital. I aspired to "climb the clinical ladder," so I joined a team whose purpose was to identify solutions to the high incidence rates of surgical site infection (SSI) in patients who had a surgical delivery or cesarean section (C-section). Our team had no formal name or structure; it included me, another staff nurse, the nursing manager, and one obstetrician. At that time, there were no formal evidence-based practice (EBP) or quality improvement (QI) teams; we came together because we had a problem and needed to solve it.
>
> All staff nurses in our unit were required to scrub and circulate during emergency C-sections. After 5:00 p.m., we had no dedicated operating room (OR) staff. To prepare a patient's abdomen for a surgical incision, a nurse would use a disposable razor to shave the patient's entire pubic area; despite this being done as carefully as possible, the patient's skin was often left nicked and bleeding. In the OR, we cleansed the abdomen with a large four-sided sponge and povidone-iodine solution. This procedure involved moving the sponge in circular motions outwards from the inner abdomen, then flipping the sponge and repeating the process until all four sides of the sponge had been used. I began to wonder whether a nick in the skin after shaving, even if well cleansed, might compromise the skin's protective function. The procedure for cleansing the abdomen was not an optimal aseptic technique, so could our preoperative preparation be causing our high SSI rate? Although I did not realize it at the time, my spirit of inquiry had kicked in.
>
> I had access to the local university library and used the single computer available there to search the CINAHL database. I do not recall the keywords or subject headings I used or whether my search contained limits or Boolean connectors (I suspect they did not). However, I found one article that examined the use of clippers and a single-application surgical skin preparation product to reduce SSI following C-section. I brought a copy of the article back to discuss with the team. We invited a representative from the surgical skin preparation company to demonstrate the product, adopted this technique, and purchased two clippers. I worked on this unit for an additional 6 years, and to my knowledge, we did not have a single SSI after implementing these two practice changes. We had successfully implemented an EBPQI initiative!
>
> Back then, we didn't have any terminology to describe what we had done. Using research evidence often meant making practice changes based on the results of a single research study (as was done in our case). Rigorous appraisal and synthesis techniques were absent). Without a systematic process for assessing the level and quality of research evidence, nurses had a limited ability to identify flaws and biases that could lead to ineffective, or even harmful, practice changes in a specific setting.

We have shared Tracy's story with you to set the focus of this chapter, which is to introduce you to the critical appraisal of quantitative research (external evidence). You will use your knowledge and skills of critical appraisal as you evaluate and synthesize the results of quantitative research studies to support confident recommendations and, ultimately, practice changes. Throughout this chapter, we will examine different types of quantitative research studies in detail, building on their introduction in Chapter 1. In later chapters, you will learn about the critical appraisal of qualitative and mixed methods research evidence (Chapter 6) as well as other types of evidence (Chapter 7).

What Is the Difference Between Critique and Critical Appraisal?

The terms "critique" and "critical appraisal" of research are often used synonymously, yet they refer to very different processes. A **critique** of research involves comprehensively analyzing the strengths and limitations of the study's design, methods, statistical analysis, and conclusions. In addition, a critique typically includes feedback and suggestions for improvement of the study (Polit & Beck, 2021). When critiquing a research article, we ask the following evaluation questions:

- What did the researcher/s aim to do?
- Did their methodology make sense in relation to what they aimed to do?
- How professionally, thoughtfully, and thoroughly was the research conducted?
- What gaps in knowledge were discovered?

As researchers designing our own projects, we critique articles to learn lessons about what has (and has not) worked well for others, as well as to identify gaps in knowledge that need to be filled.

Critical appraisal involves a systematic, stepwise approach to the evaluation of research evidence using specific tools to determine the quality and strength of findings. Critical appraisal is a skill that clinicians use to evaluate a research report's (a) worth in regard to the issue being addressed and (b) fitness to be included as part of the **body of evidence** related to that issue. Critical appraisal is to EBP what the critique of research studies is to research (Al-Jundi & Sakka, 2017).

A critical appraisal of research evidence is essential to the EBP process because it helps you to determine whether you can trust the findings to improve the care you provide your patients. Critical appraisal applies to all types of evidence. You must critically appraise individual research studies to assess their value and fitness, but you must also use critical appraisal to compare multiple studies to synthesize (combine) all the evidence you feel will provide a firm grounding for definitive recommendations for best practices (Fineout-Overholt, 2023). As previously discussed, when we appraise a quantitative research study, we attempt to determine its validity, reliability, transferability, and generalizability. Similarly, when we appraise a qualitative research study, we attempt to determine its trustworthiness, which includes its credibility, dependability, confirmability, and transferability (see Chapter 6).

As nurses, our role is to integrate research findings into practice to improve the quality and safety of patient outcomes. Study evidence that you determine is of a high level and quality relevant to your chosen problem should be synthesized and compared across studies to provide a body of evidence on which you can have sufficient confidence to base your practice recommendations. Remember that a trove of research evidence is insufficient for making safe clinical practice decisions if that evidence has not been clinically appraised! EBP clinical decision-making and practice recommendations must always be patient-centered and incorporate varying levels of appraised evidence and clinician expertise (Fernandez et al., 2015; Jones & Steel, 2018; O'Halloran et al., 2010) to ensure that patients receive the best care.

Hierarchy and Levels of Evidence

As we learned in Chapter 4, evidence hierarchies are typically illustrated with a pyramid that ranks evidence based on the research study design. Generally, studies at the top levels of the pyramid provide the most reliable and robust evidence. In contrast, studies at the bottom of the pyramid may be subject to bias and provide weaker evidence. **Bias** refers to systematic errors or deviations from truth in how a research study is designed or conducted (Polit & Beck, 2021). The more bias discovered, the poorer the research quality or validity (see the Components of Critical Appraisal section and Table 5.6 in this chapter). Numerous evidence hierarchies exist to guide clinicians as they search for evidence to answer clinical questions. The scientific community considers randomized controlled trials (RCTs) the most rigorous study design, as they have the highest probability of establishing causality between variables while minimizing bias. Although research studies using qualitative, descriptive, or nonresearch designs were not included in original evidence pyramids, they can now be found in several modifications of the pyramid used in healthcare settings (Polit & Beck, 2021; Whalen & Dang, 2022). There is no consensus on what constitutes "best evidence" in EBP, yet there is general agreement that findings from well-designed research studies are essential to best practice (Polit & Beck, 2021).

Hierarchy pyramids can offer a visual representation of the levels and available quantities of different types of evidence used in clinical decision-making, but they do not signify the quality (validity and reliability) of evidence. Consider the top segment of the evidence pyramid presented in Chapter 4 (replicated in Figure 5.1). The upper point of the pyramid represents the highest level of evidence, such as systematic reviews with (or without) a meta-analysis of RCTs. Quality of evidence can be determined only by conducting a thorough critical appraisal using a systematic approach with a standardized tool. Remember, a study situated higher on the pyramid is not necessarily of higher quality than a well-conducted descriptive study situated at the pyramid base (Murad et al., 2016).

Individual reports of research studies are considered **primary sources**. A systematic review is composed of primary studies or sources. Also included in the pyramid are secondary sources of evidence, such as evidence-based guidelines based on systematic reviews. Pre-appraised evidence can include summaries

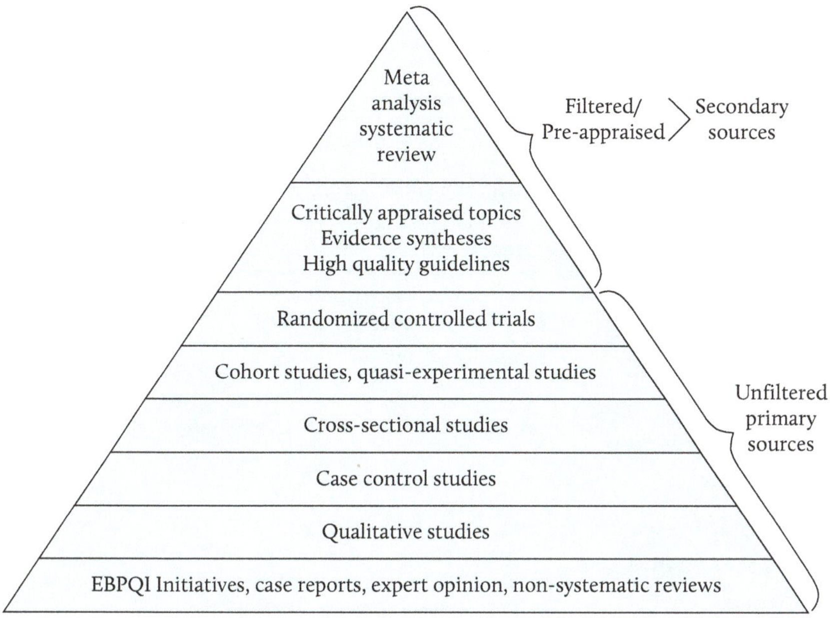

FIGURE 5.1 Hierarchy of Evidence Pyramid

and analyses of evidence derived from original research studies that authors have already appraised using a standardized tool or checklist. Examples of pre-appraised evidence are UpToDate (https://www.wolterskluwer.com/en/solutions/uptodate) and JBI Nursing (https://jbi.global/ebp). High quality pre-appraisals often inform practice recommendations, such as those from the American Academy of Pediatrics (https://www.aap.org/en/patient-care/). (See more on pre-appraised evidence in Chapter 7.)

Levels of Evidence

Assigning an evidence level refers to making an objective hierarchical rating of a research study or other source of evidence according to its design and methodology. This is the initial step in the critical appraisal process. Evidence levels are often assigned based on established guidelines or frameworks, such as the evidence hierarchy pyramid. Numerous guides and scales exist for assigning levels of evidence, with variations in the ranking of research and other evidence designs. For example, in some level ratings, Roman numerals are used to rank evidence from I to VII (Melnyk & Fineout-Overholt, 2023). In contrast, yhe Johns Hopkins evidence-based practice model *Appendix D: Hierarchy of Evidence Guide* provides a 5-level evidence hierarchy for research (Levels I, II, and III) and other evidence (Levels IV and V; Whalen & Dang, 2022).

No level of evidence rating scale or hierarchy is considered the best; however, some have corresponding critical appraisal tools. EBPQI teams should choose a single rating scale and use it consistently throughout the critical appraisal process.

TABLE 5.1 Level of Evidence Guides

Sources for level guides	Website access	Access and fee
Oxford Centre for Evidence-Based Medicine: Levels of Evidence	https://www.cebm.ox.ac.uk/resources/levels-of-evidence/oxford-centre-for-evidence-based-medicine-levels-of-evidence-march-2009	Free. A downloadable version is unavailable.
Johns Hopkins Evidence-Based Practice Model for Nursing and Healthcare Professionals Appendix D: Hierarchy of Evidence Guide	https://www.hopkinsmedicine.org/evidence-based-practice/models-tools.html	Free. Must complete a copyright permission form for access. A zipped file with all model appendices is sent via email and made available for download and use.
Hierarchy of Evidence for Interventional Studies	Fineout-Overholt, et al. (2010). Evidence-based practice step by step: Critical appraisal of the evidence: part I. *The American Journal of Nursing, 110*(7), 47–52. https://journals.lww.com/ajnonline/Fulltext/2010/07000/Evidence_Based_Practice_Step_by_Step__Critical.26.aspx	Free. The table is in the article and is available as open access.

When you first begin to read research reports, you may find it challenging to determine types of evidence or identify various research study designs. Ask a team member or available researcher who is knowledgeable in research design to assist whenever possible, and don't be afraid to ask for help from trusted resources as needed. You will find some examples of levels-of-evidence rating guides to add to your EBP resources in Table 5.1.

Critical Appraisal Process

Include or Exclude

Learning to read and appraise a research study is just like learning a new nursing skill such as giving an injection or taking vital signs: It requires exposure, a plan, and practice. After reading an article, you should first determine whether the study may help to answer your clinical question given the inclusion/exclusion criteria you created prior to searching for evidence (see Chapter 4). If the answer is "yes," move on to the next step in the critical appraisal process for assessing study quality. Figure 5.2 shows you the type of content to look for as you read various sections of articles.

Quality of Evidence

To evaluate the quality of a research study you first need to understand the various types of study designs. The following sections will describe the most common types of research study designs used in nursing. We begin at the top of the evidence hierarchy pyramid.

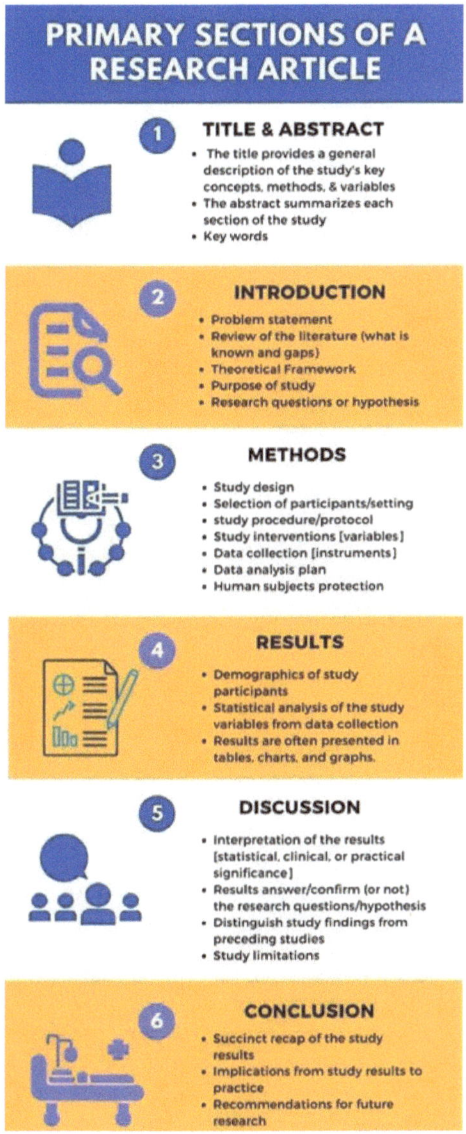

FIGURE 5.2 Infographic of Primary Sections of a Research Article

Quantitative Research Study Designs

Along with various level-of-evidence guides, numerous tools and checklists exist to help you systematically assess the quality of evidence; however, these tools vary in their complexity and applicability to evidence designs (Buccheri & Sharifi, 2017). You should understand the basic designs of quantitative research studies at the top of the pyramid, so let's get started!

Systematic Review and Meta-Analyses

A *systematic review* is a rigorous synthesis of multiple research findings that address a specific clinical question. A team of experts conducts a systematic review using a stringent protocol, including predetermined inclusion and exclusion criteria to reduce biases and errors in reporting; these criteria may be specific to the study's design, population, or setting. The Preferred Reporting Items for Systematic Reviews and Meta-Analyses (PRISMA) diagram visually represents a clear and concise summary of the selection of studies for inclusion in a systematic review or meta-analysis (Page et al., 2021; see Figure 5.3.). The team uses a standard tool to critically appraise each study's quality by determining the risk of bias and displays the findings in a chart or graph. The outcomes from all the findings are synthesized and interpreted, accounting for each study's quality and implications to practice (Rochwerg, 2022). PRISMA provides a standard guideline and checklist for authors and editors to

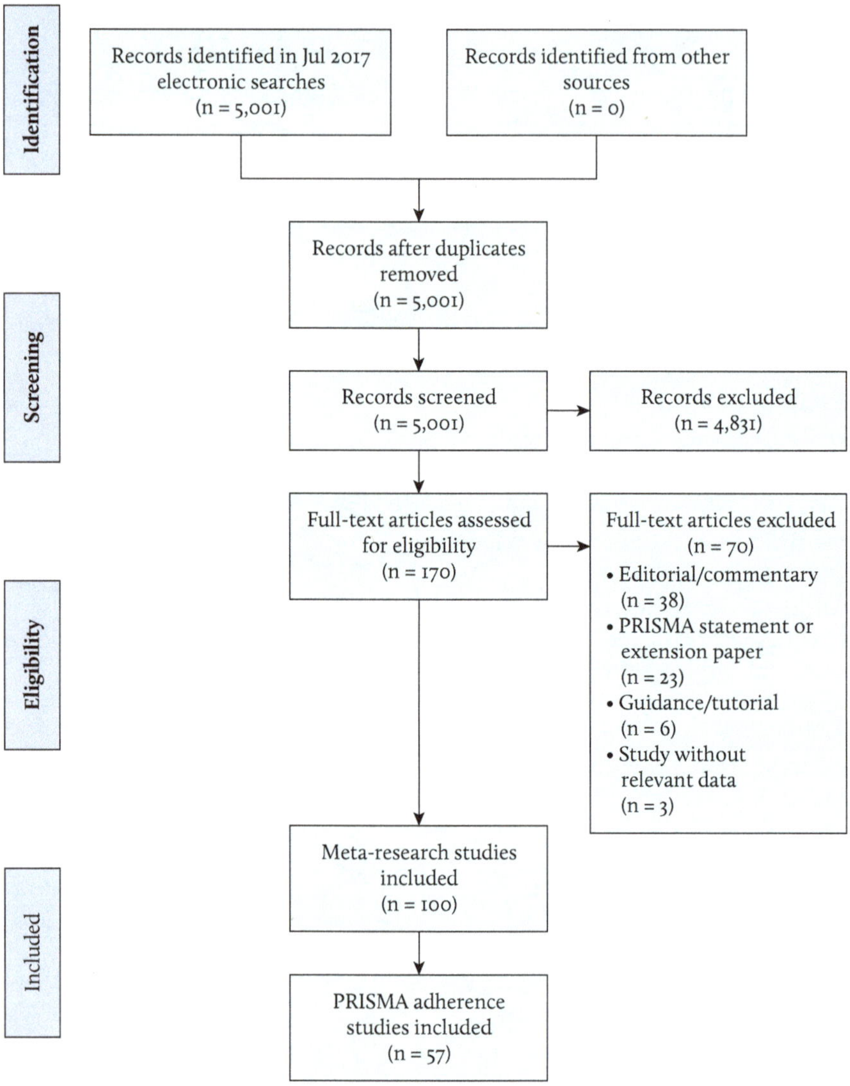

FIGURE 5.3 PRISMA Flow Diagram

ensure that the systematic review or meta-analysis is transparent, comprehensive, and reproducible for publication (Page et al., 2021).

Let's suppose that you are reading a systematic review and the findings are written in narrative form. How can you discover whether there are enough studies or similar data across studies to summarize or pool the study results for an overall statistical finding? You can use a meta-analysis to collect the multiple studies in a systematic review with similar enough interventions and outcome measures to be statistically combined (Rochwerg, 2022). The addition of a meta-analysis

TABLE 5.2 Interpretation of an Effect Size

Effect size	Cohen's d
Small	0.2
Medium	0.5
Large	0.8 or greater

allows the team to report an overall summary of the treatment effect (i.e., the strength of the relationship between the intervention and its outcomes). The *effect size* assesses the difference between the means in a study group. The higher the effect size (Table 5.2), the more confident you will be that the intervention caused the effect found in the outcomes (results) of the combined studies (Whalen & Dang, 2022). For example, an effect size of 0.9 would instill confidence that the intervention(s) affected the outcome(s).

A well-conducted systematic review with a meta-analysis is considered the highest level of evidence to answer specific clinical questions for making practice recommendations (Rochwerg, 2022). The *Cochrane Database of Systematic Reviews (CDSR)* is the leading journal and database for accessing systematic reviews and meta-analyses in healthcare. When searching for systematic reviews, always begin your search in the Cochrane Database, which is also indexed in PubMed, Web of Science, and Scopus.

Additional Types of Reviews

Many articles are published with the word "review" in the title. When searching databases, if you have applied the systematic review limit option, your results may include other types of reviews. The most common reviews are integrative, scoping, and literature (narrative) reviews. In Figure 5.4, you will recognize the overabundance of these types of reviews compared to the availability of systematic reviews and meta-analyses. Although these reviews may be useful in answering your clinical question, they lack the rigor and quality assessment performed in the systematic review process.

Approaches to Quantitative Research

Quantitative research methods measure and quantify data using statistical and numerical methods. The strength of quantitative research is that it allows you to collect objective, numerical data that you can analyze using statistics to draw meaningful conclusions about relationships between independent (intervention) and dependent (measured outcome) variables (Whalen & Dang, 2022). In EBP, the independent variable is the "I" (intervention of interest) in the PICO or the "C" (change in practice) in the PPCO, and the dependent variable is the "O" (outcome/s) in both the frameworks.

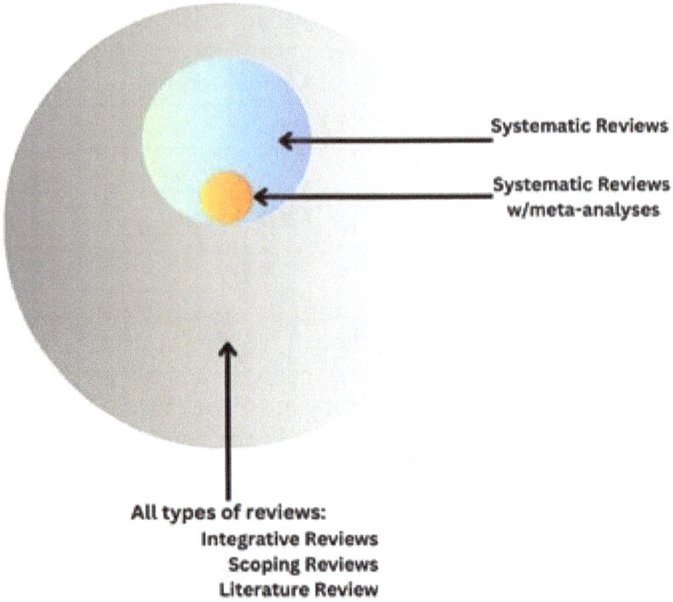

FIGURE 5.4 Comparison of the Availability of Systematic Reviews and All Reviews

Quantitative Research Designs

A study's *research design* refers to the plan or strategy its researchers used to conduct their study as well as the procedures they used to collect and analyze data based on their research question. The key components of quantitative research are a research question, a population or sample to be studied, independent and dependent variables, data collection and analysis methods and instruments, and ethical considerations. Different research designs have various strengths and weaknesses. Experimental and observational designs are common broad quantitative categories; Table 5.3 outlines these basic categories and their associated research designs, methods, and examples.

TABLE 5.3 Common Quantitative Research Designs and Features

Type	Design	Methods	Examples
Experimental	Randomized control trial	-Random sample and assignment -Blinding (when applicable) -Intervention and control intervention(s) -Manipulation of one or more variables	Recruitment of participants with high blood pressure is assigned to either the experimental group that receives a new hypertensive drug or the control group that receives a placebo. Blood pressure is monitored in each group and compared to determine if the new drug is more effective than the placebo.

Type	Design	Methods	Examples
	Quasi-experimental	-Lack random assignment -Control group not required (comparison group) -Intervention -Manipulation of variables	Participants are recruited but not randomized to groups and instead are assigned based on pre-existing characteristics or non-random factors. An example is a study of students in one class where a new teaching strategy is used and compared to a class where traditional teaching strategies are used, and academic performance is compared.
Observational	Cohort case-control (retrospective)	-No randomization of groups -No intervention or manipulation of variable -Occurs in a natural setting -Relationship between variables -Prospective or retrospective	A research study that compares an outcome (e.g., lung cancer) between groups of individuals who are alike in many ways but different in another specific way, such as a behavior like exercise (one group does not regularly exercise and the other does). -A study that compares two groups of people: those with the disease or condition under study (cases) and a very similar group of people who do not have the disease or condition (controls).
	Cross-sectional	-No randomization or control group -No manipulation of variables -Occurs in a natural setting	Research study where a group of people is observed or their information is collected at a single point in time. An example is a survey to collect information about the total number of people in a group who have or had a certain disease (such as cancer) or risk factor (such as smoking or obesity).

Note. Adapted from Denise Polit and Cheryl Beck, "Common Quantitative Research Designs and Features," Essentials of Nursing Research: Appraising Evidence for Nursing Practice. Copyright © 2021 by Wolters Kluwer.

Experimental Designs

Randomized controlled trials (RTCs) are considered the gold standard for evaluating the effectiveness of interventions because the researcher uses randomization to allocate participants to an intervention or control group by chance. Random assignment helps to ensure that the groups are similar at the outset; thus, any differences observed between them can be attributed to the intervention rather than to factors such as different characteristics. RCTs typically use "blinding" to minimize bias and to control for confounding (extraneous) variables that could influence the outcome (dependent variable) outside the intervention (independent variable) (Polit & Beck, 2021). The participants are informed before the study begins that they will not know whether they have been assigned to the intervention or the control group (see Chapter 10 for more information on consent to participate in research); in this way, they are blinded. A simple example would be a study of a new medication in which the control group is given a "placebo," perhaps just a sugar pill, while those in the intervention group receive the actual new medication. You might recall that one of the authors of this textbook decided to become a nurse after having been a participant in many such studies; she understood before participating that she would be "blinded," so she did not know whether the pill she was given was a sugar (placebo) pill or an actual active medication. Blinding participants can help to prevent the "Hawthorne effect" (named for the researcher who first described it), which is a possible tendency of some participants to change their behavior or habits because they know they are being studied. This consequence of knowing that one is participating in an intervention can mask the effects of the variables being studied.

Although considered a type of experimental design, quasi-experimental studies lack randomization and may not include a control group; therefore, they are considered much less rigorous than RCTs. Use of a control group is not always possible; in such cases, a comparison group is typically created by selecting subjects who are like the experimental group but will not receive the treatment or intervention being studied. Another way to create a comparison group is to evaluate the same participants prior to and after the intervention is implemented to achieve a "before and after" comparison. Although quasi-experimental studies can be useful for evaluating interventions when randomization is not feasible or ethical, they are more susceptible to bias and confounding variables than RCTs. As a result, the conclusions drawn from quasi-experimental studies are generally considered less certain than those from RCTs, but they may still be transferable to clinical practice (Whalen & Dang, 2022).

Observational Designs

Observational research aims to describe or understand a phenomenon, behavior, or situation in its natural setting. An *observational design* is a research method in which the researcher observes and records what is being studied as it occurs naturally, without manipulating any variables or interventions. Cohort, case-control trials, and cross-sectional studies are observational studies that investigate the relationship between an exposure or risk factor and a health outcome.

In a *cohort study*, a group (cohort) of individuals is followed over time to assess the relationship between exposure to a risk factor and the incidence of a particular health outcome. Cohort studies can be either prospective or retrospective, depending on whether the study follows the cohort forward in time (prospective) or looks back at data that has already been collected (retrospective). Prospective cohort studies are considered more reliable because they follow the individuals over time and the researcher can observe changes in exposure and health outcomes. For example, through its recruitment of nurses, the Nurses' Health Study is among the largest prospective studies investigating the risk factors for major chronic diseases in women. Nurses are selected because of their knowledge about health and ability to provide complete and accurate information regarding various diseases. Now in its third phase, the Nurses' Health Study includes nurses (both men and women) from diverse backgrounds (Barrett & Noble, 2019).

A *case-control study* compares individuals with a particular health outcome (cases) to those without the health outcome (controls). The researcher looks back in time (retrospective) and identifies potential exposures or risk factors that may have contributed to the outcome being investigated, then compares the frequency of these exposures in cases and controls to determine whether there is a relationship between exposure and the health outcome. The main difference between cohort and case-control studies is the selection of participants. In cohort studies, individuals are selected based on their exposure status and followed over time. In case-control studies, participants are selected based on their disease status and looked at retrospectively (Tenny et al., 2022). A case control study design was used in one of the first studies to identify the importance of masking to prevent the spread of SARS-CoV-2 among healthcare workers (Rodriguez-Lopez et al., 2021). In this study, 110 healthcare workers with a positive COVID-19 test and 113 healthcare workers with a negative test were randomly selected and interviewed about their infection control behaviors. Results demonstrated a strong association between wearing a high-performance filtering mask or double masking and negative COVID-19 test results.

Cross-sectional studies aim to describe, explain, or summarize a particular phenomenon or behavior without manipulating variables. In this type of study, the researchers collect data from a sample of individuals at a single point in time to describe the prevalence of a phenomenon or characteristics, such as the beliefs or health characteristics of a specific population. Cross-sectional studies have limitations, such as their inability to establish cause-and-effect relationships between variables or control for confounding factors (Polit & Beck, 2021). Researchers in Great Britain used a cross-sectional study design and a survey/questionnaire to identify factors associated with the frequency of respiratory rate measurement by nurses in hospital settings. This study included 944 nurses from nine different hospitals. The participants' perception of importance of the measurement and educational experiences were positively associated with whether or not respiratory rate was measured (Takayama et al., 2022).

Table 5.4 provides some key research terms and definitions you can reference if you need clarification to interpret research terms.

TABLE 5.4 Key Research Terms

Key terms	Definitions
Randomization	The assignment of subjects to treatment conditions in a random manner (i.e., in a manner by chance alone).
Independent variable	The variable that is believed to cause or influence the dependent variable; the variable that is manipulated (intervention).
Dependent variable	The variable that is predicted to depend on or be caused by another variable (independent variable/intervention) on the outcome of interest.
Confounding (extraneous) variable	A variable(s) that is not included in the study but possibly influences the dependent variable (outcome).
Internal validity	The degree to which observed outcomes (dependent variable) is caused by the experimental treatment or intervention (independent variable) rather than by other alternative causes.
External validity	The degree to which study results can be generalized to settings or groups other than in the study setting.

Critical Appraisal of Quantitative Research Evidence

Now that you have a basic understanding of evidence hierarchies and quantitative research, your EBPQI team is ready to complete the first step of the critical appraisal process (see Table 5.5) by evaluating the quality of evidence by systematic critical appraisal.

Critical Appraisal Tools for Assigning Quality

Various critical appraisal tools are available to appraise research evidence's validity, reliability, and applicability. The EBPQI team first determines the research study design in order to select the appropriate critical appraisal tool to determine the quality of the evidence (Buccheri & Sharifi, 2017). Rating the quality of evidence is a subjective activity that will require you and your EBP team to think critically. Table 5.5 includes valuable resources to help your team with tool selection. The table contains each tool's copyright owner, website URL, coverage of research designs, download accessibility, and cost, as well as an overview of available instructions.

TABLE 5.5 Critical Appraisal Resources

Critical appraisal tool	Website	Research study designs	Overview
Critical Appraisal Skills Programme Checklists (CASP)	https://casp-uk.net/casp-tools-checklists/	-Systematic review -Randomized controlled trial -Cohort study -Case-control study -Diagnostic study	-Includes instructions and embedded hints throughout the checklists -No level or quality rating guide -Free access -Full-text PDF, Word, or print & fill
Centre for Evidence-Based Medicine	https://www.cebm.ox.ac.uk/resources/ebm-tools/critical-appraisal-tools	-Systematic review -Randomized controlled trial -Cohort (prognostic) study -Diagnostic accuracy study	-Embedded hints throughout the form -Associated level and quality rating guide (different URL) -Free access -Full-text downloadable form

Critical appraisal tool	Website	Research study designs	Overview
JBI Global	https://jbi.global/critical-appraisal-tools	-Systematic review -Randomized controlled trial -Quasi-experimental -Cohort study -Case-control study -Diagnostic test accuracy studies -Analytical cross-sectional -Case reports -Case series -Prevalence studies	-Includes instructions with the form -No level or quality rating guide -Free access -Full-text Word
Johns Hopkins EBP Model and Tools	https://www.hopkinsmedicine.org/evidence-based-practice/models-tools.html	-Quantitative research (RCT, quasi, descriptive) -Systematic review	-Includes instructions and embedded hints throughout all forms -Level and quality guide for ratings -Strength of recommendation rating -Free access -Request permission for use and receive a zip file with all forms
Helene Fuld Health Trust National Institute for Evidence-Based Practice in Nursing and Healthcare	https://fuld.nursing.osu.edu/become-a-member	-Systematic review -Randomized controlled trial -Quasi-experimental -Cohort study -Case-control Study -Descriptive study	-Requires a fee membership to EBP HQ for access

Components of Critical Appraisal

Critical Appraisal includes the components of validity, bias, and reliability. Each one contributes to the trustworthiness of the results. All three focus on how the research study was conducted.

Validity

Determining *validity* involves deciding how credibly the research study measured the outcomes as intended. Was the study conducted using sound scientific methods? As you appraise your article for validity, your critical appraisal tool may ask common questions such as the following:

- Did the researcher/s identify what is known or unknown about the clinical issue?
- What gaps will the research study address?
- What is the purpose of the study?
- Was a literature review conducted, and if so, was the literature current?
- Depending on the design, did the researcher randomize their sample to an experimental and control group, and were the characteristics of these groups similar?

Researchers often publish a flowchart that visually displays their study's enrollment process, allocation, follow-up, and analysis of participants in the experimental and control groups. To determine the degree of a study's internal validity, it is important to note whether the researchers controlled for confounding variables that could have influenced the outcomes (dependent variable) or biased the study results. Bias occurs in the best-designed studies and is difficult to eliminate; therefore, the researcher should have attempted to limit bias when possible (Whalen & Dang, 2022). Table 5.6 lists types of bias that can affect a study's internal validity and how they can be controlled.

Additional appraisal questions may ask how the data to measure the dependent variable (outcomes) were collected and whether the instruments used were valid and reliable. Don't get overly anxious about all the questions about validity and reliability of the quality of the study; they are simply meant to help you determine whether the instrument used in the study measured the concept/outcome (dependent variable) it was intended to measure (instrument validity) and did so consistently across all participants (reliability). Remember that you are a novice and will have an expert EBP mentor on your team to help you with these new terms and questions.

TABLE 5.6 Types of Bias in Research

Type of bias	Description	Reduce bias
Selection (allocation) bias	The selection of study participants is not representative of the target population. Participants are not randomly selected. Exclusion criteria disproportionately exclude certain groups.	Random sample Criteria for inclusion/exclusion Sampling plan Sample size (power)
Detection bias	Study participants or investigators are not blinded or are aware of the treatment assignment.	Blinding or masking the investigators, group assignments, and study participants to who is receiving the intervention or control.
Attrition bias	A differential dropout or loss to follow-up among study participants.	Offer incentives or reminders. Minimize participant burden. Clear study information to participants.
Measurement bias	Outcomes are measured or assessed differently between study groups.	Definitions of measures Validity and reliability of measures Instructions for data collection

Note. Adapted from Denise Polit and Cheryl Beck, "Types of Bias in Research," Essentials of Nursing Research: Appraising Evidence for Nursing Practice. Copyright © 2021 by Wolters Kluwer.

Reliability

Reliability refers to how likely it is that the findings of the study will be generalizable to other settings (beyond that of the study). In EBPQI, you must know whether the study's findings apply to your patient population before you make recommendations based on the research evidence. Remember that experimental studies, such as RCTs, usually have high internal validity due to the rigorous nature of their methods for controlling confounding variables. However, non-experimental (quasi-experimental) and observational studies may have lower internal validity yet be more transferable to the clinical setting. You will recall that the level of the study cannot predict its quality; therefore, a high-quality observational study that applies to your setting and patient needs may be of more value to your EBPQI team than an RCT that is not as applicable outside the confines of its study setting (Whalen & Dang, 2022).

The reliability of a study's findings will help you to determine whether the effects will have a sufficient influence on practice or your patient outcomes. In other words, ask yourself, "Would these findings make a difference for the patients I serve if my EBPQI team were to implement the study?" Your team should determine whether the study's findings were statistically, practically, and/or clinically significant. A study that does not have statistical significance can still be clinically or practically significant (see Table 5.7). For example, clinical significance occurs when a patient's experience is improved (Carpenter et al., 2021). EBPQI teams should closely and thoughtfully assess significance types. It is important to know (a) whether study results were likely (or not) to occur due to chance (the statistical significance); (b) whether patients, families, and/or communities are likely to benefit from the noted effect or change (the clinical significance); and (c) the quantifiable (actual) magnitude (how much change to is estimated to occur) of the effect (practical significance).

TABLE 5.7 Brief Descriptions of Significance Types

Significance type	Description	Questions asked of the findings
Statistical	Results due to chance	-Were the results of the intervention due to chance? -What is the probability that these results occurred by chance alone?
Practical	Quantifies the impact of a treatment; estimates the magnitude of effect.	-How effective was the intervention/treatment? -How much change does the intervention/treatment cause?
Clinical	The practical or applied importance of effect and whether it make a difference to clients/subjects/patients in everyday life	-Was the intervention/treatment effective enough to improve the patient's experience (e.g., of their health or provision of care)? -Was the intervention/treatment enough to improve or eliminate a diagnostic criterion for a condition?

Source: Roger Carpenter, Julee Waldrop, and Heather Carter-Templeton, "Statistical, Practical and Clinical Significance and Doctor of Nursing Practice Projects," Nurse Author & Editor, vol. 31, no. 3-4. Copyright © 2021 by John Wiley & Sons, Inc.

Finally, beyond interpreting the study results, you must determine whether the researcher provided clinical implications and addressed study limitations. This is important information to explore as you appraise each study with your team. After you have completed the critical appraisal tool or checklist for each of the studies you included to answer your PICO or PPCO question, you and your team must conduct an evaluation of the body of evidence as a whole.

Evaluation of Research

The next step in the critical appraisal process is *evaluation*. During the evaluation phase, you will take the information from your critical appraisals and place it into an evidence table or matrix template. You will discard any evidence that you or your team found to be of low quality or inapplicable to your PICO or PPCO question, patient population, or setting. There is no magic number of research articles to add to your evaluation tables. Your confidence in the quality and consistency of your research evidence will support your confidence to make practice recommendations (Fineout-Overholt et al., 2010).

An evidence table or matrix is a tool used to summarize and organize the key information from appraising research studies to answer your clinical question. As you add each systematic review or study to an evaluation table row, you will observe similarities and differences across the study variables, outcome measures, data analyses, and findings that aid in answering your question. Fineout-Overholt et al. (2010) recommend creating headings for essential elements to extract from your critical appraisals to add to the evaluation table. The table should include the study design, sample size, intervention, outcome measures, and results. Depending on your question, you may also add other columns, such as intervention or educational methods used in each study. Once each study or systematic review has been added to an evaluation table, you will begin to synthesize the evidence for its worth to your practice (O'Mathúna et al., 2023).

You will use a synthesis table to collect the relevant aspects of the studies you plan to include in your **synthesis** of all of your evidence, not just the quantitative studies but qualitative studies and other evidence as well (see Chapters 6 and 7; see Table 5.8).

TABLE 5.8 Synthesis Table

Citation	Purpose of study	Design/ method	Sample/ setting	Major variables studied and their definitions	Measurement of major variables	Data analysis	Study findings/ results	Level of evidence	Worth to practice

Strength or Recommendation Rating

At this point, you are not ready to make a definitive recommendation for a practice change because other types of evidence remain to be appraised (Chapters 6 and 7), but as you view the key information you have placed into your evaluation and synthesis tables so far, search for consistency in quality and outcomes across studies to support a compelling case for developing your practice recommendation (Newhouse, 2022). *Practice recommendations* are "clear, definitive evidence-based statements of best practice that are expected for all clinicians" to adopt (O'Mathúna et al., 2023, p. 260). Figure 5.5 provides options for selecting a strength of recommendation rating for your body of evidence. The decision loop at the base of the EBPQI mountain reflects your determination that there is enough evidence to change practice or that more research is needed before you can pursue change safely.

Johns Hopkins uses the following categories for describing the strength of recommendation based on your synthesis:

- **Strong and compelling evidence, consistent results** > Recommendations are reliable; evaluate for organizational translation.
- **Good evidence and consistent results** > Recommendations may be reliable; evaluate for risk and organizational translation.
- **Good evidence but conflicting results** > Unable to establish best practice based on current evidence; *evaluate risk*, consider further investigation for new evidence, develop a research study, or discontinue the project.
- **Little or no evidence** > Unable to establish best practice based on current evidence; consider further investigation for new evidence, develop a research study, or discontinue the project. (Newhouse, 2022, p. 321)

Notice that the strength of the recommendation rating "good evidence but conflicting results" allows you to evaluate the risk for patient harm. If the likelihood of harm is low, using a quality improvement approach of manageable plan-do-study-act (PDSA) cycles to pilot a small change may be reasonable (see Chapter 9–11). Always remember that you must determine whether the intervention is feasible in your setting. Consideration of patient preferences and values is critical to determine the applicability of the study findings (see Chapter 8).

WRAPPING UP

In conclusion, before you can implement any recommended practice changes, you and the EBPQI team must communicate about your recommendations with the key practice-setting stakeholders based on the body of evidence you have compiled. If the practice change does not align with the organizational priorities, it may not be suitable to implement an EBPQI initiative. You will need to make certain that the recommendations are both acceptable to the organizational stakeholders and meet patients' preferences and values (more on this in Chapter 11; Newhouse, 2022). The EBPQI team will also need to explore whether the recommended practice change is feasible from a monetary and resource perspective. Leadership and stakeholder buy-in is key, and we will continue to consider this important point as our journey up the EBPQI mountain continues.

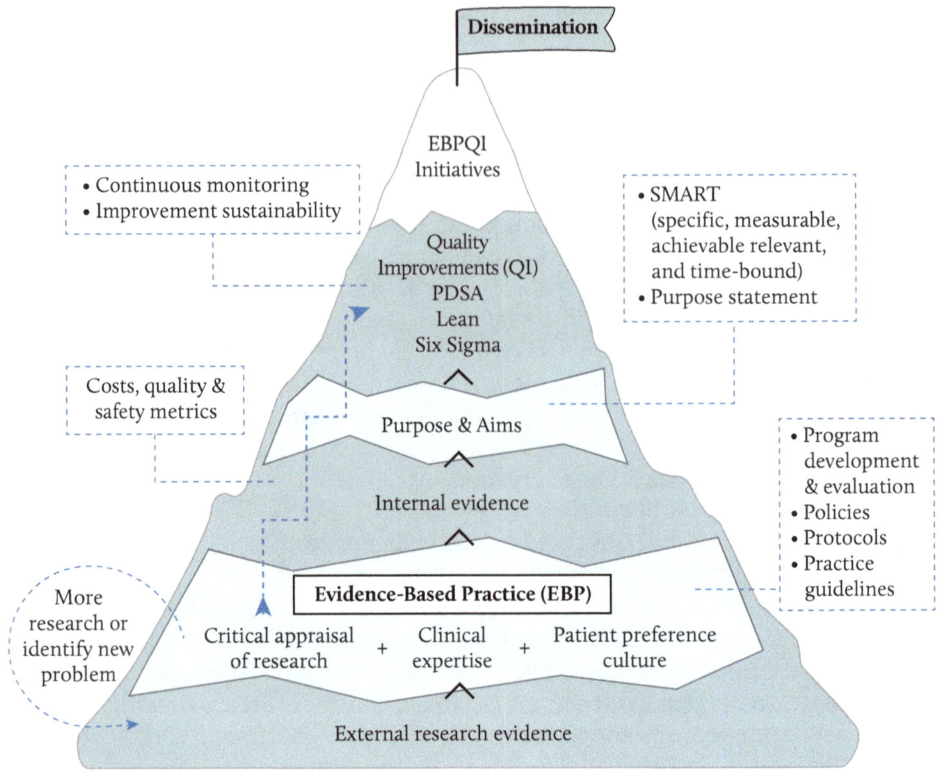

FIGURE 5.5 EBP Within the Mountain Model

Be mindful that various sources of research evidence are acceptable for nurses' clinical decision-making. Due to the complexities of healthcare delivery, several sources of evidence may be needed to answer a clinical question, including regarding clinical expertise and patient preferences. This chapter has focused on introducing quantitative evidence as it relates to EBP, but you will remember from Chapter 1 that EBP decisions are not based on research evidence alone. Patient preferences and clinical expertise are of equal importance on the second tier of the EBPQI mountain. For example, as a nurse working on the mother-baby unit, you might want to implement evidence-based interventions to support mother-infant breastfeeding, but if you are unaware of how the mothers perceive breastfeeding support, what component of EBP will you focus on to gather information to offer them the types of support they desire? You will need to understand patient preferences and values, a topic we cover in Chapter 8.

WELLNESS IN ACTION: DIGITAL WELL-BEING

Although a recent survey shows that Americans are checking their phones less in 2023 than in 2022 (a good sign!), they are still checking them on average 144 times per day and an average of 4 hours and 5 minutes a day (Dreibelbis, 2023). Excessive digital media usage can deprive us of rest and productive time, leading to decreased sleep and reduced performance and mood. As a nursing student, your time is extremely valuable, and we hope that you are motivated to allocate your time to helpful actions. Digital well-being has been suggested as a practice to reduce unproductive screen time and establish a better work-life balance through the healthy use of technology (Thomas et al., 2022). Consider engaging in one or more of the following suggested steps based on your personal level of digital use (or overuse):

1. Use a screen-monitoring app for accountability purposes and to reduce nonproductive digital media time.
2. Try a digital detox for a set period of time to give yourself healthy time to disconnect from digital distractions.
3. Notice how you feel after participating in digital media; reduce or eliminate the apps or activities that do not feel useful or beneficial to you as an individual.
4. Replace unhealthy screen time with a healthy lifestyle habit; use a tracking app to monitor physical activity or the pursuit of a hobby.
5. Be mindful and present in the moment by looking up from your screen and noticing something around you that brings you peace, calm, or excitement.

REFLECTION QUESTIONS

1. What are the differences between a systematic review and a meta-analysis?
2. What is the key difference between an experimental study design and an observational study design?

REFERENCES

Al-Jundi, A., & Sakka, S. (2017). Critical appraisal of clinical research. *Journal of Clinical and Diagnostic Research*, *11*(5), JE01–JE05. https://doi.org/10.7860/JCDR/2017/26047.9942

Barrett, D., & Noble, H. (2019). What are cohort studies? *Evidence-Based Nursing*, *22*(4), 95–96. https://doi.org/10.1136/ebnurs-2019-103183

Buccheri, R. K., & Sharifi, C. (2017). Critical appraisal tools and reporting guidelines for evidence-based practice. *Worldviews on Evidence-Based Nursing*, *14*(6), 463–472. https://doi.org/10.1111/wvn.12258

Carpenter, R., Waldrop, J., & Carter-Templeton, H. (2021). Statistical, practical and clinical significance and Doctor of Nursing Practice projects. *Nurse Author & Editor*, *31*(3–4), 50–53. https://doi.org/10.1111/nae2.27

Deng, T., Kanthawala, S., Meng, J., Peng, W., Kononova, A., Hao, Q., Zhang, Q., & David, P. (2019). Measuring smartphone usage and task switching with log tracking and self-reports. *Mobile Media & Communication*, 7(1), 3–23. https://doi.org/10.1177/2050157918761491

Dreibelbis, E. (2023). Americans check their phones an alarming number of times per day. *PC Magazine*, May 19. https://www.pcmag.com/news/americans-check-their-phones-an-alarming-number-of-times-per-day

Fernandez, A., Sturmberg, J., Lukersmith, S., Madden, R., Torkfar, G., Colagiuri, R., & Salvador-Carulla, L. (2015). Evidence-based medicine: Is it a bridge too far? *Health Research Policy and Systems*, *13*(66), 1–9. https://doi.org/10.1186/s12961-015-0057-0

Fineout-Overholt, E. (2023). Critically appraising knowledge for clinical decision making. In B. M. Melnyk & E. Fineout-Overholt (Eds.), *Evidence-based practice in nursing and healthcare: A guide to best practice* (5th ed., p. 161). Wolters Kluwer.

Fineout-Overholt, E., Melnyk, B. M., Stillwell, S. B., & Williamson, K. M. (2010). Evidence-based practice step by step: Critical appraisal of the evidence: part I. *The American Journal of Nursing, 110*(7), 47–52. https://doi.org/10.1097/01.NAJ.0000383935.22721.9c

Jones, A., & Steel, D. (2018). Evaluating the quality of medical evidence in real-world contexts. *Journal of Evaluation in Clinical Practice, 24*(5), 950–956. https://doi.org/10.1111/jep.12983

Melnyk, B. M., & Fineout-Overholt, E. (2023). Making the case for evidence-based practice and cultivating a spirit of inquiry. In B. M. Melnyk & E. Fineout-Overholt (Eds.), *Evidence-based practice in nursing and healthcare: A guide to best practice* (5th ed., pp. 20–25). Wolters Kluwer.

Murad, M. H., Asi, N., Alsawas, M., & Alahdab, F. (2016). New evidence pyramid. *Evidence-Based Medicine, 21*(4), 125–127. https://doi.org/10.1136/ebmed-2016-110401

Newhouse, R. P. (2022). Translation. In D. Dang, S. L. Dearholt, K. Bissett, J. Ascenzi, & M. Whalen (Eds.), *Johns Hopkins evidence-based practice for nurses and healthcare professionals* (4th ed., pp. 196–198, 322). Sigma Theta Tau International.

O'Halloran, P., Porter, S., & Blackwood, B. (2010). Evidence based practice and its critics: What is a nurse manager to do? *Journal of Nursing Management, 18*(1), 90–95. https://doi.org/10.1111/j.1365-2834.2009.01068.x

O'Mathúna, D. P., Finest-Overholt, E., Graham, D. B., & Canada, A. (2023). Critically appraising quantitative evidence for clinical decision making. In B. M. Melnyk & E. Fineout-Overholt (Eds.), *Evidence-based practice in nursing and healthcare: A guide to best practice* (5th ed., pp. 259–260). Wolters Kluwer.

Page, M. J., McKenzie, J. E., Bossuyt, P. M., Boutron, I., Hoffmann, T. C., Mulrow, C. D., Shamseer, L., Tetzlaff, J. M., Akl, E. A., Brennan, S. E., Chou, R., Glanville, J., Grimshaw, J. M., Hróbjartsson, A., Lalu, M. M., Li, T., Loder, E. W., Mayo-Wilson, E., McDonald, S., McGuinness, L. A., ... Moher, D. (2021). The PRISMA 2020 statement: An updated guideline for reporting systematic reviews. *BMJ, 372*(71), 1–9. https://doi.org/10.1136/bmj.n71

Polit, D. F., & Beck, C. T. (2021). *Essentials of nursing research: Appraising evidence for nursing practice.* (11th ed.). Wolters Kluwer.

Rochwerg, B. (2022). Critical appraisal of a systematic review: A concise review. *Critical Care Medicine, 50*(9), 1371–1379. https://10.1097/CCM.0000000000005602

Rodriquez-Lopez, M., Parra, B. Vergara, E., Rey, L., Salcedo, M., Arturo, G., Alarcon, L., Holguin, J., & Osorio, L. (2021). A case control study of factors associated with SARS-CoV-2 infection among healthcare workers in Columbia. *BMC Infectious Diseases, 21*(1), 878–787. https://doi.org/10.1186/s12879-021-06581-y

Takayama, A., Takeshima, T., & Nagamine, T. (2022). Factors associated with the frequency of respiratory rate measurement by hospital nurses: a multicentre cross-sectional study. *British Journal of Nursing (Mark Allen Publishing), 31*(9), 495–501. https://doi.org/10.12968/bjon.2022.31.9.495

Tenny, S., Kerndt, C. C., & Hoffman, M. R. (2022). Case control studies. StatPearls.

Thomas, N. M., Choudhari, S. G., Gaidhane, A. M., & Quazi Syed, Z. (2022). "Digital wellbeing": The need of the hour in today's digitalized and technology driven world! *Cureus, 14*(8), Article e27743. https://doi.org/10.7759/cureus.27743

Whalen, M., & Dang, D. (2022). Evidence appraisal: Research. In D. Dang, S.L. Dearholt, K. Bissett, J. Ascenzi, & M. Whalen (Eds.), *Johns Hopkins evidence-based practice for nurses and healthcare professionals* (4th ed., pp. 121–123, 142, 147–149, 130–131, 296, 298–302). Sigma Theta Tau International.

Winnick, M. (2016). *Putting a finger on our phone obsession.* dscout. https://dscout.com/people-nerds/mobile-touches 2016.

IMAGE CREDITS

Fig. 5.3: Matthew J. Page and David Moher, "Evaluations of the Uptake and Impact of the Preferred Reporting Items for Systematic Reviews and Meta-analyses (PRISMA) Statement and Extensions: A Scoping Review," Systematic Reviews, vol. 6, no. 263, p. 5. Copyright © 2017 by Matthew J. Page and David Moher (CC by 4.0) at https://systematicreviewsjournal.biomedcentral.com/articles/10.1186/s13643-017-0663-8.

Fig. 5.4: Adapted from Denise Polit and Cheryl Beck, Essentials of Nursing Research: Appraising Evidence for Nursing Practice. Copyright © 2021 by Wolters Kluwer.

CHAPTER 6

Critically Appraising Qualitative Evidence

Cynthia D. Beckett, Cindy Zellefrow, and Julee Briscoe Waldrop

KEY CONCEPTS

Qualitative research

Types of qualitative research

Critical appraisal

LEARNING OBJECTIVES

1. Define qualitative research methods.
2. Describe the importance of qualitative research in EBPQI.
3. Discuss critical appraisal strategies for qualitative methods.
4. Describe the role of qualitative research in mixed methods studies.

Sometimes I inspire my patients; more often, they inspire me.

—Unknown

Introduction

In this chapter, you will learn the basics about qualitative research. **Qualitative research** is an interpretative or naturalistic approach to research that seeks to explore or answer questions about the meanings people attribute to their experiences in the world. Qualitative data collection gathers words and/or observations that might assist you to interpret social phenomena (interactions, behaviors, and communications) through interpretative analytic methods (Denzin & Lincoln, 2018; Pope & Mayes, 2020). We use qualitative research to hear people's stories and descriptions of their lived experiences so that we can capture and analyze data in words rather than numbers. Qualitative studies add to our knowledge base in two main ways: First, if little is known about a topic, a qualitative research study is a great way to begin exploring it. For example, you might conduct a case study with someone who has contracted a rare infectious disease, after which the results can be used to inform future research of a quantitative nature. The second way in which qualitative research adds to our knowledge is by more fully describing an experience that has already been quantified. For example, when the COVID-19 pandemic erupted, quantitative studies reported the number of cases, who was getting sick, and who was dying; these reports were followed by qualitative studies on the personal experiences of persons who had contracted COVID-19.

Qualitative Research Approaches

There are multiple approaches to data collection in qualitative methodology, including personal or group interviews, audio recordings, observations, videos, or written text. A common strategy is to conduct an interview. In a structured interview, every participant is asked the same questions and no deviation occurs, whereas in a semi-structured interview, the researcher can ask questions to further explore a participant's answer and better understand their voice. Focus group interviews place participants in small groups to respond to questions and discuss answers. Interviews are frequently audio recorded and transcribed into text for analysis. Written words from any source (e.g., open-ended questions, journals, blogs, Twitter feeds) can be analyzed, and observations (either video recorded or in the form of notes taken in real time) can be transcribed, reviewed, and analyzed.

Qualitative Analysis

Qualitative analysis occurs continuously throughout the study and includes reflection and dynamic iteration—in other words, close, thoughtful, repeated consideration! *Thematic analysis* is the process of carefully synthesizing the transcripts that produce the themes you will use to develop hypothetical propositions about the experience, phenomenon, or perceptions you are researching (Creswell, 2007; Denzin & Lincoln, 2018; Meadows-Oliver & Kapaale, 2023; Pope & Mayes, 2020). You will spend substantial time with your data, and each time you analyze it further, more of a pattern may emerge. Like placing a leaf under a sheet of paper and rubbing a crayon over the top, each rubbing may reveal a more intricate picture. Let's consider an example of thematic analysis of qualitative data.

The authors of the chapters in this textbook have each provided a short (less than 250 words) answer to the question "Why did you become a nurse?" (see pp. 000) as a way of introducing themselves to you, the reader. Suppose you wanted to answer the following question: "Why did this group of nurse textbook authors decide to become nurses?" You could use their personal stories in this textbook as data on which to conduct a thematic analysis. The basic steps of thematic analysis underlie all other more complex (even software-assisted) methods. The most important of all is that the researcher must become highly familiar with the written words in the documents, so your first step will be to read through all the stories. Your second step will be to re-read them, and this time, you might highlight the key reasons the authors shared about why they chose nursing as a career. The third time you read, you might notice ways in which these reasons can be categorized into themes; and the fourth time you read, you will choose quotes to represent those themes. You can then provide an interpretation of your findings based on what is known (previous research) about why people become nurses.

Qualitative data collection can be a very interactive process. For this reason, qualitative data interpretation can be especially vulnerable to influences (or biases) in the form of researchers' personal beliefs, experiences, ideas, and prejudices (Smith & Noble, 2014). The researcher or research team becomes part of the process, so they must be aware of any bias that they may bring to the study (Creswell, 2007; Denzin & Lincoln, 2018; Meadows-Oliver & Kapaale, 2023; Pope & Mayes, 2020). If stated clearly in advance of the study, bias can be lessened. Techniques used to give credence to the results of qualitative research include the use of *thick description* (text that is rich in detail), *triangulation* (data collected in multiple ways to see whether the same themes continue to present themselves), *respondent validation* (asking the participant whether you have correctly interpreted their statements), constant comparison of data, and independent analysis of data. Putting such safeguards into place helps the reader and users of qualitative research have confidence that the work is trustworthy (Smith & Noble, 2014; Stahl & King, 2020).

Qualitative Research Samples

The sample of participants for a qualitative research study is often purposeful. Participants are usually selected or recruited based on a similarity that is a critical aspect of the study's research question. For example, participants may be included based on their experience with a specific culture or community, social process, or phenomenon of interest. Another way that participants are recruited is called *snowball sampling*. In snowball sampling, those who have participated in the study reach out to others who have similar experiences or characteristics and provide them with information about the research and how to take part. For example, in a study about the experience of having breast cancer, participants might share recruitment information with members of their cancer support group. A small sample size in a qualitative study does not indicate that the study is of lower quality or strength (Creswell, 2007; Denzin & Lincoln, 2018; Meadows-Oliver & Kapaale, 2023; Pope & Mayes, 2020).

Types of Qualitative Research

There are multiple **types of qualitative research**: General qualitative study methods include descriptive, case study, participatory action research, historical, narrative analysis, critical theory, ethnography, grounded theory, and phenomenology. Various approaches have subtle differences that allow the researchers to explore the issue/problem, experience, or social process under consideration

TABLE 6.1 General Qualitative Research Terms

Qualitative research terms
Analytic notes: notes kept by the researcher/s on their thoughts, questions, or ideas during the data collection and analysis.
Discourse analysis: a diverse approach that analyzes the structures of conversations and forms of language used in a specific context to explain how communication and language function to create meaning and influence human interactions.
Field study: a study that occurs in the informant's/participant's natural setting.
Field notes: researcher's notes about field observations.
Focus group: group interview that uses discussion and interaction to generate data on specific topics.
Narrative analysis: analysis process that focuses on the participant's story in its entirety rather than on certain sections.
Nominated/snowball sampling: when new participants are recruited with assistance from enrolled study informants.
Purposeful/purposive sampling: when recruiters use intentional judgment to select participants or events so that the sample meets the needs of the study.
Qualitative content analysis: common analysis approach that breaks down data (e.g., by coding, contrasting, comparing information) into descriptions, interpretations, or theories.
Semi-structured interviews: formal interviews with a structured question format that allows participants to answer in their own way.
Structured, open-ended interviews: formal interviews with set questions to which participants respond in their own words but without flexibility to change topics.
Thematic analysis: analysis of the data to look for specific themes, cluster ideas and details to support those themes, and answer a research question or address an issue.
Thick description: description that includes rich details of context, emotion, and social relationships that help interpret the meaning of a human experience or interaction.
Unstructured, open-ended interviews: informal conversations that allow participants to share their thoughts, feelings, and experiences in an open and flexible way.
Volunteer/convenience sampling: recruitment through advertising and/or solicitation to identify participants who meet the study inclusion criteria.

(Creswell, 2007; Denzin & Lincoln, 2018; Hsieh & Shannon, 2005; Meadows-Oliver & Kapaale, 2023; Polit & Beck, 2017, 2021)

(Creswell, 2007; Denzin & Lincoln, 2018; Meadows-Oliver & Kapaale, 2023; Pope & Mayes, 2020). Qualitative research also has specific terms that may be unfamiliar to you (see Table 6.1). Qualitative research can be synthesized in systematic review/meta-synthesis studies or combined with quantitative approaches and labeled as mixed methods studies.

Qualitative Descriptive Study

Qualitative descriptive studies are commonly used in nursing and healthcare. For example, a researcher might interview immigrants about their first experience with the local healthcare system in their new country. The interviews would be audio recorded and transcribed into a written document for analysis; the transcripts would then be read and re-read (studied) to identify similar themes or patterns, relationships, or sequences. The study's findings could be used to fill in a gap in knowledge or allow further generalizations to be made to the sample population, similar to what was described above in the nurse stories example.

A good example of a qualitative descriptive study is the article "A Qualitative Study of How Inter-Professional Teams Influence Perioperative Nursing" by Holmes et al. (2020), which aimed "to explore Norwegian operating room nurses' perceptions of how team skills in the inter-professional operating room team influence perioperative nursing in relation to patient safety" (p. 571). This great topic incorporated many concepts presented in this textbook, such as nursing as part of a team and patient safety as the focus when TeamSTEPPS is used to improve communication skills. First, nurses were interviewed (one of the standard qualitative methods for data collection), then the researchers reviewed the evidence and decided to do a qualitative study because there was not much known about the experience of operating room nurse teamwork. The researchers used a convenience sample of 10 nurses and a semi-structured interview; thus, all interviewees were asked the same questions but allowed to expand with follow-up questions to provide more detailed information and examples. The interviews were audio recorded and transcribed. Content analysis was performed and meaningful phrases related to the purpose of the study were identified and categorized into generic categories with subcategories. The three main categories were (a) influence on the quality of perioperative nursing; (b) influence on the progress of perioperative nursing; and (c) influence on OR nurses' work environment in the OR. The conclusions of this study support prior quantitative results that team skills improve nurses' work environment and patient safety. The authors recommend future studies that explore intraoperative adverse events and their association with team skills, so quantitative research might be a good way to follow this study and explore the following question: "What is the association between team skills (TeamSTEPPS training) and OR adverse events?" For an example of using a critical appraisal tool with this report, see Appendix B.

Case Study

A *case study* approach is an intensive investigation of an individual or group experiencing a specific issue or event. This approach allows a case or an issue to be considered in its uniqueness and complexity so that the researcher can understand and appreciate the complex factors involved (Creswell, 2007; Denzin & Lincoln, 2018; Meadows-Oliver & Kapaale, 2023; Pope & Mayes, 2020). The researcher explores the case to determine why an instance of an event occurred as it did and what might be essential to note or watch for in future similar cases. Research questions are focused on the issue represented by the case (Creswell, 2007; Denzin & Lincoln, 2018; Meadows-Oliver & Kapaale, 2023; Pope & Mayes, 2020). For example, in the referenced study "The Assessment and Management of Pain in an Orthopedic Outpatient Setting: A Case Study" (Hall & Gregory, 2016), the "issue" is pain management in the outpatient orthopedic setting. The "case" of one patient and their experience illustrates how pain was identified and managed, including by seeking additional expert help. The care team addressed the importance of understanding all the factors influencing the patient's perception of pain and their impact on the patient's quality of life, and thus changes in practice were initiated to improve future care based on this one case experience.

Historical

A *historical qualitative study* approach allows researchers to describe and explore past events to better comprehend the potential impacts of a phenomenon in the present or future. The researchers analyze data from historical documents and/or interviews. This method can provide an in-depth review of an event, but it is challenging to validate the data if those with first-hand knowledge are no longer living or available. In a study by Vierira et al. (2019) that used historical documents (nurses' dissertations and theses from 1999 to 2017, $n = 50$), researchers aimed to understand more about recommended best nursing practices in the context of Brazil's current evidence-based practice movement. Content analysis was performed on the documents, revealing four categories of best practices: (a) care and assistance, (b) institutions and organizations, (c) education and research, and (d) other. Isn't it interesting that these are still topics that impact nursing care today all over the world? Nurses have always been interested in best practices to provide high-quality care for patients.

Other Qualitative Methods

There are many other qualitative methods that are not as commonly used in nursing research (Table 6.2). You might come across some of them in your search for evidence because, as you know, the research question should always guide the method.

TABLE 6.2 Other Qualitative Research Methods

General qualitative study methods	Participatory action research	Participatory action research is a method that seeks context-appropriate actions for research by including the voices of the community or group members who are asked to participate in the study. Participants collaborate to identify the problem and plan and conduct, reflect on, and evaluate the study. Participatory action research empowers community participants by using their knowledge to raise consciousness and promote social action. The study includes one community (no matter the size), and the analysis of the data is provided back to the community.
	Narrative methods	This approach allows the researcher to deeply comprehend the experiences and perspectives of individuals or small groups. Data is pulled from observations, interviews or focus groups, documents, and other types of information. Narrative methods result in rich, in-depth stories of lived experiences and situations. They can identify historically significant information and provide a voice to individuals, including marginalized people. A limitation of this approach is the "Hawthorne effect." If participants know that they are being studied, they may unconsciously change what they say or do.

	Critical theory methods	Critical theory is the umbrella term for many theoretical points of view (Marxism, feminism, oppression) that explain how power operates in society. This approach helps researchers to understand how hierarchies and relationships that support the power of one group over another are created and maintained in diverse groups or populations. The method can support the liberation or emancipation of people and may align with participatory or action research designs.
Ethnographic study methods		Ethnography is a qualitative approach in which the researcher or team becomes immersed within the group or culture being studied for an extended period to comprehend their cultural practices/traditions, beliefs, and behaviors. The research question could be phrased as "What is it like to live in ...?" or "What is it like to live with ...?" Sample sizes vary depending on the group. Data collection strategies may include interviews, observations, field notes, record reviews, and life histories, leading to a detailed and rich description of what was studied.
Grounded theory methods		Grounded theory goes beyond describing an experience, phenomenon, or social process because its purpose is to develop a theory rather than describe the phenomenon. Sample sizes vary to allow a full understanding of all aspects of the phenomenon, including beliefs, practices, and processes in the group or community. The researcher is part of the data collection, analysis, and interpretation of the findings for theory development. Data is collected from various sources, such as audio- or video-recorded interviews, observations, and reviews of notes taken by the researcher, and any additional questions that emerge can be included in subsequent interviews. This is a dynamic process, and participant/group confirmation of themes is vital.
Phenomenology	Descriptive and/or interpretive methods	Phenomenology seeks to understand specific lived experiences or phenomena from the point of view of a person or group of interest. The researcher wants to comprehend and explore how the experience in question affected the individual's or group's feelings, responses, and thoughts. Research questions may include "What is it like to have this experience?" or "What does it feel like to ...?" Data is collected and continuously analyzed for themes. The study is completed once no new themes emerge, so the sample is often small, with just six to eight participants.

Creswell, 2007; Denzin & Lincoln, 2018; Meadows-Oliver & Kapaale, 2023; Pope & Mayes, 2020; Strauss & Corbin, 1998

As with quantitative studies, qualitative studies can be synthesized. A synthesis of qualitative results is called a *meta-synthesis* and is like a meta-analysis of quantitative study results.

Meta-Synthesis

Systematic reviews provide a synthesis of evidence. The reviews may include quantitative, qualitative, or mixed methods articles. Researchers use a rigorous approach to identify, appraise, and synthesize studies to address a specific research question. Studies are only included if they meet predetermined inclusion criteria. As with meta-analyses, the authors must assess qualitative studies for quality and risk of bias. A rigorous analytic process of thematic analysis is completed to interpret meaning from the results of all the studies' data. The conclusion of a systematic review summarizes the meta-synthesis results (Creswell, 2007; Denzin & Lincoln, 2018; Meadows-Oliver & Kapaale, 2023; Sandelowski & Barroso, 2003).

An example of a meta-synthesis is the research report titled "Exploring Nurse Perceptions and Experiences of Resilience: A Meta-Synthesis Study" by Kim and Chang (2022). In this study, the researchers wanted to understand nurse resilience and what is already known about nurse resilience–related experiences to inform future research on this vital topic. The research questions were "How do nurses overcome adversity?" and "What are the characteristics of nurses' resilience experiences?" The researchers searched five databases using strategies you learned about in Chapter 4 and identified 16 studies that met their inclusion and exclusion criteria. They critically appraised these studies for quality using the CASP checklist (see Table 6.3) and used a meta-ethnography process for data synthesis (one variation of meta-synthesis). The resulting themes were (a) self-development based on one's inner self, (b) fostering a positive attitude toward life, (c) developing personal strategies for overcoming adversity, and (d) building professionalism to become a better nurse. Each theme contained subthemes that supported the primary theme; the researchers used quotes from the different studies in the synthesis to explicate each theme and subtheme. This study demonstrated what all nurses know in their hearts: that we are problem solvers and find ways to develop our own resources and resiliency to meet our patients' needs!

Mixed Methods Research (Quantitative AND Qualitative Combined)

Studies that incorporate both quantitative and qualitative strategies are called *mixed methods*, although there are separate and clearly defined means of data collection and analysis for each approach. An example of mixed method research would be a study of nurses working in acute care settings that has a cross-sectional component requiring the nurses to first complete a questionnaire. After analyzing the data from the questionnaire, the researchers might hold focus groups to further explore key concepts identified from the nurses' answers. This study would apply both quantitative and qualitative methods in its design; however, analyzing the written responses to an open-ended question from a questionnaire used in a cross-sectional study does not, in itself, constitute a mixed methods study (Creswell, 2007; Denzin & Lincoln, 2018; Meadows-Oliver & Kapaale, 2023).

Mixed method studies provide researchers with a deeper understanding of the topic by applying both strategies. In appraising these studies, the level of evidence will usually align with the qualitative strategies. The quality, however, will be determined by the strength of both methods used for the study (Creswell, 2007; Denzin & Lincoln, 2018; Meadows-Oliver & Kapaale, 2023).

An example of a mixed methods study is presented in the article "Safety Culture in Healthcare: Mixed Method Study by Lorenzini et al. (2021), which aimed to explore patient safety culture within an interprofessional team in a neurosurgery center to better understand why previous studies had consistently reported healthcare workers' low perception of management's effectiveness in achieving safety culture. The study design began with a cross-sectional survey using a validated safety attitudes questionnaire. The researchers used the results of the survey to identify the lowest-rated areas and explore those areas further with focus groups. They analyzed the data from components separately, then together as a whole, and presented the results to the institution so it could further consider recommendations to improve the patient safety culture.

Critical Appraisal of Qualitative Research

Once you have found articles that address your PICO or PPCO, it is essential to do a **critical appraisal** of them to determine the quality and strength of each article. Determining the quality and strength of a qualitative study requires a review of its key components. Table 6.3 provides examples of some tools available to appraise qualitative research studies. You will need to ask questions: Did the researchers tell the story clearly? What were the purpose, sample, and data collection strategies? Did the researchers clearly articulate the participant voices in identifying themes, subthemes, categories, or theories in the thematic analysis? Did they describe the rigor used to ensure that the data collection and analysis steps were consistent across the study? Did they describe using an audit trail to validate their process and observations? Just like with quantitative studies, there are resources available to help you with critically appraising qualitative studies.

Qualitative and quantitative research employ different types of appraisals. In quantitative research, we critically appraise for *validity* (how accurately the results reflect what they are supposed to measure), *reliability* (whether the results can be reproduced in similar settings or conditions), and *generalizability* (whether the results can be applied to the general population; see Chapter 5). In qualitative research, we critically appraise for credibility, dependability and confirmability, and transferability to determine a study's trustworthiness. Both quantitative and qualitative research, however, are appraised for *applicability* (whether the results from the work can be applied to your setting and/or population). See Tables 6.4 and 6.5 for definitions and comparison of concepts in critical appraisal of quantitative versus qualitative research (Stahl & King, 2020).

TABLE 6.3 Qualitative Critical Appraisal Tools

Critical appraisal tool	Website	Research study designs	Overview
Critical Appraisal Skills Programme Checklists (CASP)	https://casp-uk.net/casp-tools-checklists/	Qualitative studies checklist	-Includes instructions and embedded hints throughout the checklists -Free access -Full-text PDF, Word, or print & fill
JBI Global	https://jbi.global/critical-appraisal-tools	-Qualitative research -Qualitative synthesis	-Includes instructions with the form -Free access -Full-text Word
Johns Hopkins EBP Model and Tools	https://www.hopkinsmedicine.org/nursing/center-nursing-inquiry/_documents/Appendix_E_2022_Final.pdf	-Critical Appraisal Toolkit for all study types, including qualitative	-Includes instructions and embedded hints throughout all forms -Level and Quality Guide for ratings -Strength of recommendation rating -Free access
Helene Fuld Health Trust National Institute for Evidence-Based Practice in Nursing and Healthcare	https://fuld.nursing.osu.edu/become-a-member	-Qualitative research	-Requires a fee membership to EBP HQ for access

TABLE 6.4 Comparison of Concepts of Critical Appraisal in Quantitative Versus Qualitative Research

Quantitative terminology	Qualitative terminology
Validity	Credibility
Reliability	Dependability and confirmability
Generalizability	Transferability
Applicability	

TABLE 6.5 Definitions of Concepts of Critical Appraisal of Qualitative Research That Lead to Trustworthiness

Credibility: The study includes accurate, valid, true descriptions of a particular reality (internal validity) that can be compared to other groups (external validity). "Can you believe the description is accurate?"
Dependability: Findings are consistent and repeatable (have reliability) between researchers and study data. "Would the results be the same if the study were repeated with the same subjects in a similar context?"
Confirmability: (objectivity) Study findings reflect the participants' voices and not the researcher's perspectives. "Was the study object neutral and free from bias?"
Transferability: Results can be transferred to other contexts or settings. "Can the results of the study be transferred to my population?"

Denzin & Lincoln, 2018; Lincoln & Guba, 1985; Meadows-Oliver & Kapaale, 2023

WRAPPING UP

Qualitative research is a valuable addition to the body of evidence in EBP. Whereas quantitative research helps us to understand the outcomes of an intervention in a controlled environment, qualitative research helps us to understand such lived experiences as administering or receiving an intervention, weathering the challenges of a situation, or being subjected to a particular condition/ phenomenon. This is particularly important in EBP, where preferences and values are a significant consideration when making decisions. Remember, when engaging in EBPQI, it is paramount that we consider the best available evidence (external and internal) in conjunction with clinical expertise and patient preferences and values when making decisions. As you grow in your role as a nurse, be sure to embrace exploration with curiosity and wonder, and let the evidence guide your decisions.

WELLNESS IN ACTION: PRAYER AND MEDITATION

Meditation involves focused concentration on being present in the moment; prayer involves connection and communication with a higher power. Both intentional practices can calm your sympathetic nervous system and promote mindfulness, connection, and guidance while reducing stress and anxiety. Prayer and meditation can bring calm and comfort; integrate the mind, body, and spirit; and increase attention, memory, and mood (Basso et al., 2019). Engagement in either or both activities can be spontaneous, planned, or ritualistic. If you decide to use meditation or prayer to improve and support your personal well-being, we suggest that you choose a time and place with minimal distractions. You may prefer a specific space: Some people have prayer closets, some enjoy being outside in nature, and some pray or meditate on the go.

Consider engaging in the following steps:

1. Disengage from your mental voice and any pressing thoughts.
2. Pause and listen to your breathing.
3. Wait for inner quietness.
4. Be present in the quiet.

Pay attention to how this practice impacts you, and adjust as appropriate. As holistic experts caring for patients, we encourage you to nurture your spiritual health.

REFLECTION QUESTIONS

1. What are the differences between quantitative and qualitative research study methods?
2. Consider the following questions and what research study method would best answer them:
    a. Does structured breathwork for 5 minutes twice a shift improve emotional exhaustion among nurses who work in the ICU?
    b. What practices do nurses who provide hospice care use to provide support to family members of the patient?
    c. What motivates nurses to leave practice and go into teaching?

REFERENCES

Basso, J. C., McHale, A., Ende, V., Oberlin, D. J., & Suzuki, W. A. (2019). Brief, daily meditation enhances attention, memory, mood, and emotional regulation in non-experienced meditators. *Behavioural Brain Research, 356*, 208–220. https://doi.org/10.1016/j.bbr.2018.08.023

Creswell, J. W. (2007). *Qualitative inquiry & research design: Choosing among five approaches* (2nd ed.). SAGE.

Denzin, N. K., & Lincoln, Y. S. (2018). *The SAGE handbook of qualitative research* (5th ed.). SAGE.

Hall, G., & Gregory, J. (2016). The assessment and management of pain in an orthopaedic out-patient setting: A case study. *International Journal of Orthopaedic and Trauma Nursing, 22*, 24–28. https://doi.org/10.1016/j.ijotn.2015.10.001

Holmes, T., Vifladt, A., & Ballangrud, R. (2020). A qualitative study of how inteprofessional teamwork influences perioperative nursing. *Nursing Open, 7*(2), 571–580.

Hsieh, H. F., & Shannon, S. E. (2005). Three approaches to qualitative content analysis. *Qualitative Health Research*, 15, 1277–1288. https://doi.org/10.1177/1049732305276687

Kim, E. Y., & Chang, S. O. (2022) Exploring nurse perceptions and experiences of resilience: A meta-synthesis study. *BMC Nursing, 21*, Article 26. https://doi.org/10.1186/s12912-021-00803-z

Lincoln, Y. S., & Guba, E. G. (1985). *Naturalistic inquiry.* SAGE.

Lorenzini, E., Oelke, N. D., & Marck, P. B. (2021). Safety culture in healthcare: Mixed method study. *Journal of Health Organization and Management, 35*(8), 1080–1097. https://doi.org/10.1108/JHOM-04-2020-0110

Meadows-Oliver, M., & Kapaale, C. (2023). Critically appraising qualitative and mixed methods evidence for clinical decision making. In B. M. Melnyk & E. Fineout-Overholt (Eds.), *EBP in nursing & healthcare: A guide to best practice* (5th ed., pp. 266–301). Wolters Kluwer.

Polit, D., & Beck, C. (2017). Qualitative research design and approaches. In D. Polit & C. Beck (Eds.), *Nursing research: Generating and assessing evidence for nursing practice* (10th ed.). Wolters Kluwer.

Polit, D. F., & Beck, C. T. (2021). *Nursing research: Generating and assessing evidence for nursing practice* (11th ed.). Wolters Kluwer.

Pope, C., & Mayes, N. (2020). *Qualitative research in health care* (4th ed.). Wiley Blackwell.

Sandelowski, M. (2000). Whatever happened to qualitative description? *Research in Nursing & Health, 23*(4), 334–340. https://doi.org/10.1002/1098-240X(200008)23:4<334::AID-NUR9>3.0.CO;2-G

Sandelowski, M., & Barroso, J. (2003). Classifying the findings in qualitative studies. *Qualitative Health Research, 13*(7), 905–923. https://doi.org/10.1177/1049732303253488

Smith, J., & Noble, H. (2014). Bias in research. *Evidence-Based Nursing, 17*(4), 100–101.

Stahl, N., & King, J. (2020). Expanding approaches for research: Understanding and using trustworthiness in qualitative research. *Journal of Developmental Education, 44*(1), 26–28. https://files.eric.ed.gov/fulltext/EJ1320570.pdf

Strauss, A. L., & Corbin, J. (1998). *Basics of qualitative research. techniques and procedures for developing grounded theory* (2nd ed.). SAGE.

Vierira, A. N., Petry, S., & Padilha, M. I. (2019). Best practices in historical studies of nursing and health (1999–2017). *Revista Brasileira de Enfermagem, 72*, 973–978.

CHAPTER 7

Appraising Other Types of Evidence to Inform Best Practices

Melissa Hessock, Tracy L. Brewer, Julee Briscoe Waldrop, and Jayne Jennings Dunlap

KEY CONCEPTS

Clinical practice guidelines (CPGs)
Position statement
Consensus statement
Literature review
Scoping review
Integrative review
Economic evaluation
Expert opinion
Non-research

LEARNING OBJECTIVES

1. Describe other types of evidence that can contribute to EBPQI initiatives and improvement in healthcare.
2. Identify resources and tools that nurses may use to search for and appraise other types of evidence used in EBPQI.
3. Discuss the rationale for critical appraisal of other types of evidence.

> The important thing is not to stop questioning. Curiosity has its own reason for existing.
>
> —Albert Einstein

Introduction

In Chapter 4, you learned how to use a clinical question as a starting point in your search for the best available evidence. In Chapters 5 and 6, you learned about quantitative and qualitative research study designs, the types of evidence they provide, and how to critically appraise the level and quality of these research studies. Research evidence is not the only type of evidence, however. This chapter will focus on the appraisal of several other types of evidence that contribute to the body (compilation) of evidence you can use to answer clinical questions.

You are probably more familiar with these other types of evidence than you realize. Anytime you observe or hear about someone else's experience and consider it information you might use, you are encountering a type of evidence called *anecdotal evidence*. Anecdotal evidence is based on personal accounts or opinions rather than research, so it is not necessarily reliable or factual, but it is still evidence. The quality of anecdotal evidence is not generally considered to be as high as the quality of research-based evidence. As we progress through this chapter, you will gain a deeper understanding of the role of other types of evidence in EBP.

Let's look at an example. Jayne's story:

I noticed that many children diagnosed with autism spectrum disorder (ASD) had not been screened for autism as currently recommended by the Centers for Disease Control and Prevention (CDC, 2022) and American Academy of Pediatrics (AAP, 2023; Hymen et al., 2020) in my primary care clinical practice. Several of these children had parental concerns noted in their medical records, and yet no specialist referral or evaluation had been completed and there was no documentation of anticipatory guidance or a follow-up plan. I looked at the literature and found that a lack of developmental screening was common across healthcare settings (Hirai et al., 2018). Motivated by the increasing number of individuals diagnosed with ASD, currently 1 in 36 children (Maenner et al., 2023) at the time of this writing, I decided to explore how nurses could support this vulnerable group through the use of evidence.

While strong research evidence supports early detection and treatment for ASD is associated with best outcomes, care gaps continue to exist. After appraising the current literature base, I contacted Dr. Temple Grandin, arguably the world's most well-known individual with autism. Temple is an ASD ambassador and early intervention recipient who was one of the first people to widely verbalize her experience as a person on the autism spectrum. Her journey was documented in an award-winning movie titled *Temple Grandin*, which is based on her life.

Temple is an advocate for early ASD intervention, and during one phone call while we discussed the limitations of research and the importance of early ASD detection, she said, "Jayne, at some point anecdotal becomes evidence!" (Temple Grandin, personal communication, May 2020). Temple also stated that if a toddler was not talking, "Don't wait, get help immediately." This anecdotal evidence led me to partner with a leading neurologist and ASD expert to build evidence-based continuing education focused on screening and early action recommendations for nurses (Dunlap & Filipek, 2020). In our work, we used clinical practice guidelines and expert opinion to complement research evidence in making EBP actionable recommendations for nurses when ASD is suspected. One practical piece of information highlighted in this work that incorporated other sources of evidence was the importance of nurses not dismissing parental concerns for ASD.

Best Available Evidence and the Hierarchy of Evidence

You have learned that EBP is informed by three primary components: the best available evidence, clinical expertise, and patient preferences and values. One particular strength of EBP is that it incorporates various types of evidence and knowledge (Dang et al., 2022). You should explore all relevant evidence that can inform practice recommendations for the best quality of care.

In some discussions of EBP, you may find "best scientific evidence" used synonymously with "best available evidence"; however, the best evidence may comprise both research (scientific) evidence and other evidence (Dang et al., 2022). Although neither type of evidence is necessarily more important, some types of evidence do offer a higher level of reliability and support for EBP recommendations

Pre-Appraised Evidence

Pre-appraised evidence includes summaries based on high-quality evidence sources, such as single randomized control trials (RCTs) of a specific clinical topic. Authors appraise the quality of these studies and include a narrative report of the findings. As a nurse, you are likely to use pre-appraised sources of evidence in your daily practice because they offer a time-saving benefit. Clinical practice guidelines (CPGs) and professional consensus or position statements are examples of pre-appraised evidence. *Clinical practice guidelines* contain practice recommendations based on research evidence, including the benefits and harms of interventions, to optimize patient care and outcomes (Grinspun et al., 2023). CPGs are often based on high-quality research evidence. For example, the American Academy of Pediatrics has several CPGs available with open access (e.g., Hampel et al. [2023]).

As you learned in previous chapters, specific types of evidence are assigned different levels on the evidence pyramid based on their study design (see Figure 7.1). We are now going to focus on the lower segment of the pyramid (which includes individual research studies of various types of design) and, more specifically, on the bottom tier of the pyramid (which includes non-research and other types of evidence). Note the broadness of the pyramid's base compared to its top tier; this broadness signifies the surplus of various types of evidence you may find there, depending on your topic of EBPQI interest.

Other Types of Evidence

Simply stated, *other evidence* means evidence that is presented or generated without using scientific methods. This type of evidence generally fits into one of two broad categories: (a) evidence-based summaries of scientific (research) evidence and (b) evidence gained through practice experience, typically at an

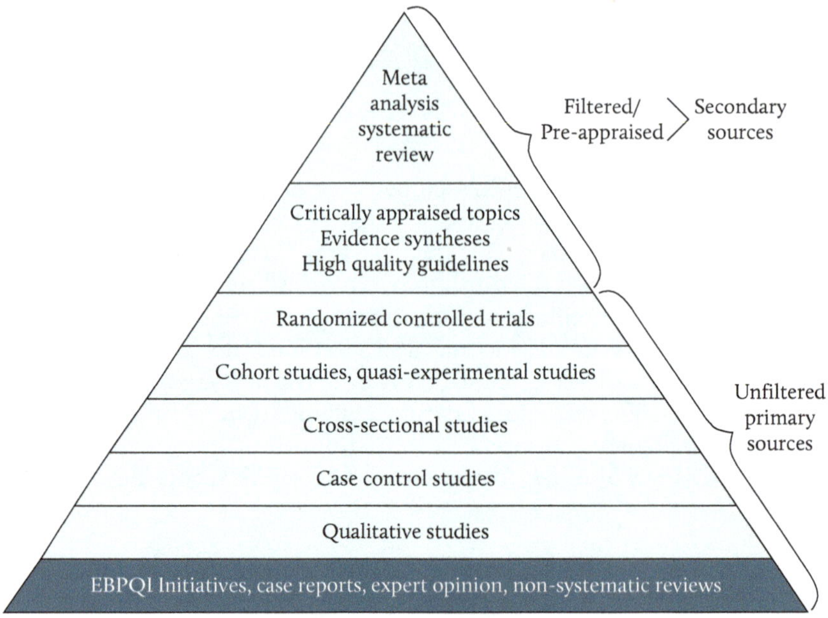

FIGURE 7.1 Hierarchy of Evidence Pyramid

organizational level (often simply referred to as *practice-based evidence*; Dang et al., 2022; Fineout-Overholt, 2023). At the highest level of other evidence is the evidence generated by systematic synthesis or a summary of existing scientific research (e.g., CPGs). Evidence that is not a synthesis of research can fill gaps in knowledge when there is limited research available and help bridge the translation of research into patient care. When findings and outcomes across a variety of types of evidence are in agreement (e.g., EBPQI-generated evidence and research as well as anecdotal evidence), it can provide a more holistic understanding of the body of evidence available to support clinical decision-making and recommendations (Fineout-Overholt, 2023).

Summaries of Evidence

Clinical Practice Guidelines, Consensus Statements, and Position Statements

Clinical practice guidelines, consensus statements, and position statements are sometimes viewed interchangeably, but they are different. Although each provides practice recommendations, these recommendations have been developed based on different degrees of evidence and rigor; therefore, they do not provide the same level of evidence.

Quality **clinical practice guidelines (CPGs)** provide the highest level of evidence and are the most trustworthy among clinical practice recommendations because (a) they are systematically developed with transparent methods and (b) the

TABLE 7.1 Universal Terminology for Practice Recommendation Types

Term	Definition
Clinical practice guideline	Systematically developed documents created with a validated methodology that includes identifying the literature on specific clinical question(s), using explicit methods of searching and selecting literature, and grading the available evidence. Following this process, recommendations are developed and the strength of each recommendation is graded.
Consensus statement	Recommendations developed based on a collective opinion or consensus of an expert panel. Often presented when available evidence is limited or conflicting or the intervention's risk versus benefit is not obvious.
Position statement	Comprehensive document that explains, justifies, and recommends a particular approach to a clinical problem.

Note. Adapted from Joshi, G. P., Benzon, H. T., Gan, T., J., & Vetter, T. R. (2019). Consistent definitions of clinical practice guidelines, consensus statements, position statements, and practice alerts. Anesthesia & Analgesia, *129(6), 1767–1770. https://doi.org/10.1213/ane.0000000000004236*

strength of their recommendations is graded. **Position statements** may provide a high level of evidence if their development is based on a systematic review of research evidence. You must appraise these statements as carefully as you would research evidence so you can understand how the positions taken were determined. **Consensus statements** reflect the collective opinion of an expert panel; thus, they may be based on limited, new, or conflicting evidence. As they have the most risk for bias, consensus statements provide a lower level of evidence.

CLINICAL PRACTICE GUIDELINE EXAMPLE

The Registered Nurses Association of Ontario has several open access clinical practice guidelines to explore, including *Promoting Smoking Reduction and Cessation With Indigenous Peoples of Reproductive Age and Their Communities* (Registered Nurses Association of Ontario, 2022; https://rnao.ca/bpg/guidelines/promoting-smoking-reduction-and-cessation-indigenous-peoples-reproductive-age-and). This guideline is the nursing organization's first CPG to focus on Indigenous people.

Reviews of the Literature Other Than Systematic Reviews

As you learned in Chapter 5, systematic reviews of research involve a rigorous search, appraisal, and synthesis of scientific evidence. Because they use a systematic methodology and are typically based on numerous research studies, systematic reviews inherently have a lower risk for bias and, therefore, are considered a higher level of evidence. However, there are other approaches to exploring the literature on a particular topic, problem, or question, as well as many types of reviews, including literature reviews, scoping reviews, and integrative reviews. You may have noticed that even review types with very similar methodologies have different names (Carter-Templeton et al., 2023).

Literature review is a generic term that describes the examination and summary of available evidence on a topic, sometimes including both research and other types of evidence. There is no standard methodology for conducting literature reviews, so various approaches may be taken (Bowden & Purper, 2022). A **scoping review** aims to identify and map the amount and type of evidence available on a particular topic, identify and analyze gaps in knowledge, and clarify key concepts associated with a topic. A scoping review does not include a critical appraisal or seek to answer a clinical question (Munn et al., 2018), but it can be very rigorous and follow a strict methodology, such as the PRISMA reporting guide for scoping reviews (PRISMA, 2024). **Integrative reviews** aim to provide a comprehensive and holistic understanding of a healthcare problem by considering a variety of evidence and knowledge sources. A high-quality integrative review will follow a specific framework for development, including five stages: problem identification, literature search, data evaluation, data analysis, and presentation of findings (Oermann & Knafl, 2021).

Practice-Based Evidence (Experiential or Organizational)

Evidence-Based Practice and Quality Improvement Projects or Initiatives

Reports of EBP and quality improvement (QI) projects or initiatives are increasingly found in the literature. Both EBP and QI projects are conducted at an organizational level. *Evidence-based practice projects or initiatives* aim to (a) search and appraise the best available evidence, (b) synthesize it with clinical expertise as well as patient preferences and values, and (c) subsequently recommend and support practice changes that improve healthcare. *Quality improvement projects or initiatives* aim to improve a process or outcome related to an identified problem using a systematic approach, but they may not include a rigorous search for and appraisal of evidence (HQ Solutions, 2024). Given the recognized value of basing practice change on the best evidence and of using a systematic process to apply and sustain change, there has been a movement toward combining these two processes and calling them "evidence-based quality improvement" (Levin et al., 2010; Melnyk et al., 2015) or "evidence-based practice quality improvement" (EBPQI; Waldrop & Dunlap, 2024). Although it is understood that outcomes related to EBPQI are not generalizable, the information found in reports of these projects is transferable and can contribute to the body of evidence used to answer a clinical question. You learned in Chapter 1 that *transferability* is the degree to which an effective intervention and outcome in one context (a specific population and organization) can be applied and achieved in a different context (a different population and organization; Schloemer & Schröder-Bäck, 2018). Transferability will be discussed further in Chapter 12.

Economic Evaluation

Economic evaluations in healthcare are used to determine the monetary costs and value of interventions or programs. These evaluations use a variety of analyses, which may include program cost analysis, cost of illness analysis, cost-effectiveness

TABLE 7.2. Definitions of Economic Evaluation Terms

Term	Definition	Example
Cost analysis	A breakdown of a cost summary by individual factors	Evaluation of all expenses and revenues
Cost of illness	The total cost of resources expended because of a health problem	Patient's decreased/lost productivity (indirect costs) and cost of pain and suffering (intangible costs)
Cost-effectiveness analysis	A comparison of one intervention to another (or the current status quo) by estimating cost to gain a particular health outcome	Death prevented or year of life gained
Cost utility Analysis	A form of cost-effectiveness analysis using quality-adjusted life years as a health outcome	Improved quality of life
Cost-benefit analysis	A summation of the potential benefits expected from the practice change followed by the subtraction of the total associated costs, with both expressed in monetary units	The cost of a program to help persons with diabetes learn self-management versus the costs of care provision to these patients if they do not manage their own care

analysis, cost utility analysis, and cost-benefit analysis (CDC, 2021; Turner et al., 2021). See Table 7.2.

As healthcare resources are not unlimited, economic evaluations can provide an organization with valuable decision-making insights regarding how best to fund interventions and programs, prioritize expenditures, or allocate limited resources. EBPQI teams should incorporate known cost information whenever possible to inform decision-making for necessary practice changes (Conner et al., 2023).

Expert Opinion

An **expert opinion** is a recommendation or stated point of view based on the knowledge and experience of an individual who is recognized as an expert on a particular subject. Common sources of expert opinion are opinion-editorials, commentaries, editorials, and personal communications (with or from an expert; Dang et al., 2022). Consensus statements by experts, although not based on scientific evidence, may also be considered expert opinion. Because expertise is subjective, expert opinion is subject to bias, yet it can offer information that is particularly useful for bridging the gap between research and the provision of direct care to patients. Evidence from various types of expert opinion can provide valuable contributions to the body of evidence needed to answer clinical questions and guide clinical decision-making.

Searching for Other Types of Evidence

You have learned that EBP relies on various evidence types to make appropriate recommendations for best practice changes. Searching for evidence to answer a clinical question requires a systematic approach as well as knowledge of available resources. In Chapter 4, you learned to use the components of your clinical question (PICO, PPCO), database-specific language such as MeSH terms, and Boolean connectors to start and refine your search in research databases. Many other types of evidence we have discussed can be found using these same search strategies and databases. The tools and techniques you learned in Chapter 4 will be your foundation for finding all relevant evidence.

Your search of terms associated with the population, intervention, comparison, and outcome of your PICO question (or with the problem, population, change, and outcome of your PPCO question) will yield various types of publications beyond research evidence. As you screen each record found in your literature search, you will often find that its title or the methods section of the abstract will provide an indication of the type of study or initiative it is. Initially, your search may focus on higher levels of evidence, such as systematic reviews and RCTs; however, the screening process offers a valuable opportunity to capture other evidence by looking for titles, terms, or information in the abstract that includes wording such as "evidence-based project/initiative," "quality improvement project/initiative," "literature review," "case report," or "economic evaluation." As you turn your focus to other types of evidence, you can narrow your results by adding this same wording (e.g., "quality improvement," "economic evaluation") to your PICO-based or PPCO-based search terms.

Searching for Clinical Practice Guidelines

Searching for clinical practice guidelines can be challenging because CPGs, unlike research studies and QI reports, are not centrally located in specified databases and thus easily revealed by traditional searches; rather, CPGs are more likely to be found in an exhaustive number of professional, governmental, and independent databases, repositories, and websites. Your search for CPGs will be more efficient and effective if you begin with a specific intention and an awareness of the variety of evidence-based or practice-focused databases and resources.

Literature Databases: Practice Guideline Filters

You have been introduced to the search CINAHL and PubMed databases. To find CPGs in these databases, start your search as you would for research evidence. In CINAHL, enter your search terms, then scroll down through the search options; from the "Publication Type" dropdown menu, select "Practice Guidelines" to search for CPGs. To search for CPGs in PubMed, you must first enter your search terms, select the search button, then navigate to the filter menu on the left and select "Practice Guideline" under the "Article Type" filter. Sum Search (https://sumsearch.org/) is another database that can be used to search for CPGs. After entering your search terms in Sum Search and selecting submit, simply click the "Guidelines" tab to narrow your search. Remember that some databases provide free complete articles but others require a subscription (See Table 4.2 in Chapter 4).

Evidence-Based Clinical Decision-Making Resources

Evidence-based clinical resources intended for use at the point of care to aid in clinical decision-making are another link to accessing clinical practice guidelines. These sites provide access to various evidence-based tools, materials, and systematically conducted appraisals/syntheses of topics that address clinical questions, and they are generally similar in their accuracy and use (Bradley-Ridout et al., 2021). The downside to these resources is that they require paid access; however, many universities and healthcare facilities provide access through their library.

Professional Nursing and Medical Organization Websites and Journals

Professional healthcare organizations are the most common developers of CPGs. Professional organization sites and journals are common places to find consensus or position statements. To get started looking for CPGs (or other statements), find the professional organization in the specialty that

TABLE 7.3 Clinical Decision-Making Resources

Resource	Focus	Guidance
DynaMed www.dnynamed.com	Healthcare providers (nurse practitioners, physicians, and physician assistants)	Enter the general condition or concern related to your clinical question. Select the relevant result. Navigate to the left side menu and select "Guidelines and Resources." There is also an option to select "Prevention and Screening" to search for preventive practice guidelines if this is relevant to your clinical question.
Clinical Key for Nursing https://beta.elsevier.com/products/clinicalkey/nurses	Nurses and other allied health clinicians	Enter the general condition or concern related to your clinical question. Select the relevant result.
UpToDate www.uptodate.com	Physicians and pharmacists	Enter the general condition or concern related to your clinical question. Select the relevant result. Navigate to the left menu options and select "Society Guideline Links" to search for CPGs.

encompasses your clinical issue and questions. For example, if you are interested in clinical practice guidelines for managing patients in labor, you could consider searching websites for organizations such as the Association of Women's Health, Obstetric, and Neonatal Nurses; the American College of Nurse-Midwives; or the American College of Obstetricians and Gynecologists. Some organizations restrict access to members only, but many provide free access to CPGs on their website, and most publish their CPGs in their associated professional journals, thus allowing access through literature database searches through CINAHL or PubMed.

Evidence-Based Practice and Guideline Databases

Although there is no central repository for clinical practice guidelines, there are resources for searching and accessing quality CPGs: Some are sponsored by governments, some are dedicated guideline databases, and some are larger organizations or databases with dedicated searchable sections for evidence-based recommendations and guidelines. A significant benefit of CPG databases is that most allow open access or access by creating a free account.

One of the most widely recognized CPG sources is the Emergency Care Research Institute (ECRI) Guidelines Trust, which has a mission to advance effective evidence-based healthcare globally. The ERCI catalogs high-quality CPGs that are vetted with transparent and rigorous criteria for inclusion in their database (Sender, 2019). Guideline Central is another robust repository option; it provides a multilayer filtered search for CGP summaries, pocket guides, and full-text links and is touted as the largest free access site for current CPGs. An additional feature of Guideline Central is the availability of a free, easy-to-navigate app version. If you want to broaden your search to include international CPGs, the Guidelines International Network has an extensive database of CPGs offered without cost to promote high-quality standards for CPG development, sharing, and implementation to encourage best practice. Lastly, the United States Preventive Services Task Force (USPSTF) website is a critical starting point if your clinical question is focused on preventive care. The USPSTF (n.d.) is a panel of experts in preventive and evidence-based care who use a systematic, rigorous approach to developing practice recommendations based on current evidence. Table 7.4 provides some examples of resources to assist your search for CPGs related to your clinical question. Please keep in mind that other specialty nursing/medical organizations may have additional or updated CPGs available.

It is vital to seek other forms of evidence as part of your search for information and knowledge to answer a clinical question and fully synthesize the body of evidence. At times, research evidence may be limited, and other sources may provide the best available evidence with which to make decisions or recommendations. Finding other evidence is sometimes less straightforward than finding pertinent research evidence. However, using the resources and practical tips we discussed will help you get off to a good start in collecting a varied body of evidence to support EBP recommendations.

TABLE 7.4 Resources for Clinical Practice Guidelines Searches

Type	Name	Location
Government/ global agencies	• Centers for Disease Control and Prevention (CDC) • Healthy People 2030 • United States Preventive Services Task Force (USPSTF) • World Health Organization (WHO)	https://www.cdc.gov/infectioncontrol/guidelines/index.html https://health.gov/healthypeople/tools-action/browse-evidence-based-resources https://www.uspreventiveservicestaskforce.org/uspstf/ https://www.who.int/publications/who-guidelines
Guideline repositories	• Emergency Care Research Institute (ECRI) Guidelines Trust • Guidelines Central • Guidelines International Network • Veterans Affairs/ Department of Defense (VA/DoD) CPG	https://www.ecri.org/solutions/ecri-guidelines-trust https://www.guidelinecentral.com/guidelines/ https://g-i-n.net/international-guidelines-library https://www.healthquality.va.gov/
Medical reference site with dedicated guidelines section	• Medscape	https://reference.medscape.com/features/guidelines
Professional organizations	• Registered Nurses' Association of Ontario • American Academy of Pediatrics (AAP) • American College of Physicians • American Diabetes Association (ADA) • American Heart Association (AHA) • National Comprehensive Cancer Network (NCCN)	https://rnao.ca/bpg/guidelines https://publications.aap.org/pediatrics/collection/523/Clinical-Practice-Guidelines https://www.acponline.org/clinical-information/clinical-guidelines-recommendations https://professional.diabetes.org/content-page/practice-guidelines-resources https://professional.heart.org/en/guidelines-and-statements/guidelines-and-statements-search https://www.nccn.org/guidelines/category_1

Appraising Other Types of Evidence

When you find additional relevant evidence, you must critically appraise it with your EBPQI team. Remember from Chapter 4 that all critical appraisal involves a series of sequential steps: (1) assigning level and quality ratings to each piece of evidence and discarding evidence of low quality, (2) evaluating and summarizing each piece of evidence, (3) synthesizing the individual summaries into a body of evidence, and (4) making a practice recommendation (Fineout-Overholt, 2023). The use of standardized appraisal checklists or tools to guide your appraisal will enhance its objectivity and transparency and reduce individual bias (Buccheri & Sharifi, 2017; Tod et al., 2021); moreover, this process should be completed in teams to improve the appraisal accuracy (Dang et al., 2022).

Step 1: Assessing Level and Quality of Other Types of Evidence

At the beginning of this chapter, we discussed the hierarchy of evidence, an essential guide for ranking levels of different evidence types, but you should avoid an unchecked reliance on the hierarchy of evidence because the level of evidence will not necessarily predict its quality (Harris et al., 2014). For example, a poorly designed and executed randomized control trial does not carry the same weight or strength as a well-designed one simply because both are RCTs. Similarly, the expert opinion of an unrecognized expert will not carry the same strength as that of a nationally recognized expert. A thorough consideration of both the level and quality of your evidence will ensure its strength as well as your confidence to make practice recommendations (Melnyk, 2016). As such, it is imperative that you use a systematic approach to assess and determine quality as you decide on the best evidence upon which to build a body of evidence to answer your clinical question and make a practice recommendation.

As discussed in Chapters 5 and 6, as you assess the quality of research studies, you must determine whether each study is valid, reliable, and applicable (Fineout-Overholt et al., 2010). *Applicability* describes how well the evidence informs your clinical question in the context of your population and can be universally assessed among different evidence types. Traditional elements used to determine validity and reliability may not apply to other evidence because it is not based on the scientific method; however, traditional concepts can be applied through a non-research lens while appraising this evidence. For example, when considering an EBPQI initiative, you could appraise validity by looking for a rigorous and systematic literature search, appraisal, and synthesis or appraise reliability by ensuring that measured outcomes are clearly defined and clinically meaningful (O'Mathuna et al., 2023). **Non-research** or other evidence appraisal tools assess validity, reliability, and applicability in a meaningful manner specific to the type of evidence. Most of these tools do not result in scoring quality directly; rather, they serve as a guide to highlight critical components associated with quality, thus allowing appraisers an overview from which to make consensus decisions about quality. Appraisal tools intended for use with non-research or other evidence can provide a clear and standardized approach to asking the right questions to determine quality.

Clinical Practice Guidelines

As you now know, clinical practice guidelines are practice recommendations made with the goal of optimizing patient care and are formulated based on a systematic review of scientific evidence and an assessment of the benefits and harms of related interventions (Institute of Medicine, 2011). It is important to note, however, that not all CPGs are created with the same level of rigor, which can result in varying quality.

There are several tools available that have been explicitly developed to appraise rigor and adherence to quality standards for CPG development; the AGREE II tool (https://www.agreetrust.org/agree-ii/) is the most widely used and can serve as a framework for CPG development and reporting. For example, your EBPQI team could use this tool to evaluate a CPG that you are considering as potential evidence to support your practice change. The AGREE II tool comprises six quality-related domains: scope and purpose, stakeholder involvement, the rigor of development, clarity of presentation, applicability, and editorial independence. A group of raters (like your team) score the CPG in each domain. An aggregate score is not used, but domain scores of > 70% typically indicate a high-quality CPG. Additionally, the tool prompts the appraiser to rank the overall quality of the CPG and indicate whether they would recommend using the guideline (AGREE Next Steps Consortium, 2017).

EBP and QI Initiatives

EBPQI initiatives are increasingly being published in the literature, so researchers must have the ability to determine the quality of these reports. As EBPQI findings are not research, they are not generalizable. Still, they can inform your clinical question and provide important information transferable to your EBPQI initiative population, organization, and process. To demonstrate quality in development and reporting, EBPQI reports should (a) show the use of a process or model to guide the project, (b) have a clear purpose or aim, (c) align with the evidence (external and internal), and (d) have outcome measurements that are clearly defined and discussed. As with CPGs, guidance has been developed to promote standardized reporting and appraisal of EBPQI initiatives.

Appraisal and reporting tools specific to EBP projects and initiatives are somewhat limited in availability. The Evidence-Based Practice Process Quality Assessment (EPQA) guideline was developed as an appraisal tool and guide to planning and reporting EBP projects (Lee et al., 2013); it uses a checklist format to identify key markers expected in quality EBP projects and initiatives. The Evidence-Based Practice Dissemination Guide can also be used in the appraisal of EBP projects (Dean et al., 2021).

QI projects and initiatives have historically been used and reported among a wider audience of healthcare professionals, so there is a widely used standard for reporting these projects called the Standards for Quality Improvement Reporting Excellence (SQUIRE). SQUIRE 2.0 is a flexible framework for reporting QI initiatives done at a systems level with measurable intervention-related outcomes (SQUIRE, 2020). Considered the gold standard for reporting QI initiatives, these reporting standards provide clear sections and items to be included in reports for publication.

There are several options for QI appraisal tools, such as the Quality Improvement Minimum Quality Criteria Set (QI-MQCS) tool (https://qualitysafety.bmj.com/content/qhc/24/12/796.full.pdf?with-ds=yes) and the Rapid Critical Appraisal of a Quality Improvement Project Tool by the Fuld Institute (https://fuld.nursing.osu.edu/sites/default/files/va_facilitator_files/3_Wednesday_Critical_Appraisal_Session/RCA_Tool_Set_folder/11_Quality_Improvement_Project.pdf). A nice feature of the QI-MQCS is that it provides a checklist format that states the minimum criteria for quality for each of the 16 domains (Hempel et al., 2015). See Appendix B for an example of using the QI-MQCS tool.

Additional Types of Evidence

As discussed earlier in this chapter, there are many types of non-research evidence besides CPGs and EBPQI projects or initiatives, including position or consensus statements, literature reviews, case reports, and expert opinions. Only some types of non-research evidence will have a specific appraisal tool; however, you can begin your appraisal by considering the validity (accuracy), reliability (consistency), and applicability in the context of the type of evidence. The Johns Hopkins EBP Non-Research Evidence Tool (https://www.cvph.org/data/files/Appendix%20F%20Nonresearch%20evidence%20appraisal%20tool%202022.pdf)is an appraisal tool tailored to several different types of evidence and a great tool to use for consistency in determining quality for a variety of evidence types. The JHEBP Non-Research Appraisal Tool is a short checklist form with sections for different types of evidence; criteria for assigning quality are included in the tool (Dang et al., 2022). A summary of select resources for various non-research appraisal tools can be found in Table 7.5.

TABLE 7.5 **Resources for Non-Research Appraisal Tools**

Type	Name	Location
Non-research evidence (general, may be used with any type of non-research evidence)	Johns Hopkins Evidence-Based Practice (JHEBP) Non-Research Evidence Appraisal Tool	https://www.hopkinsmedicine.org/evidence-based-practice/_docs/appendix_f_nonresearch_evidence_appraisal_tool.pdf
Clinical practice guidelines	AGREE II instrument	https://www.agreetrust.org/agree-ii/
EBPQI projects and initiatives	-Fuld National Institute for Evidence-Based Practice* -Evidence-Based Practice Process Quality Assessment (EPQA) -Quality Improvement Minimum Quality Criteria Set (QI-MQCS)	https://fuld.nursing.osu.edu/ebphq/rcatools https://pubmed.ncbi.nlm.nih.gov/23387900/ https://www.ncbi.nlm.nih.gov/pmc/articles/PMC4680162/ (in supplemental materials)
Other non-research evidence (case reports, economic evaluations, expert opinion)	-Joanna Briggs Institute (JBI) -Critical Appraisal Skills Programme (CASP) economic evaluation checklist -Fuld National Institute for Evidence-Based Practice*	https://jbi.global/critical-appraisal-tools https://casp-uk.net/casp-tools-checklists/ https://fuld.nursing.osu.edu/ebphq/rcatools

*Note. *= requires membership subscription.*

Appraising non-research evidence for the level and quality of evidence can sometimes feel daunting due to the numerous types of evidence and tools available. Although it is essential to use an appropriate appraisal method or tool for the type of evidence, the specific tool used is less important than a systematic and consistent team approach. As a new nurse or an experienced nurse new to EBP, you are not expected to be able to undertake or lead this task alone. Working with an established EBP mentor is crucial to effective learning and implementing EBP. Remember that critical appraisal is a team sport!

After assigning a level and quality grade to each piece of non-research or other type of evidence, you will discard low-quality evidence and move to the next step of the critical appraisal process: evaluation.

Step 2: Evaluating Other Evidence

Evaluation is the process of reviewing each piece of evidence and pulling out information that is relevant to your clinical question. This step is typically reserved for research evidence and includes research components such as study design, variables, data analysis, and findings. However, some types of evidence that measure outcomes, such as EBP and QI initiatives, may also be appropriate to include in the evaluation and can be included in your evaluation table.

Steps 3 and 4: Synthesizing the Body of Evidence and Making Recommendations for Practice

As you consider the final steps of critical appraisal, you may wonder what the difference is between summarizing and synthesizing. In the context of EBP, *summarizing* involves evaluating, then briefly stating or recording in an evaluation table the key information from each *individual* piece of evidence, as discussed in Chapter 6. *Synthesis* involves combining, contrasting, and interpreting the evidence, using your summaries as individual puzzle pieces to build a complete picture or conclusion about what is known about your clinical question (O'Mathuna et al., 2023).

By synthesizing all the relevant evidence from your literature search that you determined to be of quality during your critical appraisal, including both research and non-research or other types of evidence, you should be able to gain an understanding of the body of evidence, which will allow you to answer clinical questions and make recommendations for practice. Recommendations for practice change are best made when the body of evidence has quantity, consistency, and strength (Dang et al., 2022). When there is no clear answer to the clinical question or if an appropriate body of quality evidence does not exist, then a recommendation for practice change should not be made. As demonstrated in the mountain model, after all the available evidence has been critically appraised, you may conclude that you must conduct more research before making a recommendation for practice change. Once an initial practice recommendation has been made, your team will move to the next step of EBP, which is to integrate clinician expertise and patient values and preferences into the recommendation formulated. You will be introduced to this step in the next chapter.

WRAPPING UP

You must search for and appraise various types of evidence to fully develop and synthesize a body of evidence that allows you to answer a clinical question and make evidence-based practice recommendations. Common non-research and other types of evidence used to inform a body of evidence include clinical practice guidelines, practice statements, consensus statements, EBP and QI projects/initiatives, economic evaluations, and various types of reviews. Given the diversity of other evidence types, a variety of search techniques and resources may be needed to find the best available evidence. Regardless of evidence type, systematic critical appraisal is vital to determining the level and quality of evidence. Higher levels and quality of evidence strengthen our confidence in making sound EBP recommendations. Although considered a lower level of evidence than research evidence, other types of evidence can provide important contributions, especially when research evidence is limited or more information is needed to fill gaps or bridge what is known from research to provide safe, quality patient care.

WELLNESS IN ACTION: NUTRITIOUS EATING

The United States is currently facing an obesity epidemic and associated health problems. Poor food choices present a significant risk factor for premature death, yet shifting dietary trends tend to focus primarily on weight loss rather than health and nutrition (Locke, 2018). As nurses, we can be role models for our patients, loved ones, and communities by making evidence-based nutritional choices. During nursing school, students may often experience stress, frequent on-the-go eating, or other factors that can compound mindless eating and unhealthy eating habits, such as binging and restriction. We challenge you to invest in healthy dietary habits and practice *mindful eating*, which involves using your physical and emotional senses to explore and enjoy wholesome food choices and your overall eating experience (Tapper, 2022). Evidence has demonstrated that mindful eating is associated with healthier food choices and a healthier diet (Farrar et al., 2022; Sala et al., 2020). As you work on integrating nutritional wellness into your dietary choices, we encourage you to plan nutritional, mindful eating experiences. Eating should be nutritious and enjoyable. At your next mealtime, try to:

- Choose a variety of nutritious foods prepared in healthy ways.
- Select a setting that is pleasing to your eyes and ears (e.g., outdoors).
- Avoid distracting devices or study materials while you are eating.
- Savor your delicious, healthy meal (with good company as a bonus!).

Note: If you are experiencing symptoms of an eating disorder, seek professional help, evidence-based programs, and community recovery support. Unlike most addictions, abstinence is not an option with disordered eating, and we urge you to secure help immediately. The National Association of Anorexia Nervosa and Associated Disorders can be contacted at 1-888-375-7767.

REFLECTION QUESTIONS

1. Using the resources and tips discussed, start a search for other non-research evidence on a topic of your choice using PubMed (https://pubmed.ncbi.nlm.nih.gov) and Guideline Central (https://www.guidelinecentral.com/guidelines) or the USPSTF (https://www.uspreventiveservicestaskforce.org/uspstf/topic_search_results).
2. Remember the clinical question about sleep in adolescents? Find a clinical practice guideline, consensus statement, or other recommendation on this topic. Using the AGREE II tool with your group, appraise the document you have found. You can use the online AGREE II tool (https://www.agreetrust.org/) by creating a free account, then selecting "My AGREE PLUS" and then the orange "Start New" button. Alternatively, you can download the pdf version (https://www.agreetrust.org/wp-content/uploads/2017/12/AGREE-II-Users-Manual-and-23-item-Instrument-2009-Update-2017.pdf).

REFERENCES

AGREE Next Steps Consortium. (2017). *Appraisal of guidelines for research and evaluation II: AGREE II instrument.* https://www.agreetrust.org/wp-content/uploads/2017/12/AGREE-II-Users-Manual-and-23-item-Instrument-2009-Update-2017.pdf

American Academy of Pediatrics (2023). Autism spectrum disorder, https://www.aap.org/en/patient-care/autism/#:~:text=The%20AAP%20recommends%20that%20all,through%20screening%20and%2For%20surveillance.

Bowden, V. R., & Purper, C. (2022). Types of reviews—Part 3: Literature review, integrative review, scoping review. *Pediatric Nursing, 48*(2), 97–100.

Bradley-Ridout, G., Nekolaichuk, E., Jamieson, T., Jones, C., Morson, N., Chuang, R., & Springall, E. (2021). UpToDate versus Dynamed: A cross-sectional study comparing the speed and accuracy of two point-of-care information tools. *Journal of the Medical Library Association, 109*(3). https://doi.org/10.5195/jmla.2021.1176

Buccheri, R. K., & Sharifi, C. (2017). Critical appraisal tools and reporting guidelines for evidence-based practice. *Worldviews on Evidence-Based Nursing, 14*(6), 463–472. https://doi.org/10.1111/wvn.12258

Carter-Templeton, H., Wrigley, J., Nicoll, L. H., Owens, J. K., Oermann, M. H., & Ledbetter, L. S. (2023). A bibliometric analysis of review types published in the nursing scientific literature. *Advances in Nursing Science, 46*(1), 28–40. https://doi.org/10.1097/ANS.0000000000000424

Centers for Disease Control and Prevention. (2021, March 3). *Economic evaluation overview.* https://www.cdc.gov/policy/polaris/economics/index.html#:~:text=Print-,Economic%20 Evaluation,of%20different%20public%20health%20interventions.

Centers for Disease Control and Prevention (2022). Screening and diagnosis of autism spectrum disorder. https://www.cdc.gov/ncbddd/autism/screening.html

Connor, L., Dean, J., McNett, M., Tydings, D. M., Shrout, A., Gorsuch, P. F., Hole, A., Moore, L., Brown, R., Melnyk, B., & Gallagher-Ford, L. (2023). Evidence-based practice improves patient outcomes and healthcare system return on investment: Findings from a scoping review. *Worldviews on Evidence-Based Nursing, 20*(1), 6–15. https://doi.org/10.1111/wvn.12621

Dang, D., Dearholt, S., Bissett, K., Ascenzi, J., & Whalen, M. (2022). *Johns Hopkins evidence-based practice for nurses and healthcare professionals: Models and guidelines* (4th ed.). Sigma Theta Tau International.

Dean, J., Gallagher-Ford, L., & Connor, L. (2021). Evidence-based practice: A new dissemination guide. *Worldviews on Evidence-Based Nursing, 18*(1), 4–7. https://doi.org/10.1111/wvn.12489

Dunlap, J. J., & Filipek, P. A. (2020). CE: Autism spectrum disorder: The nurse's role. *The American Journal of Nursing, 120*(11), 40–49. https://doi.org/10.1097/01.NAJ.0000721236.69639.e3

Farrar, S. T., Plagnol, A. C., & Tapper, K. (2022). The effect of priming on food choice: A field and laboratory study. *Appetite, 168*, 105749. https://doi.org/10.1016/j.appet.2021.105749

Fineout-Overholt, E. (2023). Critically appraising knowledge for clinical decision making. In B. M. Melnyk & E. Fineout-Overholt (Eds.), *Evidence-based practice in nursing & healthcare: A guide to best practice* (5th ed., pp. 153–170). Wolters Kluwer.

Fineout-Overholt, E., Melnyk, B., Stillwell, S. B., & Williamson, K. M. (2010). Evidence-based practice, step by step: Critical appraisal of the evidence: Part II. *AJN, 110*(9), 41–48. https://doi.org/10.1097/01.naj.0000388264.49427.f9

Hampel, S. E., Hassink, S. G., Skinner, A. C., Armstrong, S. C., Barlow, S. E., Bolling, C. F., Avila Edwards, K. C., Eneli, I., Hamre, R., Joseph, M. M., Lunsford, D., Mendonca, E., Michalsky, M. P., Mirza, N., Ochoa, E. R., Sharifi, M., Staiano, A. E., Weedn, A. E., Flinn, S. K., … Lindros, J. (2023). Clinical practice guidelines for the evaluation and treatment of children and adolescents with obesity. *Pediatrics, 151*(2), Article e2022060640. https://doi.org/10.1542/peds.2022-060640

Harris, M., Taylor, G., & Jackson, D. (2014). *Clinical evidence made easy: The basics of evidence-based medicine.* Scion.

Hempel, S., Shekelle, P. G., Liu, J. L., Sherwood Danz, M., Foy, R., Lim, Y.-W., Motala, A., & Rubenstein, L. V. (2015). Development of the Quality Improvement Minimum Quality Criteria Set (QI-MQCS): A tool for critical appraisal of quality improvement intervention publications. *BMJ Quality & Safety, 24*(12), 796–804. https://doi.org/10.1136/bmjqs-2014-003151

Hirai AH, Kogan MD, Kandasamy V, Reuland C, Bethell C. (2018). Prevalence and variation of developmental screening and surveillance in early childhood. *JAMA Pediatrics*,172(9):857–866. doi:10.1001/jamapediatrics.2018.1524

Hyman et al., (2020). Identification, evaluation and management of children with autism spectrum disorder. *Pediatrics, 154*, 1, https://publications.aap.org/pediatrics/article/145/1/e20193447/36917/Identification-Evaluation-and-Management-of

Institute of Medicine. (2001). *Crossing the quality chasm: A new health system for the 21st century.* National Academies Press. https://doi.org/10.17226/10027

Institute of Medicine. (2011). *Clinical practice guidelines we can trust.* National Academies Press. https://doi.org/10.17226/13058

Joshi, G. P., Benzon, H. T., Gan, T. J., & Vetter, T. R. (2019). Consistent definitions of clinical practice guidelines, consensus statements, position statements, and practice alerts. *Anesthesia & Analgesia, 129*(6), 1767–1770. https://doi.org/10.1213/ane.0000000000004236

Lee, M., Johnson, K. L., Newhouse, R. P., & Warren, J. I. (2013). Evidence-based practice process quality assessment: EPQA guidelines. *Worldviews on Evidence-Based Nursing, 10*(3), 140–149. https://doi.org/10.1111/j.1741-6787.2012.00264.x

Levin, R. F., Keefer, J. M., Marren, J., Vetter, M., Lauder, B., & Sobolewski, S. (2010). Evidence-based practice improvement: Merging 2 paradigms. *Journal of Nursing Care Quality, 25*(2), 117–126. https://doi.org/10.1097/NCQ.0b013e3181b5f19f

Locke, A., Schneiderhan, J., & Zick, S. M. (2018). Diets for health: Goals and guidelines. *American Family Physician, 97*(11), 721–728.

Melnyk, B. (2016). Level of evidence plus critical appraisal of its quality yields confidence to implement evidence-based practice changes. *Worldviews on Evidence-Based Nursing, 13*(5), 337–339. https://doi.org/10.1111/wvn.12181

Melnyk, B., Buck, J., & Gallagher-Ford, L. (2015). Transforming quality improvement into evidence-based quality improvement: A key solution to improve healthcare outcomes. *Worldviews on Evidence-Based Nursing, 12*(5), 251–252. https://doi.org/10.1111/wvn.12112

Munn, Z., Peters, M. J., Stern, C., Tufanaru, C., McArthur, A., & Aromataris, E. (2018). Systematic review or scoping review? Guidance for authors when choosing between a systematic or scoping review approach. *BMC Medical Research Methodology, 18*(1). https://doi.org/10.1186/s12874-018-0611-x

NAHQ (2024) HQ Solutions. https://nahq.org/products/hq-solutions-resource-for-the-healthcare-quality-professional-fifth-edition/

Oermann, M. H., & Knafl, K. A. (2021). Strategies for completing a successful integrative review. *Nurse Author & Editor, 31*(3–4), 65–68. https://doi.org/10.1111/nae2.30

O'Mathuna, D. P., Finest-Overholt, E., Graham, D. B., & Canada, A. (2023). Critically appraising quantitative evidence for clinical decision making. In B. M. Melnyk & E. Fineout-Overholt (Eds.), *Evidence-based practice in nursing and healthcare: A guide to best practice* (5th ed., pp. 189–265). Wolters Kluwer.

PRISMA for scoping reviews (2024). http://www.prisma-statement.org/Extensions/ScopingReviews?AspxAutoDetectCookieSupport=1

Registered Nurses Association of Ontario. (2022). *Promoting smoking reduction and cessation with Indigenous peoples of reproductive age and their communities*. https://rnao.ca/bpg/guidelines/promoting-smoking-reduction-and-cessation-indigenous-peoples-reproductive-age-and

Sala, M., Rochefort, C., Lui, P. P., & Baldwin, A. S. (2020). Trait mindfulness and health behaviours: A meta-analysis. *Health Psychology Review, 14*(3), 345–393. https://doi.org/10.1080/17437199.2019.1650290

Schloemer, T., & Schröder-Bäck, P. (2018). Criteria for evaluating transferability of health interventions: A systematic review and thematic synthesis. *Implementation Science, 13*(1). https://doi.org/10.1186/s13012-018-0751-8

Sender, J. (2019). ECRI Institute Guidelines Trust. *Journal of the Medical Library Association, 107*(3). https://doi.org/10.5195/jmla.2019.693

SQUIRE. (2020). *Revised standards for quality improvement reporting excellence: SQUIRE 2.0*. http://www.squire-statement.org/index.cfm?fuseaction=Page.ViewPage&pageId=471

Tapper, K. (2022). Mindful eating: What we know so far. *Nutrition Bulletin, 47*(2), 168–185. https://doi.org/10.1111/nbu.12559

Tod, D., Booth, A., & Smith, B. (2021). Critical appraisal. *International Review of Sport and Exercise Psychology, 15*(1), 52–72. https://doi.org/10.1080/1750984x.2021.1952471

Turner, H. C., Archer, R. A., Downey, L. E., Isaranuwatchai, W., Chalkidou, K., Jit, M., & Teerawattananon, Y. (2021). An introduction to the main types of economic evaluations used for informing priority setting and resource allocation in healthcare: Key features, uses, and limitations. *Frontiers in Public Health*, *9*. https://doi.org/10.3389/fpubh.2021.722927

United States Preventive Services Task Force. (n.d.). *About the USPSTF.* Retrieved February 28, 2023, from https://uspreventiveservicestaskforce.org/uspstf/about-uspstf

Waldrop, J. & Dunlap, J.J. (2024). The Mountain Model for Evidence-Based Practice Quality Improvement Initiatives, *American Journal of Nursing,* in press.

CHAPTER 8

Patient Preferences and Values

Elizabeth Miller Walters, Francisco Ayala, and Kathleen Ellis

KEY CONCEPTS

Patient engagement
Family engagement
Shared decision-making (SDM)
Clinical expertise
Cultural competence
Health literacy

LEARNING OBJECTIVES

1. Discuss the importance of incorporating patient preference with EPB.
2. Identify benefits and barriers to shared decision-making.

Change is the end result of all true learning.

—Leo Buscaglia

Introduction

Imagine your best friend bringing you coffee in the morning. However, the coffee is not your usual caffeine concoction but rather over-sweetened and of a distinct creamer that is not appealing to your palate. While you appreciate the good gesture, you silently would have appreciated it if your input would have been considered. Your friend meant well. She previously knew that you enjoyed coffee and used her expertise, experience, and even went to a location that you frequent with them. In the future, their ability to get you coffee may be compromised! If you would have been involved or if they would have asked you what you would like in your coffee, then you would have thoroughly enjoyed your drink and been prepared to seize the day! This analogy is akin to patients who want to be involved in their care and not merely recipients of a unilateral decision made by their healthcare professional.

It is best practice to incorporate patient preference into nursing care. Like the example above, you had a different preference for coffee than your colleague ordered and brought for you. Your patients would also like to have input into their healthcare, much like you would like a say in the type of coffee that you drink. When patient preference is incorporated into EBP, there are better patient outcomes. Research shows us that patients who have a say in their healthcare options are more likely to initiate and continue that treatment (King et al., 2005; Swift et al., 2017, 2018).

Patient Preference and EBP

Personalizing healthcare interventions is important for evidence-based practice. If you remember from Chapter 2, the Quintuple Aim in healthcare focuses on enhancing the patient experience, improving population health, reducing healthcare costs, and improving caregiver well-being and equity (Nunday, 2022; see Chapter 2). When connecting the Quintuple Aim with incorporating patient preference in their healthcare, research has shown a positive impact on patient experiences, like patient satisfaction and reduction in unmet needs (Haverfield et al., 2020).

Further, there is a correlation between patient health outcomes like depression, adherence, and quality of life. There is also a correlation between improved healthcare professional well-being, stress, and communication between healthcare professionals and patients (Haverfield et al., 2020). Personalizing healthcare interventions and improving patient engagement has a direct effect on the Quintuple Aim.

Many factors influence **patient engagement**. It is important to personalize healthcare interventions according to the patient's values and preferences. Patient commitment is another key factor in patient engagement. Finally, the therapeutic alliance between the healthcare provider and the patient is essential for engaging patients (Hickmann et al., 2022).

Patient preference relies on understanding our patients' values and preferences. We cannot assume their values and preferences. We must incorporate patient preference into our care because it is imperative to respect patients' rights and dignity. *Patient-centered care* means understanding our patients' values and preferences and incorporating this into our nursing care (Gooberman-Hill, 2012). *Values* are a patient's attitude and perception about their healthcare, and *preferences* are their choices regarding healthcare when incorporating their values (Llewellyn-Thomas & Crump, 2013). For example, you may encounter a patient who has not been taking their prescribed medication for anxiety. This decision by the patient may seem like the wrong one to you based on your values and preferences, but the patient may have different values and preferences than you, and these need exploring. Patients have a right to a say in their care.

Patient commitment or willingness to participate in their healthcare is key to patient engagement (Higgins et al., 2017). Understanding patients' motivation and commitment to health is very important for nurses and all healthcare providers. Going back to the patient with anxiety, we understand from further communication that the patient desires a medication-free approach to helping with their anxiety because of previous negative experiences with anxiety medication side effects. The patient is committed to improving their anxiety, and because you took the time to explore this more with the patient, you now understand their decision-making is related to past experiences with medications.

The alliance between healthcare professionals and patients is key to patient engagement (Higgins et al., 2017). Forming relationships with patients is a cornerstone of patient engagement. Relationships are built on trust. Be honest with your patients about their health and healthcare. Answer their questions openly and honestly. Set the stage for a trustworthy alliance by actively listening. With your anxious patient, you listened to the patient and heard their desire for a medication-free approach to anxiety treatment and that avoiding potential medication side effects is important for the patient. The patient felt heard and thus strengthened their therapeutic alliance with you.

Family Engagement

Patient engagement is simple compared to the incorporation of the family unit in the discussions about the patient's care. There are, however, instances where **family engagement** is required (e.g., end-of-life care, pediatric patients, serious illness). But the stakes do not always need to be high for the involvement of the family unit. In some cultures, communicating treatment plans with the entire family or with specific family members is a cultural norm and a sign of respect. More will be discussed regarding cultural competence and cultural humility later in this chapter.

Regardless of your intent when involving the patient's family, you need to remember that you are an advocate for the patient and need to avoid the possibility of a loss of trust, embarrassment, or psychological discomfort from discussing the patient's health problems with their family (Haines et al., 2017). It is essential that the patient's wishes to share information with the family are respected to prevent not only damages to the nurse–patient relationship but also litigation risks from HIPAA violations (Haines et al., 2017).

Communication

It is important that when soliciting patient preference you use therapeutic communication. Therapeutic communication is a cornerstone of nursing care, and you are likely well on your way to becoming good at this type of communication. *Therapeutic communication* is a collection of communication techniques that ensure patients are supported physically, mentally, and emotionally (Nightingale College, 2022). Therapeutic communication includes using specific communication techniques, such as building a relationship, active listening, silence, focusing, asking open-ended questions, clarifying, exploring, paraphrasing, reflecting, restating, summarizing, acknowledging, and offering oneself (Nightingale College, 2022).

Let's use the above therapeutic communication techniques in an example. When you are a nurse, people around you will likely ask for your advice for anything and everything medical. Imagine that your neighbor with three small children at home asks you about giving up breastfeeding her 3-month-old. She explains that breastfeeding is difficult and painful and causes her a lot of stress and anxiety because she doesn't know how much milk her baby is getting and he's smaller than her other two children were at age 3 months. She asks for your advice. You know that breastfeeding reduces conditions like ear infections and childhood obesity. But your neighbor is stressed and anxious, which is also not good for her family. Let's use this scenario as an example of incorporating evidence-based recommendations, both using and not using therapeutic communication techniques.

REAL-WORLD EXAMPLE

Neighbor: I think I'll stop breastfeeding because my life is so stressful with three little kids.

You: Do you think that's a good idea? Breastfeeding is the *best* option for your baby. He needs you to breastfeed so he won't get ear infections and be obese.

Neighbor: It's just so hard and painful, and he's not gaining weight like my other kids did. He's so much tinier.

You: All the research shows that breastfeeding is superior to bottle feeding. Don't you want to do the best thing for your child? If it were me, I'd breastfeed my children for the recommended 1 full year to be the healthiest they can be!

Neighbor: (Sighs) I guess you're right since you're a nurse.

In this example, the neighbor walks off feeling guilty for wanting to stop breastfeeding and frustrated that she wasn't heard. The nurse feels good because she used the evidence to tell her neighbor about the benefits of breastfeeding. What are some ways that the nurse could have used therapeutic communication skills with her neighbor? Now, let's see how things turn out between the nurse and her neighbor using therapeutic communication techniques:

Neighbor: I think I'll stop breastfeeding because my life is so stressful with three little kids.

Nurse: Tell me more about why you're considering stopping breastfeeding. [Open-ended question]

Neighbor: Because it's very painful, and my child isn't growing as well as his siblings. I'm afraid I'm not producing enough. I'm also scared that my anxiety about this issue is really hard on our family.

Nurse: (Is actively looking at her neighbor and thoughtfully stays silent) [Active listening, silence]

Neighbor: I'm so anxious that I'm getting snappy with my toddlers and partner. All I can think about is making sure that my baby is getting enough milk. I dread going to the primary care provider because I'm afraid he didn't gain enough weight.

Nurse: It sounds like you're experiencing a lot of anxiety about breastfeeding and are concerned about how that anxiety affects your family. [Paraphrasing] I understand that this is a very stressful situation for you and your family. [Acknowledgment] Has your primary care provider mentioned that your son's weight is concerning? [Clarifying]

Neighbor: The nurse practitioner we see isn't concerned about his weight gain. And at our most recent appointment, she reminded me of all of the benefits of breastfeeding. But I can't seem to control these worries.

Nurse: What do you think the best decision is for your family? [Exploring]

Neighbor: I think that switching to bottle feeding will certainly ease my anxiety and allow my partner to help with feedings too so that we can divide the night feedings and I could get a little more sleep. That would help a lot too. Thank you for listening to me and helping me sort this out. Sometimes, I feel like my concerns aren't heard by my medical providers.

Nurse: I'm here anytime you need to talk. [Offering of oneself]

Shared Decision-Making

Shared decision-making (SDM) is a process in which the nurse and the patient both participate in the decision-making process for a patient's care. SDM is a tool utilizing therapeutic communication techniques to solicit patient preferences and incorporate them with evidence for joint healthcare decision-making (Truglio-Londrigan & Slyer, 2018). SDM is a growing phenomenon as patients are becoming more proactive consumers of their healthcare (Elwyn et al., 2021). Involving patients in their care has shown positive effects, including improved nurse–patient relationships and increased compliance to treatment (Deniz et al., 2021). A key concept in shared decision-making is that patients and healthcare providers, including nurses, have different but equally valuable viewpoints and roles in the decision-making encounter. SDM is a bidirectional exchange between a patient who provides their goals, values, and preferences and the healthcare professional or nurse who discusses the risks, benefits, and uncertainties of options for care, which are based on their knowledge, experience, and best available evidence (Frerichs et al., 2016). Various factors influence the success of shared decision-making, both on the side of the patient and the healthcare professional.

TABLE 8.1 Factors Influencing Shared Decision-Making

Healthcare provider	Patients
Knowledge	Resources
Experiences	Experiences
Skills	Health literacy

(Waddell et al., 2021)

SDM can be utilized for any healthcare decisions (e.g., medication or treatment, managing a chronic disease, end-of-life treatment in palliative care). The uniqueness of each case calls for an individualized approach to care. On one hand, as the nurse, you are well versed on the appropriateness of the medication for the condition that is being treated. This is based on your education, experience/expertise, and relevant evidence. However, a patient may be more concerned about being able to afford the medication, the side effects of the medication, and the overall effect of the medication on their daily life. Think back to the patient earlier in this chapter who was anxious and preferred a medication-free approach to anxiety treatment. The nurse knows that the research evidence shows that both medication and therapy are good options. Using therapeutic communication techniques, the nurse discusses the options with the patient. The patient decides to move forward with therapy because they prefer to avoid medication side effects. SDM is a tool that can be used to incorporate research-based evidence and the nurse's **clinical expertise** with patient preference.

Healthcare Provider Factors

Nurses use their knowledge, experiences, and skills when participating in shared decision-making with patients. Thinking back on the patient with anxiety, the nurse's education and experience brought knowledge to them about the disease process of anxiety and the mechanism of actions of medications and therapy on this disease process. The nurse's knowledge allows them to understand the diagnosis of anxiety and which treatments are best.

Nurses' experiences also influence shared decision-making. Experiences with past patients and personal experiences may influence the nurse's side in shared decision-making. For example, with the patient with anxiety, the nurse may have recently had a patient who was started on anti-anxiety medication who did experience a rare but serious side effect of suicidality. This experience may have influenced the provider's recommendations for this patient. Or thinking back to the nurse and her neighbor, the nurse may have successfully breastfed all of her children, which could influence her recommendations to her neighbor.

Another essential component of successful SDM includes the healthcare professional's experiences in cultural competence and humility. *Culture* refers to specific patterns in behavior, beliefs, language, symbols, rituals, and other characteristics specific to a group of people (Brown et al., 2016). **Cultural competence** is the ability to work respectfully with people from diverse cultures while recognizing one's own cultural biases (Agner, 2020). The uniqueness of someone's beliefs can alter their lifestyle, diet, healthcare practices, and medical preferences. This uniqueness can contradict the beliefs of accepted Western society, and this contrast may create discomfort, disagreement, and conflict in the nurse–patient relationship.

Your nursing skills certainly influence shared decision-making. Your therapeutic communication skills and your skills in evidence-based practice (i.e., the ability to find high-quality evidence for best practice) affect your ability to participate in SDM successfully. Nurses must use all their knowledge, experiences, and skills when participating in SDM with patients.

Patient Factors

To have an effective SDM encounter, your knowledge, experience, and skills need to be considered in the context of patient factors that influence SDM. Patients' resources, experiences, and health literacy affect their engagement in SDM (Waddell et al., 2021). In SDM, the patient should be able to have multiple diagnostic and treatment considerations while simultaneously considering patient factors to optimize health outcomes.

Resources

A patient's resources must be considered when participating in SDM (Hickmann et al., 2022; Higgins et al., 2017). Financial resources and access to transportation are two areas that can directly affect the patient's ability to participate in their healthcare. As our patient with anxiety values a medication-free approach to treating their anxiety and opts for therapy, the patient must be able to access that therapy. Questions you should consider related to the patient's preference and decision related to treatment are:

- Does this patient have adequate healthcare insurance or resources to pay for therapy?
- Does this patient have transportation to access therapy?
- Is there a therapist in this patient's community?

Ensuring patients have accessible resources does not include just the cost of healthcare.

Health Literacy

Other patient factors can hinder the positive effects of SDM. A patient's **health literacy** taps into a specific domain of literacy concerned with whether or not the patient possesses literary skills and knowledge-based tasks that can be used together in the proper context to make appropriate health decisions (Nutbeam et al., 2018). Health literacy is important in shared decision-making. For example, how would you approach your patient with anxiety if they were a fellow nurse? Would your approach be different if the patient was someone who dropped out of high school, is currently unemployed, or uninsured? How can you tailor your conversation to ensure patients both understand their treatment options and can make an informed decision? The Agency for Healthcare Research and Quality (2020) has a tool kit that provides support for answering these questions (https://www.ahrq.gov/health-literacy/professional-training/shared-decision/tool/resource-4.html)

Experiences

Patients' experiences also affect their participation in shared decision-making. It is important to be aware that these experiences affect how they may interact with a healthcare professional who is perceived to hold more power in the healthcare decision-making than they feel they do. It is important to consider the cultural norms that may affect patients' decision-making. It is also vital to understand patients' past experiences with medical decision-making. For example, your patient with anxiety may not be comfortable opening up about their mental health struggles due to the cultural stigma of mental health in their community. Or they could have had a past experience with a healthcare provider ignoring their concerns or not presenting them with any options for treatment beyond medication (Abelson et al., 2022).

Diversity is an important consideration in patients' experience. Diversity is often considered to be a synonym for race or ethnicity. While these categories are important, we must consider a broader, more robust definition. Individuals come to us for care with various attributes, including gender, socioeconomic status, geographical location, and history of trauma. During the assessment, it is also important to note that none of these categories are entirely homogeneous. Individuals have unique attributes within categories. By asking patients about their experiences, concerns, and preferences, nurses can show respect and interest in them as individuals. Questions should focus on the patient. What is their preferred language? What are their preferred pronouns? Taking a person-centered approach can help develop a trusting relationship, as opposed to making assumptions based on appearance. A person-centered approach transcends the immediate healthcare interaction and creates an atmosphere of respect (Nava et al., 2022).

Intersectionality is an important consideration when discussing diversity. This focuses on the additive impact of personal attributes that have historically been marginalized. For example, a person who identifies as Hispanic and transgender may face greater marginalization than a Hispanic male (Ruiz et al., 2021). Using an intersectional approach can help you understand some of the complexities facing patients. It can also help inform you in ways to evaluate literature and incorporate EBP into practice.

As we learned in Chapter 3, historically, research has undersampled racial and ethnic minorities and people who identify as female. People from historically marginalized groups may decline to participate in research due to historical issues (e.g., experimentation without the consent of participants, inadequate access to available treatments), bias (e.g., inadequate recruitment, stereotyping), and lack of resources (e.g., limited ability to translate recruitment materials, consent forms, and instruments). Studies that sample participants in patterns that do not reflect the population at large can result in decreased generalizability (Syder & Elbuluk,

2023). Recent efforts have shown improvement for some groups (such as those identifying as female), but many groups remain underrepresented. Transgender participation is particularly low. A systematic review of 5,388 clinical trials showed that only three trials (0.10%) reported the participation of transgender people. Of these three trials, only five participants were described as transgender (Buffenstein et al., 2023). These disparities in research participation highlight the need for a careful analysis of the studies you select as evidence for your interventions.

Essential Elements of Shared Decision-Making

Now that we have reviewed the "why" of SDM, how do we, as nurses, participate in shared decision-making? Going back to the example of our patient with anxiety, let's review the steps in SDM in Table 8.2.

TABLE 8.2 Essential Elements of Shared Decision-Making

Steps in SDM	Example: Anxious patient
Defining and explaining the problem	Review the patient's symptoms and the healthcare provider's diagnosis. Explain them to the patient using plain language, such as: "Your symptoms are consistent with anxiety, a condition that causes your natural fight-or-flight response to turn on in situations in which it does not need to, like riding in elevators, new social situations, or getting a blood draw."
Evaluating available options	Search for the best available evidence for the management of anxiety. Look for clinical practice guidelines, available evidence-based tool kits, and research studies.
Discussing pros and cons of options	Use an available tool kit to review the pros and cons of treatment options to help with anxiety, including medication, therapy, or a combination of both.
Clarifying patient values and preferences	Ask the patient what their preference is for managing their anxiety. The patient states, "I really want to avoid medications because I have had a bad experience with anxiety medication side effects. Plus, my family doesn't like the idea of medications for anxiety."
Discussing patient's self-efficacy and abilities	Once a shared decision is made, further discussion needs to occur to be sure that that decision can be implemented. Ask the patient questions about their resources and abilities. For example: Nurse: "Tell me about your ability to attend regular therapy." Patient: "I usually have Wednesdays off from my job, and my health insurance covers 'in-network' providers, so as long as I can go to an in-network provider on Wednesdays, it should be OK." Nurse: "We will work hard to find a therapist in your network with openings on Wednesdays."
Describing healthcare provider's professional knowledge and recommendations	Clearly state the decision that has been made. For example: "The research shows us that therapy is a great option to help manage anxiety. I have had many patients who have been successful in managing their anxiety symptoms with the tools that they learn in therapy. That is a great treatment option based on your preference to avoid medications."

Steps in SDM	Example: Anxious patient
Clarifying the patient's understanding	Confirm the patient's understanding. For example: "Please review your plan for anxiety management with me."
Making or deferring decision	After a decision is made, follow through with the next step. Either make an appointment for the patient or be sure the patient makes an appointment. Many times this is the point where the ball is dropped and patients end up not getting the care they need.
Keeping the conversation going	Follow-up is critical. It helps ensure patients move forward with their decisions and demonstrates that you care about their health and want to continue to support them.

WRAPPING UP

Incorporating patient preference with the best available evidence shows improved patient satisfaction and treatment adherence (King et al., 2005; Swift et al., 2017, 2018). Therapeutic communication techniques can aid in understanding your patients' preferences regarding their healthcare. Shared decision-making is a model to incorporate the best evidence and your clinical expertise with your patient's preference. There are multiple factors, both on the healthcare provider's side and the patient's side, that affect the success of shared decision-making. When patients feel heard and their values and preferences are considered and respected, the chances increase for successful management of their health condition. This is the final and third component of evidence-based practice. You are now ready to add quality improvement strategies in the next chapter to EBP to optimize practice improvement.

WELLNESS IN ACTION: ARTS

Participation in the arts, including music, can increase personal health and well-being, especially as we age (Hanna-Pladdy & MacKay, 2011; Johnson et al., 2017; National Institutes of Health, 2019). Establishing habits that involve meaningful engagement in art and music may promote stress reduction and social connectedness. Think about giving some or all of the following a try as inclined and desired:

1. Play an instrument or sing (solo or collectively with others) on a regular basis that works for you.
2. Challenge yourself to become better at your craft through personal or group lessons.
3. Pursue a variety of art forms that you find aesthetically pleasing, mentally stimulating, and/or relaxing as opportunities arise.

REFLECTION QUESTIONS

1. Consider how a patient's health literacy impacts healthcare decision-making. What do the recommendations from AHRQ (2020) say about how you might approach SDM conversations depending on a patient's level of health literacy? List three strategies that you could use and the rationale for using them.

See: https://www.ahrq.gov/health-literacy/professional-training/shared-decision/tool/resource-4.html

2. What is the difference between cultural competency and cultural humility? Why are both important to patient engagement in their care?
3. When planning to discharge a patient, you find out they do not have a car and there is no public transportation available where they live. The nurse practitioner has ordered a follow-up appointment in 2 weeks. What will you do to help the patient address this resource issue?

REFERENCES

Abelson, J., Canfield, C., Leslie, M., Levasseur, M. A., Rowland, P., Tripp, L., Vanstone, M., Panday, J., Cameron, D., Forest, P. G., Sussman, D., & Wilson, G. (2022). Understanding patient partnership in health systems: Lessons from the Canadian Patient Partner survey. *BMJ, 12*(9), Article e061465. https://doi.org/10.1136/bmjopen-2022-061465

Agency for Healthcare Research and Quality. (2020, November). *The SHARE Approach—Health literacy and shared decisionmaking: A reference guide for health care providers.* https://www.ahrq.gov/health-literacy/professional-training/shared-decision/tool/resource-4.html

Agner, J. (2020). Moving from cultural competence to cultural humility in occupational therapy: A paradigm shift. *American Journal of Occupational Therapy, 74*(4), 7404347010p1–7404347010p7. https://doi.org/10.5014/ajot.2020.038067

Brown, E. A., Bekker, H. L. Davison, S. N., Koffman, J., & Schell, J. O. (2016). Supportive care: Communication strategies to improve cultural competence in shared decision making. *Clinical Journal of the American Society of Nephrology, 11*(10), 1902–1903. https://doi.org/10.2215/CJN.13661215

Buffenstein, L., Kaneakua, B., Taylor, E., Matsunaga, M. Choi, S. Y., Carrazana, E., Viereck, J., Liow, K. K., & Chaffari-Rafi, A. (2023). Demographic recruitment bias of adults in United States randomized clinical trials by disease categories between 2008 to 2019: A systematic review and meta-analysis. *Scientific Reports, 13*(1), 42. https://doi.org/10.1038s41598-022-23664-1

Deniz, S., Akbolat, M., Cimen, M., & Unal, O. (2021). The mediating role of shared decision-making in the effect of the patient-physician relationship on compliance with treatment. *Journal of Patient Experience, 8,* Article 23743735211018064. https://doi.org/10.1177/23743735211018066

Elwyn, G., Frosch, D., Thomson, R., Joseph-Williams, N., Lloyd, A., Kinnersley, P., Cording, E., Tomson, D., Dodd, C., Rollnick, S., Edwards, A., & Barry, M. (2012). Shared decision making: A model for clinical practice. *Journal of General Internal Medicine, 27*(10), 1361–1367. https://doi.org/10.1007/s11606-012-2077-6

Frerichs, W., Hahlweg, P., Müller, E., Adis, C., & Scholl, I. (2016). Shared decision-making in oncology: A qualitative analysis of healthcare providers' views on current practice. *PloS One, 11*(3), Article e0149789. https://doi.org/10.1371/journal.pone.0149789

Gooberman-Hill, R. (2012). Qualitative approaches to understanding patient preferences. *The Patient: patient Centered Outcomes Research,* 5(4), 215–223. https://doi.org/10.2165/11633720-000000000-00000

Haines, K. J., Kelly, P., Fitzgerald, P., Skinner, E. H., & Iwashyna, T. J. (2017). The untapped potential of patient and family engagement in the organization of critical care. *Critical Care Medicine, 45*(5), 8990906. https://doi.org/10.1097/CCM.0000000000002282

Haverfield, M. C., Tierney, A., Schwartz, R., Bass, M. B., Brown-Johnson, C., Zionts, D. L., Safaeinili, N., Fischer, M., Shaw, J. G., Thadaney, S.Piccininni, G., Lorenz, K. A., Asch, S. M., Verghese, A., & Zulman, D. M. (2020). Can patient-provider interpersonal interventions achieve the Quadruple Aim of healthcare? A systematic review. *Journal of General Internal Medicine, 35*(7), 2107–2117. https://doi.org/10.1007/s11606-019-05525-2

Hickman, E., Richter, P., & Schlieter, H. (2022). Al together now—patient engagement, patient empowerment, and associated terms in personal healthcare. *BMC Health Services Research, 22*(1), 116. https://doi.org/10.1186/s12913-022-08501-5

Higgins, T., Larson, E., & Schnall, R. (2017). Unraveling the meaning of patient engagement: A concept analysis. *Patient Education and Counseling, 100*(1), 30–36.

King, M. Nazareth, L., Lampe, F., Bower, P., Chandler, M., Morou, M., Sibbald, B., & Lai, R. (2005). Impact of participant and physician intervention preferences on randomized trials: A systematic review. *Journal of the American Medical Association, 203*(9), 1089–1099. https://doi.org/10.1001/jama.293.9.1089

Llewellyn-Thomas, H. A., & Crump, R. T. (2013). Decision support for patients: Values clarification and preference elicitation. *Medical Care Research and Review, 70*(Suppl. 1), 50S–79S. https://doi.org/10.1177/1077558712461182

Makoul, G., & Clayman, M. L. (2006). An integrative model of shared decision making in medical encounters. *Patient Education and Counseling, 60*(3), 301–312. https://doi.org/10.1016/j.pec.2005.06.010

Nava, A., Estrade, L., Gerchow, L., Scot, J., Thompson, R. & Squires, A. (2022). Grouping people by language exacerbates health inequities: The case of Latinx/Hispanic populations in the US. *Research in Nursing & Health, 45*(2), 142–147. https://doi.org/10.1002/nur.22221

Nightingale College. (2022, February 24). Are you ready to employ therapeutic communication techniques in your nursing practice? https://nightingale.edu/blog/therapeutic-communication/

Nunday, S., Cooper, L. A., & Mate, K. S. (2022). The Quintuple Aim for health care improvement: A new imperative to advance health equity. *JAMA, 327*(6), 521–522. https://doi.org/10.1001/jama.2021.25181

Nutbeam, D., McGill, B., & Premkumar, P. (2018). Improving health literacy in community populations: A review of progress. *Health Promotion International, 33*(5), 901–911. https://doi.org/10.1093/heapro/dax015

Ruiz, A. M., Luebke, J., Klein, K., Moore, K., Gonzalez, M., Dressel, A., & Mkandawire-Valhmu, L. (2021). An integrative literature review and critical reflection of intersectionality theory. *Nursing Inquiry, 28*(4), Article e12414. https://doi.org/10.1111/nin.12414

Swift, J. K., Callahan, J. L., Cooper, M., & Parking, S. R. (2018). The impact of accommodating client preference in pasychotherapy: A meta-analysis. *Journal of Clinical Psychology, 74*(11, 1924–1937. https://doi.org/10.1002/jclp.22680

Swift, J. K., Greenberg, R. P., Tompkins, K. A., & Parking, S. R. (2017). Treatment refusal and premature termination in psychotherapy, pharmacotherapy, and their combination: A meta-analysis of head-to-head comparisons. *Psychotherapy, 54*(1), 47–57. https://doi.org/10.1037/pst0000104

Syder, N. C., & Elbuluk, N. (2023). Vitiligo and makeup: Analyzing interest and usage trends in the 21st century. *International Journal of Dermatology*. Advance online publication. https://doi.org/10.1111/ijd.16600.

Truglio-Londrigan, M., & Slyer, J. T. (2018). Shared decision-making for nursing practice: An integrative review. *The Open Nursing Journal, 12*, 1–14. https://doi.org/10.2174/1874434601812010001

Waddell, A., Lennox, A., Spassova, G., & Bragge, P. (2021). Barriers and facilitators to shared decision-making in hospitals from policy to practice: A systematic review. *Implementation Science, 16*(1), 74. https://doi.org/10.1186/s13012-021-01142-y

CHAPTER 9

Fundamentals of Quality Improvement for Nurses

Staci S. Reynolds and Bradi B. Granger

KEY CONCEPTS

Quality improvement (QI)
PICK chart
SMART aim statement
Plan-do-study-act (PDSA)
Run charts
Statistical process control charts

LEARNING OBJECTIVES

1. Explore the background and definition of QI.
2. Identify the practicing nurse's role as a QI team member.
3. Discuss how to measure improvements in QI.

> In the world of improvement, everybody has two jobs. They have their job, then they have the job of improving their job.
>
> —Don Berwick

Introduction

The philosophy that undergirds this chapter is summarized in the epigraph quote from Dr. Don Berwick, one of the founders of the Institute for Healthcare Improvement (IHI, 2018). Dr. Berwick's words emphasize that **quality improvement** (**QI**), or, more precisely, the process of improving the quality of care, is the responsibility of everyone on the healthcare team, from novice to expert. Nurses who understand the importance of QI are committed not only to performing their job (e.g., caring for patients during a shift) but also to improving their job through QI initiatives. Quality improvement, also known as process improvement (PI), is a framework used to systematically improve care at the local level (National Academies of Sciences, Engineering, and Medicine et al., 2018).

In Chapters 1–3, you were introduced to the concepts of quality and safety and the steps of the EBP process. In this chapter, we provide you with an introduction to QI that covers its background as well as various models, frameworks to guide initiatives, and strategies to successfully measure improvements found during EBPQI initiatives. We hope that as a future nurse beginning your clinical journey, you will find the tools and practical information in this chapter useful as you commit to improving and sustaining the quality of patient care.

Defining Quality Improvement

Within the nursing profession, there are three levels of clinician inquiry: research, EBP, and QI, as we explained in Chapter 1 (Carter et al., 2021; Roe-Prior, 2022). Each of these levels seeks to improve the quality of care provided to patients, but they approach that aim in different ways. Nursing research is inquiry driven and seeks to generate new knowledge using a systematic problem-solving approach and a formal research design (Melnyk & Fineout-Overholt, 2022); EBP is a systematic problem-solving approach driven by evidence (hence the term *evidence*-based practice), which seeks to translate research findings into clinical practice (Melnyk & Fineout-Overholt, 2022); and quality improvement is a data-driven problem-solving approach that seeks to improve workflow processes that are specific to the local area (Provost & Murray, 2011). Additionally, a primary goal of QI is to reduce variation in a process and achieve predictable results so that care is equitable, consistent, and reliable across patients. For example, suppose that you and your nursing colleagues use various methods of obtaining blood cultures based on your personal preferences. The variations in practice could lead to inconsistent care and result in some patients not receiving optimal, evidence-based care. A QI initiative could provide structure and step-by-step instructions for how to best obtain a blood culture, thus reducing the variation between nurses and improving the overall quality and rigor of blood culture acquisition.

Although the three levels of clinical inquiry in nursing are distinct, they can overlap. For example, projects can integrate best evidence from research with EBP to improve local workflow processes (i.e., QI). Throughout this textbook, we have referred to this synergy between levels as EBPQI, depicted by the mountain model (Waldrop & Dunlap, 2024). Combining EBP and QI can significantly enhance a project's impact on the quality of patient care (Reynolds & Granger, 2023). Let's consider again the example from the previous paragraph about variation in obtaining blood cultures. Suppose you are a nurse who seeks to explore this issue. You might begin by looking in the literature to identify best practices for drawing a blood culture specimen (i.e., EBP). Next, you could review the current process (or processes) used by nurses in your work setting to obtain blood cultures (i.e., QI). Let's further suppose that you find that the variation in nurses' practices is the result of having different supplies located in separate places. You, or perhaps a team that you form, could create several "blood culture kits" with all the necessary supplies to appropriately collect blood cultures, and you could place these kits conveniently in areas where they are likely to be needed. You have now used both EBP and QI (EBPQI) to provide a more effective strategy and improve patient care!

Background of Quality Improvement

Providing quality care to patients has been an essential principle of care practice since the time of Hippocrates. As we discussed in Chapter 1, clinicians have been working for hundreds of years to improve the quality of care practice. During the Crimean War, Florence Nightingale notably highlighted improvements in basic sanitation measures that nurses could implement to reduce mortality (Nightingale, 1863). Nightingale began with meticulous data collection to identify variation in the processes of care provided to soldiers. When variability in handwashing was reduced, the health outcomes for soldiers improved significantly.

As mentioned in Chapter 2, educational entities and professional organizations have developed programming and curricula to provide clinicians with the knowledge, skills, and resources needed to improve the quality-of-care delivery. In addition, numerous accreditation and regulatory organizations have enacted guidelines and laws to hold clinicians accountable for implementing knowledge and have authorized penalties for failing to provide evidence-based care.

One international organization that has been a leader in quality improvement is the Institute for Healthcare Improvement (IHI), founded by Dr. Don Berwick. Although IHI was officially established in 1991, its work began in the late 1980s as part of the National Demonstration Project on Quality Improvement in Health Care (IHI, n.d.). The goal of IHI is to redesign healthcare in a way that decreases errors, waste, delays, and unnecessary healthcare costs through use of practical QI methods. IHI has many resources that provide clinicians with the knowledge and skills needed to conduct QI initiatives (see Chapter 13 for continuing education opportunities through IHI).

Identifying Quality Improvement Opportunities

Now that we have reviewed how QI began and why it is important, we can discuss how to conduct QI initiatives in healthcare settings. The first question we often hear from nurses is "How do I know what to focus on for a quality improvement project?" Ideas for identifying a problem were presented in Chapter 2. Once you have chosen a problem on which you want to focus, you should begin by describing the current status. For this initial phase in the process, strategies and tools such as benchmarking and balanced scorecards are useful. *Balanced scorecards* are tools that help you and your team visualize how your unit or organization is performing compared to other units or organizations; they are used to identify areas for improvement, communicate strategies for improvement, and track progress toward specific improvement goals. These tools provide data that can serve as a baseline: a quick snapshot of the level of quality being generated by current care processes and the areas in which improvement is needed. *Benchmarking* involves comparing characteristics of hospitals or units to see how your setting compares with similar settings on quality metrics. Benchmark data routinely comes from external agencies, such as the following:

- The National Healthcare Safety Network (NHSN), a national infection tracking system within the Centers for Disease Control and Prevention (CDC, 2021), reports healthcare-associated infections (e.g., catheter-associated urinary tract infections [CAUTIs], central line-associated bloodstream infections [CLABSIs], surgical site infections [SSIs]).
- The National Database for Nursing Quality Indicators (NDNQI), a part of Press Ganey, measures nurse-sensitive indicators such as healthcare-associated infections, falls, and pressure injuries; readmissions; and nursing turnover (Montalvo, 2007).
- The Joint Commission, an independent, nonprofit organization that provides voluntary evaluation and accreditation for hospitals and healthcare organizations, also provides disease-specific quality metrics (e.g., a Comprehensive Stroke Center has numerous quality metrics that relate to quality of stroke care).

Balanced scorecards are often used to examine internal data and perhaps to benchmark units against their previous performance. For example, a medical/surgical unit's fall rate may be benchmarked against performance the prior calendar year. Balanced scorecards, or a similar type of unit-based "report card," should be viewed regularly because they typically contain important quality metrics that can help nurses to easily determine areas in need of QI.

Most often, your desire to engage in quality improvement will be fueled by data. You may look at benchmarked data or the data on your unit's balanced scorecard and realize that processes are not as effective or efficient as they could be. You may have a clinical experience of a process that is inefficient or ineffective and resolve to improve it.

BOX 9.1: BALANCED SCORECARD EXAMPLE FOR THE MEDICAL INTENSIVE CARE UNIT (MICU) AT NATIONAL HOSPITAL

This example of a balanced scorecard for a MICU reveals multiple areas of opportunity for QI. Based on the provided metrics, instances of falls, CAUTIs, and CLABSIs are way over their target rates. As such, you should focus your nursing QI efforts on these areas (rather than on SSIs or falls with injury).

Quality metric	Target rate	Current rate
Falls per 1,000 patient days	1.0	1.5
Falls with injury per 1,000 patient days	1.0	0.5
Hospital-acquired pressure injuries per 1,000 patient days	2.0	2.0
CAUTIs per 1,000 indwelling urinary catheter days	1.3	5.5
CLABSIs per 1,000 central line days	0.8	3.5
SSIs per 1,000 patient days	1.0	0.95

Blue:
Exceeds expectations

Green:
Fully achieves/meeting targets

Yellow:
Between prior year's average performance (or similar) and fully achieves

Red:
Below prior year's average performance

Prioritizing Quality Improvement Projects

Your examination of data from balanced scorecards and benchmarks as well as your clinical practice experiences will likely provide several potential QI initiative ideas. As shown in Box 9.1, our hypothetical MICU has more than one metric that is underperforming. On which metric(s) will you focus? As you decide, you must think through these key questions:

- Is this topic a recurring or chronic issue?
- Is it specific and measurable?
- Does it have an operational or financial impact?
- Does the topic align with the organization's goals?

There are several tools available to help you narrow down your topic list and focus on specific QI initiatives. The first option is a **PICK chart**, which is a lean Six Sigma tool used to prioritize improvement ideas. It has four quadrants, measured in terms of "payoff" (low or high) and "difficulty" (easy to hard). These quadrants represent four categories into which ideas are sorted: **P**ossible idea (low payoff and easy), **I**mplement idea (high payoff and easy), **C**hallenge idea (high payoff and hard), and **K**ill idea (low payoff and hard). To identify priority topics, team members sort ideas into the most suitable quadrants. The ideas in the "Kill" quadrant

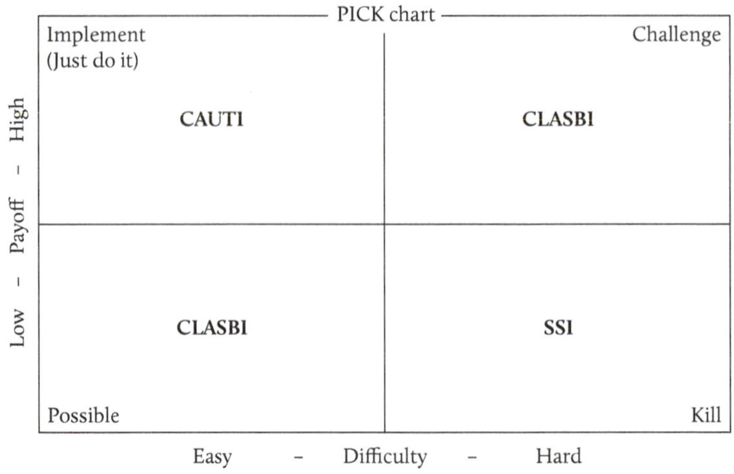

FIGURE 9.1 PICK Chart

should generally not be considered. The ideas in the "Possible" quadrant are not a priority to pursue. The team may consider whether some of the ideas in the "Challenge" quadrant might be worth pursuing in the future, given the high payoff, if the effort can be made easier. The ideas in the "Implement" quadrant, however, are easy to implement and yield a high payoff, so they are likely your best choices.

Another option for prioritizing your ideas is the aptly named *prioritization matrix* (Granger, 2008; IHI, 2016). There are numerous templates available online, but you can make your own matrix with criteria that are important to your organization. Solving a problem or achieving an improvement goal can require time, effort, and perhaps funding. A prioritization matrix can help you to calculate which competitive projects are most urgently needed, will be most beneficial or impactful, can be addressed with available resources, and are of greatest interest to your team members. The criteria (ideally developed by your team) could result from your consideration of the key questions we mentioned earlier or from your answers to other questions, such as the following:

- Resources: Are needed resources readily available?
- Feasibility: Is the opportunity actionable/feasible?
- Urgency: How soon does this issue need to be addressed?

You will want to consider and discuss questions such as these with your team in order to determine your criteria. After you have determined the criteria, devise a useful rating scale (e.g., 1–5, 1–10) and rate each item as a team in terms of its importance to address. Total the scores and make your final selection(s) after a full discussion to ensure consensus within your team. The selections do not necessarily need to be the items with the highest rating, although higher scores often indicate higher priority.

BOX 9.2: PRIORITIZATION MATRIX FOR THE MEDICAL INTENSIVE CARE UNIT AT NATIONAL HOSPITAL

A prioritization matrix can help healthcare institutions identify priority areas. In the MICU at National Hospital, three areas of opportunity were identified. Box 9.2 provides an example of the prioritization matrix. Each of the criteria was rated by the multidisciplinary team on a scale of 1 (*not at all a priority*) to 5 (*extremely high priority*). When the scores were added, CLABSI received the highest score. As such, the leadership team may consider focusing their EBPQI efforts on CLABSI.

	Fall rate	CAUTI rate	CLABSI rate
Does the topic align with the organization's goals?	5	5	5
Is there a large financial impact?	3	4	5
Is the opportunity actionable (e.g., areas of opportunity are available)?	3	3	4
Are needed resources readily available?	3	4	5
Total:	14	16	19

Writing an Aim Statement

After a QI initiative topic has been identified, your team should develop a **SMART aim statement** (as discussed in Chapter 3). Clinicians are often excited and want to begin implementing changes and improvements immediately; however, before beginning an EBPQI initiative, it is important to clarify a solid aim that you and the team are attempting to accomplish. A well-written aim statement can be (although it need not be) a formal document, sometimes referred to as a *charter* (IHI provides a clear template for this to guide you). A clear aim is an effective and valuable way of letting leaders know the goals of your project and defining the timeframe of the initiative. It can aid your selection of team members and help the team to avoid unwanted variations from the original purpose that can waste time and resources. A SMART aim statement is the generally accepted standard for writing aims or goals that are effective, measurable, and useful for focusing team efforts (Bjerke & Renger, 2017).

Let's return to the MICU example from National Hospital. In Box 9.3, the team has prioritized working on the CLABSI rate as their QI project. Their aim statement may look something like this: "Reduce CLABSI rates by 20% in the MICU at National Hospital within 6 months." As you develop your aim, take time to consider your wording carefully, work as a team, and be prepared to refocus the aim if necessary. Create a solid aim statement that will contribute to a successful project. Remember that a problem well stated is a problem half solved!

An aim statement is different from a PICO or PPCO question, which is used for discovery of evidence, as described in Chapter 3. An aim statement guides the EBPQI initiative, but PICO or PPCO questions provide a framework to guide the literature search. As you will recall, not all elements of the PICO format need be used. A PICO question for the MICU project might look something like this: "For patients admitted to the MICU (P), what evidence-based practices (I) could reduce CLABSI rates (O)?" A PPCO question might be a better choice in this instance; the first "P" could refer to the general problem of CLASBIs, and the PPCO question might look something like this: "For patients admitted to the MICU (P), what evidence-based practices (C) address CLASBI rates (O)?" Using these questions, the team would identify search strategies and terms (e.g., medical intensive care unit, evidence-based practices, central line–associated bloodstream infections) to guide the literature review. PICO questions do not contain measurable aims and outcomes. An aim statement, on the other hand, should follow the SMART format and include the overall outcome of interest to the team that is measurable (e.g., reducing CLABSIs by 20% within 6 months).

Models of Quality Improvement

Once a priority topic has been identified, your QI initiative can begin. There are many different models for improvement in healthcare. Although they all have the same goal (to improve quality of care), each model works to accomplish this goal in a slightly different way. In this chapter, we discuss several QI models commonly used in health systems. You will want to find out what model your healthcare organization uses so that you can align your project with it.

Lean

The lean model for quality improvement focuses on efficiency and waste reduction. The methodology is based on five principles: (a) define value, (b) map value stream, (c) create flow, (d) establish pull, and (e) pursue perfection. The goal of the first principle is to define the value of a process from the perspective of the recipient of the value (e.g., the patients, the staff, the organization). The goal of mapping the value stream is to identify all the activities that contribute to the defined value; activities that do not add value are considered waste. The lean model describes eight types of waste (see Box 9.3). After all waste has been removed from the value stream, the goal of the third principle is to ensure that the processes in the remaining steps flow together smoothly. The goal of the fourth principle is to establish a pull-based system in which products are provided (pulled) only when they are needed and in just the quantities needed. This principle ensures that needed materials are always available or delivered quickly but that unneeded inventory is limited, thus reducing waste (e.g., overcrowded stock space, ineffective use of staff time, expired or defective products).

The fifth step, pursuit of perfection, is the most important of all. Unlike the first four steps, which focus on value and preventing or removing waste, the fifth step seeks to make lean thinking (i.e., continuous problem solving and process improvement) part of the organizational culture at every level. This mode of thinking encourages every employee to strive toward perfection in delivering care based on changing patient needs, outcomes, and values (Lawal et al., 2014).

TABLE 9.1 Eight Types of Waste Described in the Lean QI Model

Type of waste	Examples
Defects	Hospital-acquired conditions (falls, infections, pressure injuries); avoidable readmissions
Overproduction	Duplication of laboratory tests; unnecessarily lengthened hospital stays
Waiting	Patients spending time in waiting rooms between provider consultations and blood collection in the lab
Transportation	Transport of patients between various departments; nurses gathering supplies and moving between rooms for one procedure
Inventory	Surplus supplies and medications; stockpiling outdated forms
Motion	Increased walking by hospital staff due to poor building design
Overprocessing	Patients entering repetitive information on multiple forms; nurses inputting repetitive data into multiple areas of the electronic health record
Untapped human potential	Healthcare personnel not working at the top of their license/scope of practice

BOX 9.3: LEAN PROCESS FOR THE MICU CLABSI PROJECT

For the MICU CLABSI project, the value (or aim) has been identified. The team can now map the value stream. Let us suppose that they want to map the process of nurses completing appropriate hand hygiene and daily chlorhexidine gluconate (CHG) baths. The image below identifies value-added and non-value-added steps.

Based on the value stream map, the team identifies several areas of opportunity for improvement in the CHG bath process. For example, to create flow, the team may decide to stock the CHG clothes closer to the point of use so the nurse is not required to walk 100 yards to gather the stock. They may consider moving the hand sanitizer dispensers so there is one right outside each patient's room. The team can also work with the supply department to establish pull by ensuring that the correct number of clothes are stocked in the warmer and that each hand sanitizer dispenser is refilled before it empties.

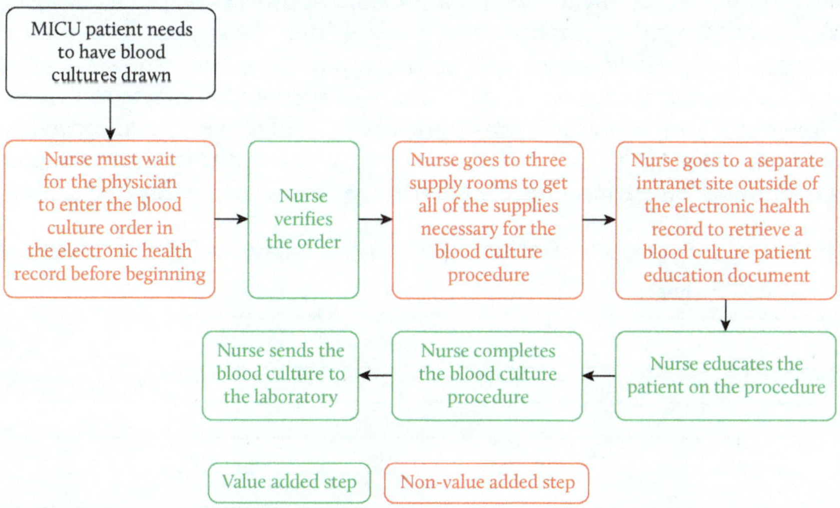

FIGURE 9.2 Value Stream Map

Define, Measure, Analyze, Improve, and Control (DMAIC)

Another type of QI model is Six Sigma, also referred to as define, measure, analyze, improve, and control (DMAIC). This commonly used approach includes steps to identify the problem, measure a baseline state, analyze the data received in the baseline state, and then implement and evaluate improvements. The model ends with a control, a unique feature of DMAIC, which requires putting in place sustainability measures (Shankar, 2009).

Plan-Do-Study-Act (PDSA)

The model for improvement, developed by IHI (2018), is one of the most common QI models available and incorporates iterative **plan-do-study-act (PDSA)** cycles. This model is the simplest approach to exploring QI processes: The first step is to plan and identify what the team aims to accomplish (this step is similar to the define phase in DMAIC).

Let's suppose that the MICU CLABSI project uses the PDSA model for improvement (see Box 9.4). The team's first step (plan) is to identify a goal. That's easy because the answer to "What are we trying to accomplish?" is the same as the aim statement: "Reduce CLABSI rates by 20% in the MICU at National Hospital within 6 months." The next step is to figure out how the team will know whether a change is an improvement. To do this, the team must identify measures to obtain feedback on whether changes are having a desired impact. Using the rates provided by the hospital's infection prevention department on the MICU balanced scorecard (Box 9.1), the outcome measure that will determine whether a change has made an improvement will be "CLABSI rate per 1,000 central line days." To help the team visualize whether improvements are being made, measures should be displayed on run charts or statistical process control charts to facilitate learning. Unlike simple pre- and post-implementation data, run and statistical process control charts provide feedback on measures throughout the initiative.

The next question in the model for improvement process is "What change can we make that will result in improvement?" Sometimes the answer is obvious, and the team easily identifies interventions that can address the issue successfully. Unfortunately, potential interventions or changes are not always apparent. In such cases, it is not uncommon for teams to resort to ineffective ways of developing change, such as using "more of the same" (e.g., more training, more people) or trying to develop "one perfect fix." Teams can get stuck as they search for an idea

TABLE 9.2 Comparison of the Six Sigma DMAIC and the Model for Improvement PDSA

DMAIC	PDSA
Define	Plan
Measure	Do
Analyze	Study
Improve	Act
Control	

or try to understand the problem(s) in the current process. This is why we suggest using known tools and strategies rather than brainstorming.

There are many tools to assist with identifying changes; for example, you could use a fishbone diagram, flowchart, histogram, Pareto chart, or driver diagram. A *fishbone diagram*, also known as a *cause-and-effect diagram*, displays possible causes and effects of a problem on a graph, along with the potential factors responsible (e.g., people, the environment, materials, methods, equipment).

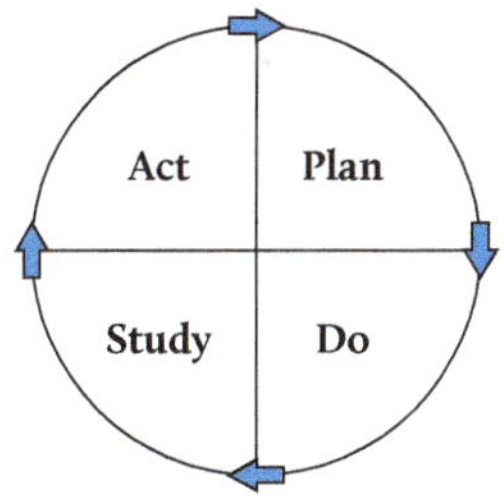

What are you hoping to achieve?
How will you know that what you changed worked?
What practice change can you make that will lead to improvement?

FIGURE 9.3 Institute for Healthcare Improvement's Model for Improvement

See Box 9.4 for an example of a fishbone diagram related to the MICU CLABSI project.

BOX 9.4: EXAMPLE OF A FISHBONE DIAGRAM

Here is an example of a fishbone diagram for the MICU's CLABSI project. Each "fishbone" represents an area that could affect the problem (i.e., CLABSIs, as noted at the far right). This display allows the team to identify various areas of opportunity that they can target for a QI project.

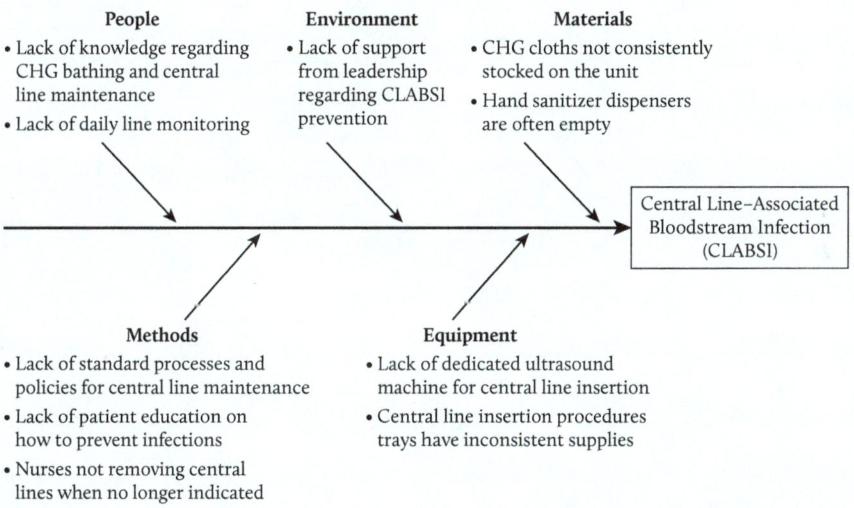

FIGURE 9.4 Fishbone Diagram

A *flowchart*, also known as a *process map*, visually represents the sequences of steps of a process. Laying out a process as it currently operates can help the team identify points at which inefficiencies regularly occur. See Box 9.5 for an example of a process flowchart.

BOX 9.5: EXAMPLE OF A PROCESS FLOWCHART

This process flowchart displays the process for inserting, maintaining, and removing a central line for a patient in our MICU example. Diamond shapes typically signify a decision point within the process. Outlining a process from beginning to end allows the team to identify potential roadblocks and areas for improvement.

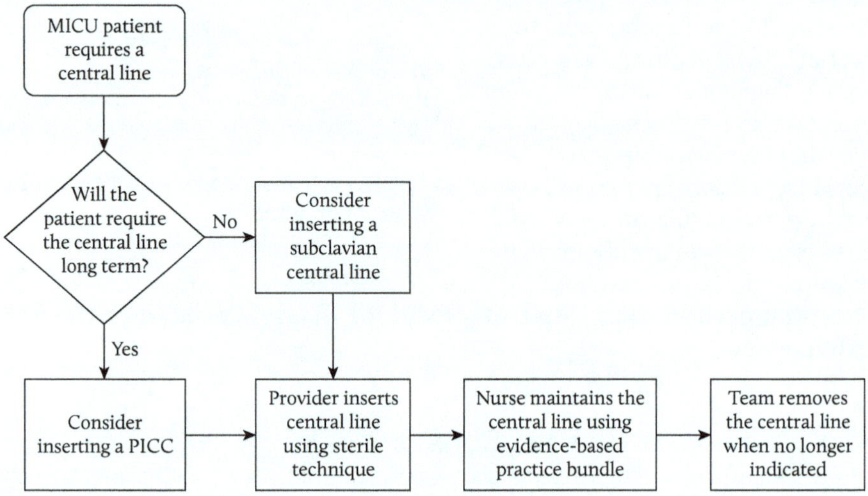

FIGURE 9.5 Process Flowchart 1

PICC = peripherally inserted central catheter

Here is another example of a process flowchart; this one outlines the steps a nurse would need to take to complete a daily CHG bath. Areas noted in red are opportunities for improvement within the process.

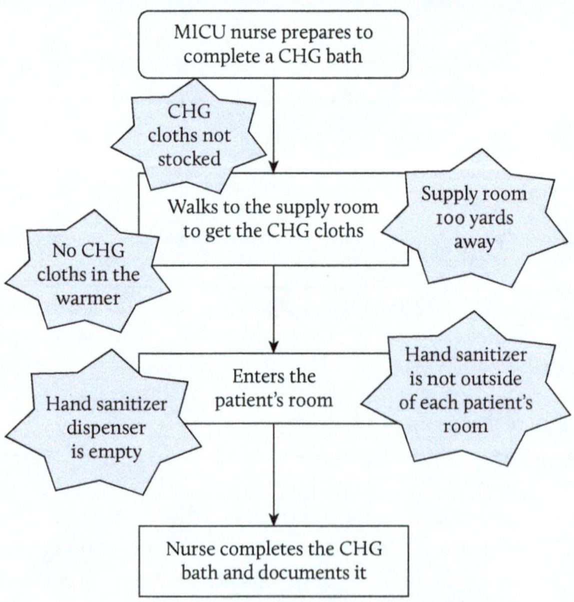

FIGURE 9.6 Process Flowchart 2

Histograms and Pareto charts both allow teams to recognize and analyze patterns that may be hiding in tables. A *Pareto chart*, which is a type of bar chart, displays contributing factors in order (from the largest to the smallest effect), thus allowing viewers to easily identify factors that are having the largest effect and warrant the most attention. A Pareto chart is an effective tool that can help your team target their improvement efforts to have the greatest impact (Provost & Murray, 2011). For example, let's say that nurses in the MICU regularly complete CLABSI prevention bundle audits. When put into a Pareto chart, this data can show the nursing staff the process areas with the most opportunity for improvement (Box 9.6).

BOX 9.6: PARETO CHART EXAMPLE FOR THE MICU CLABSI PROJECT

A Pareto chart provides a visual display of areas of opportunity. Various data categories are plotted on the *x*-axis, and frequency is plotted on the *y*-axis. The bars are ordered from left to right according to frequency (from highest to lowest). According to the Pareto principle (also known as the 80/20 rule), in any group of factors that contribute to an overall effect, roughly 80% of the effect is attributable to 20% of the causes. The Pareto chart in Box 9.5 provides CLABSI prevention bundle audit results; CHG bathing has the most "no" responses, which indicates areas of opportunity accounting for about 20% of the issues (orange line that represents the cumulative percentage). As such, the team may consider focusing their CLABSI prevention efforts on improving compliance with CHG bathing.

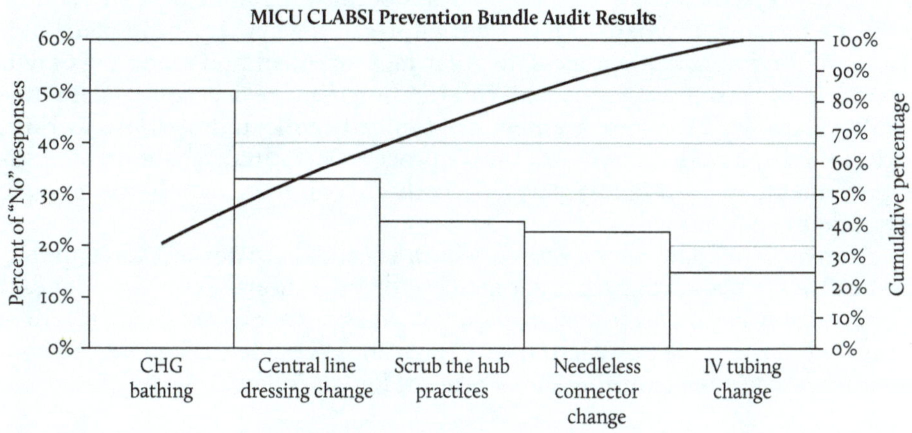

CHG = chlorhexidine gluconate; IV = intravenous

FIGURE 9.7 MICU CLABSI Prevention Bundle Audit Results

When the first three questions of the model for improvement have been answered, the team can move on to conduct PDSA cycles, which begin with planning the changes that will be implemented and tested. During the *planning phase*, the team ensures that the problem is well defined and that metrics are in place to measure the outcome; these metrics should be directly related to the aim statement.

In the *doing phase*, which follows the planning phase, the team implements the test of the change that was identified from Question 3. During this phase, data should be collected and initial analysis should occur. Beginning data collection and analysis at the start of the change allows the team to see whether the change is making an improvement or modifications need to be made (in the acting phase).

Next, in the *studying phase*, the team reviews the impact and outcomes of their test of change. Data is analyzed in more detail to see whether a change or improvement has occurred and, if so, to determine its magnitude. The use of run charts or statistical process control charts can help the team to monitor trends in performance and detect changes in outcomes quickly. In the *acting phase*, which is the final phase, the team determines whether the changes can be implemented as they are or further modifications are needed to refine the approach. If the change has been successful, the team must develop a long-term monitoring and evaluation plan to sustain the gains made. Ongoing monitoring can alert the team if performance begins to deteriorate (which is common after an initial QI project wraps up). If the change has not been successful (i.e., data show no improvements), then another approach or test of change should be implemented and another PDSA cycle begun.

Measuring Data for Quality Improvement

A common QI saying is "What gets measured gets done." Data is used ubiquitously in healthcare, which is fortunate for nurses because QI in healthcare requires feedback to show us where to focus our efforts and whether our implemented changes have improved a process. Regular measurement and reporting of data keeps teams focused, as they use this information to make decisions and improve results. Data used for improvement are typically collected by those working within the healthcare system to observe process performance, obtain ideas for improvement, and test changes to see whether an improvement has been made and is being maintained.

To ensure that data are measured accurately and consistently by members of the healthcare team, your team should develop operational definitions for each of their metrics. An *operational definition* is an agreement that a metric will be measured in the same way each time. There should be a definition, agreed upon by your team at the beginning of the project, for the following:

- What data will be collected?
- When will this data be collected (e.g., daily, weekly, monthly)?
- How will the data be collected (e.g., from the electronic health record, through patient surveys)?
- Who will collect this data?
- Where will this data be collected?

Often, an operational definition is converted into a checklist or form that delineates what is meant by "appropriate" or "complete" and helps multiple data collectors remain consistent in their use of the operational definition. To ensure consistency, it is helpful to create a checklist form for data collection.

Family of Measures

Now that you have determined how your team will measure data, you must think about developing a family of measures, including outcome, process, and balancing measures. Because healthcare systems are extremely complex, a single measure is inadequate to determine improvement. Multiple measures are necessary to best evaluate the impact of changes to improve a practice or process. Creating a family of measures will help you to answer Question 2 of the PDSA model for improvement: "How will we know whether a change is an improvement?" An overall project aim, as described previously, usually includes the main outcome measure, or what the aim is for the overall project. All improvement activities should include one or more outcome measures.

Continuing with our MICU example, the outcome measure of interest would be CLABSI rates. However, the project should also include some process and balancing measures. *Process measures* are useful because they are connected to the process of achieving the outcome measure(s) and typically show improvement before the outcome measure does. They provide early indicators of whether the changes being made are improvements. In the Pareto chart in Box 9.5, the biggest area of opportunity for CLABSI prevention is CHG bathing. Measuring compliance with CHG bathing over time would be a good process metric. Appropriately completing this process (CHG bathing) will help improve the outcome (CLABSI rates).

Balancing measures aid in detecting unintended consequences (e.g., skin reactions in patients who are allergic to CHG bathing). In a QI initiative, you want to ensure that while you are focusing on improving one aspect, the team does not inadvertently negatively impact another area of care.

Typically, a set of three to eight measures are recommended for improvement initiatives. Do not include too many measures, especially process measures, because collecting data for too many measures can reduce the time your team has to test changes and can make the project's data collection process overwhelming. For each measure, your team should include what they are measuring, the operational definition of the measure, and the data source for the measure. If helpful, the team can consider putting this information in a table to keep it organized, as in Table 9.3.

TABLE 9.3 Family of Measures for the MICU QI Project

Type of measure	Measure	Operational definition	Data source
Outcome	CLABSI rate	The number of CLABSIs that occurred in the MICU each month per 1,000 central line days	Hospital's infection prevention department
Process	CHG bathing documentation compliance	The percentage of patients who received a daily CHG bath per documentation divided by the total number of patients	Weekly audits conducted by QI team members using a standard audit form
Balancing	Skin reactions to CHG bathing	The number of patients who report having a skin reaction to the CHG cloths	Incident reports that have been entered by nurses after patients have reported skin reactions to CHG bathing

CLABSI = central line associated bloodstream infections; CHG = chlorhexidine gluconate

Run Charts

Once your team has identified a family of measures and operational definitions for each measure, it is time to plot the data on a run chart or control chart. Charts provide a visual display of data that are usually hidden within tables or text. A **run chart**, also known as a *trend chart*, is easy to construct and simple to interpret, and it provides a visual tool that allows the team to learn about the change process. Additionally, run charts can help the team determine whether a change has resulted in improvement and if gains are sustained. Although run charts can be developed on paper, it is most common to use a spreadsheet software program, such as Microsoft Excel® (using the line graph feature). Time should be displayed on the *x*-axis (e.g., in weeks, in months); the *y*-axis will display the unit of measurement (e.g., CLABSI rate, CHG compliance). The following data points should be plotted on the chart: the metric's data, median, and target. It is helpful to give the graph a title and label the *x*- and *y*-axis appropriately. Plotting data on run charts should begin as soon as you have your first data point; if available, you can plot prior baseline data (Provost & Murray, 2011).

BOX 9.7: BASELINE FAMILY OF MEASURES FOR THE MICU CLABSI PROJECT

Each of these run charts provides a quick visualization of the MICU's progress toward targets. For example, their target CLABSI rate is 0.8 CLABSIs per 1,000 central line days, based on information found in the balanced scorecard (Box 9.1); however, the unit's rate is much higher than this, with a median of 3.5. Similarly, the unit's target compliance for CHG bathing documentation is 95%, yet the median is only 54%. On the bright side, a relatively low number of patients (3; median 0, target of 0.3) have reported a skin reaction to CHG bathing over the past 10 months.

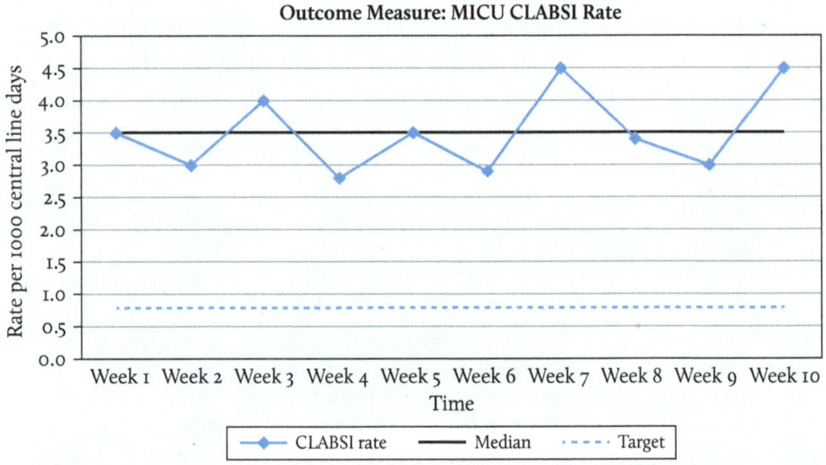

FIGURE 9.8 Outcome Measure: MICU CLABSI Rate

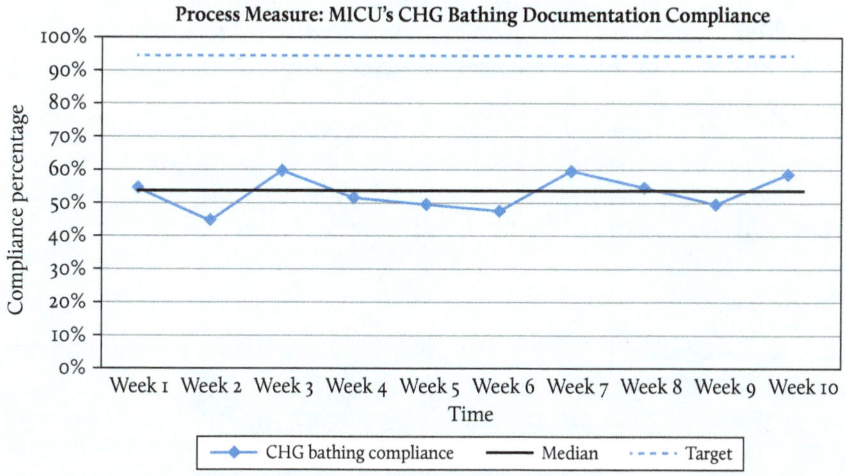

FIGURE 9.9 Process Measure: MICU's CHG Bathing Documentation Compliance

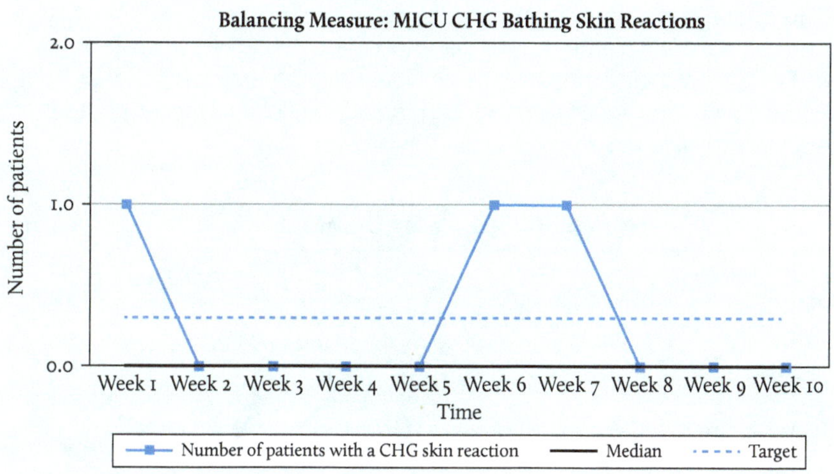

FIGURE 9.10 Balancing Measure: MICU CHG Bathing Skin Reactions

Once PDSA cycles begin, the median should be frozen and extended into the future, which will allow the team to identify improvements. Sometimes improvement is visually obvious; however, when this is not the case, probability-based "rules" for interpreting a run chart can be used to determine "signals" of improvement, or non-random evidence of change. Whereas a run chart can be developed from the beginning of the initiative, to use probability-based rules, at least 10 data points should be used to create the median. If one or more rules are identified, this indicates a signal of improvement. The two most common rules are the following:

- *Shift*: six or more consecutive points, either all above or all below the median; values that fall on the median do not add to or break a shift.
- *Trend*: five or more consecutive points, all going up or down.

It is important to review the run chart critically to determine whether a signal is an improvement (rather than a variation) and to avoid misinterpretation. For example, five data points all going up in the CLABSI run chart could be identified as a trend, although in the opposite direction of the target.

BOX 9.8: RUN CHARTS OF THE FAMILY OF MEASURES FOR THE MICU CLABSI PROJECT AFTER PDSA CYCLES BEGAN

After the PDSA cycles began in Week 10, the median was frozen and extended into the future (noted with a dashed median line). It is visually obvious that there have been improvements in both CLABSI rates and CHG bathing documentation compliance. Signals of improvement were also noted using probability-based rules. After PDSA cycles began, there were eight data points below the median for CLABSI, with 10 data points above the median for CHG bathing documentation compliance, indicating a shift. Additionally, both measures saw a trend, with five or more data points all going up or down. For the balancing measure, there were relatively no changes, indicating that increased compliance with CHG bathing did not lead to higher numbers of patients with skin reactions.

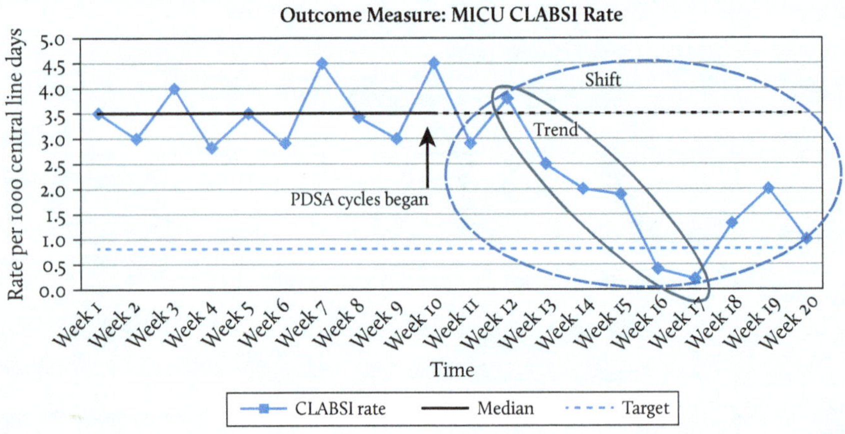

FIGURE 9.11 Outcome Measure: MICU CLABSI Rate

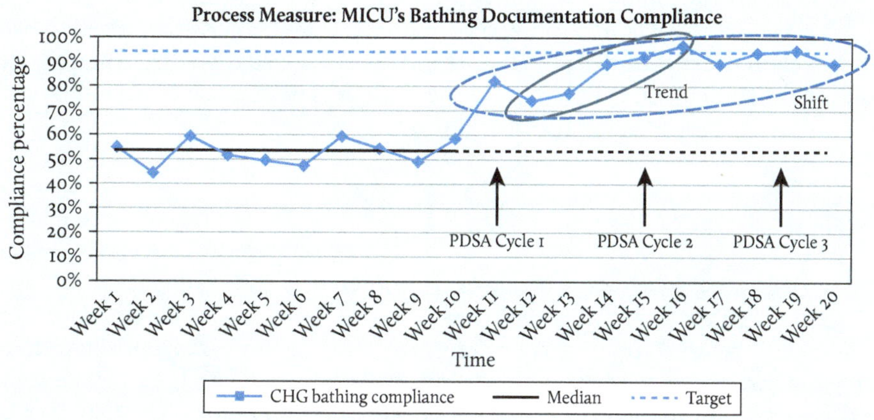

FIGURE 9.12 Process Measure: MICU's CHG Bathing Documentation Compliance

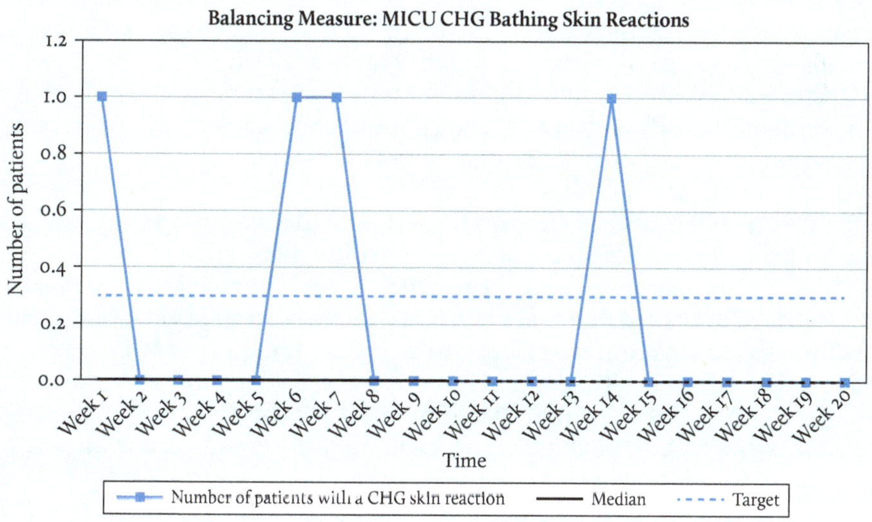

FIGURE 9.13 Balancing Measure: MICU CHG Bathing Skin Reactions

When tests of change result in improvements, it may be useful to create a new, second median for the new data representing improved performance. Some judgment is required to decide whether the improvement has been sustained long enough to warrant a new median. For example, in the CHG bathing compliance graph, improvement began immediately following the start of the PDSA cycles and was sustained; as such, the team may consider calculating a new median with data from Weeks 11–20.

Data collection should continue until the gains are sustained; once sustained, the frequency of data collection can be reduced (e.g., from once a week to every other week or every month). It is important to continue data collection long term and plot the data on the run chart; if the data gets worse, the team will see this and can act quickly to remedy the situation.

Statistical Process Control Charts

A **statistical process control chart** (also known as a SPC chart, control chart, or Shewhart chart) is another tool that can help teams visualize improvements in their data related to process characteristics. There are common variations present in any process; a control chart is useful because it can identify the source of process variation and process changes over time. In addition to the data line and target, a control chart contains three additional lines: mean, upper control limit (UCL), and lower control limit (LCL). The UCL is calculated by taking the mean *plus* 3 times the standard deviation; the LCL is calculated by taking the mean *minus* 3 times the standard deviation (also known as *three sigma deviations from the mean*). The UCL and LCL help determine whether variation in the data is in "control" (within the two lines) or out of control (outside the two lines), thus allowing the team to monitor the stability and variation within a process and alerting them to problems that might need to be corrected. Similar to "signals of improvement" identified in run charts, a control chart can detect "special causes of variation" (e.g., causes that are uncommon or unpredictable) in the data due to the addition of the UCL and LCL.

Both run charts and control charts are useful and provide valuable data for a QI project, but they have some important differences. Control charts are more rigorous but require more data. A run chart requires at least 10 baseline data points to calculate the median to use probability-based rules, but a control chart requires at least 20 baseline data points to calculate the mean, UCL, and LCL. Teams that do not have 20 baseline data points can use a run chart, but if enough baseline data is available, the team should consider using a control chart. If 20 baseline data points are available and the UCL and LCL have been calculated, the team should lock these limits and extend them into the future; this will help the team to judge the process moving forward and identify indicators of special cause variation (Provost & Murray, 2011).

Similar to the rules for interpreting a run chart, there are also rules for appropriately interpreting a control chart. The occurrence of any one rule is an indication of special cause variation. Rules can provide evidence of an improvement to a process or show "losing" gains made previously. Below are the most common rules:

- *Shift*: eight or more data points, all above or below the mean.
- *Trend*: five or more consecutive data points, all increasing or decreasing.
- *Out of UCL or LCL*: a single data point is outside of the control limits.

BOX 9.9: STATISTICAL PROCESS CONTROL CHARTS FOR THE MICU CLABSI PROJECT AFTER PDSA CYCLES BEGAN

Box 9.9 uses control charts rather than run charts to present data similar to that presented in Box 9.8. Note that the CLABSI rate, in addition to a shift and a trend, shows four data points outside of the LCL, indicating special cause variation. Similarly, the CHG bathing control chart shows a shift with all data points falling above the UCL, also indicating special cause variation.

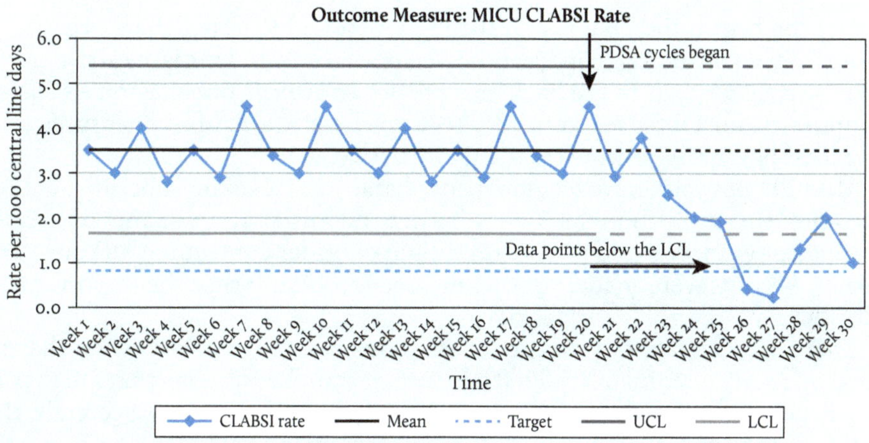

FIGURE 9.14 Outcome Measure: MICU CLABSI Rate

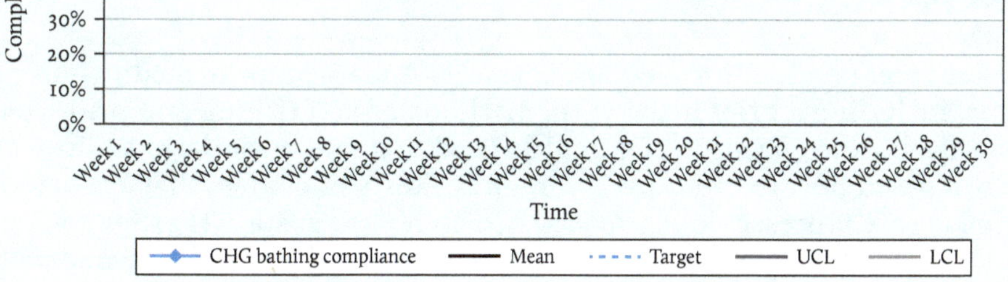

FIGURE 9.15 Process Measure: MICU's CHG Bathing Documentation Compliance

To monitor progress in EBPQI initiatives, it is essential to display the data visually so you can identify when improvements are being made. Whether your team chooses run charts or statistical process control charts, data visualization tools should be used. Once charts are made, information should be continuously fed back to your frontline team (those who are making the change in practice) so they can view their progress and either celebrate successes or discuss future tests of change.

Sustainability in Quality Improvement

During the beginning phases and throughout a QI initiative, there is generally enthusiasm when gains are made; however, once the initial initiative drive is over, it can be easy for staff to fall back into previous patterns of behavior. As such, it is important for QI teams to think about future sustainability measures, even when first beginning to construct a QI initiative.

After PDSA cycles have been instituted and your team has obtained data on outcomes, the team should review whether the initial aim was met. If the aim was not achieved, you and your team should consider continuing on your PDSA journey. If gains were made, your team needs to ensure that the improvements will "stick."

There are several key points that QI teams need to consider when they are thinking about sustainability. First, they must stabilize systems that are in place or, in other words, hardwire them into the culture and workflow. Secondly, they must avoid the pitfall of person-dependent systems so that if one person leaves the healthcare system, the sustained gains can be maintained. Whereas it is helpful to have a "project leader," the team needs to ensure that this person is not responsible for all aspects of the project. Lastly, the team should consider long-term monitoring of the process and outcome measures. For our MICU CLABSI initiative, this would entail continuously monitoring CLABSI rates and CHG bathing documentation compliance long term and plotting the data on either a run chart or statistical process control chart. Plotting the data on a chart will help the team readily identify times when gains are not being sustained (Granger, 2020).

WRAPPING UP

This chapter provided an overview of (a) the fundamentals of quality improvement, including a brief history; (b) methods of identifying and prioritizing QI projects; and (c) various QI models used to guide initiatives. Additionally, we discussed how to measure and monitor tests of change that are made to improve care processes and provided tips on how to sustain these gains. Don't forget that improving the quality of patient care is the job of everyone on the healthcare team!

WELLNESS IN ACTION: DANCING

At a recent retreat for authors of this book, after a long day of work and writing, some of us gathered around a campfire and made s'mores while others put on a new playlist of songs and danced. All of us instantly experienced relaxation and joy as we engaged in wellness activities to promote positive health effects on our brains and bodies.

Dancing has several documented health benefits. It can boost memory and support cognition (Predovan et al., 2019; Verghese et al., 2003); increase mindfulness and enhance life quality (Laird et al., 2021); and improve heart, muscle, and bone health through physical movement such as twisting and turning (CDC, 2023). The next time you feel stress or desire a change in energy level after a mentally taxing experience (maybe that moment is right now and you are ready to celebrate getting to the end of this chapter), consider dancing out your stress/energy. Just find a comfortable place, crank up your favorite song (or playlist), and start moving!

If you enjoy your dance experience, you might schedule a regular dance session into your life plan or just continue to use this wellness activity spontaneously (or maybe both). Dance can be a solo or group activity, so you get to pick your desired place and the people who will join you. The goal is to make you feel better during dancing, after dancing, and as you improve your health. No matter the dancing style you choose, try to make dance a part of your overall wellness routine, and have fun doing it!

REFLECTION QUESTIONS

1. As a nurse interested in completing a EBPQI initiative, how will you prioritize a topic on which to focus when numerous areas of improvement are needed?
2. Your team is interested in improving efficiency and reducing waste. Which quality improvement models should you discuss using?
3. Why is a blending of EBP and QI an optimal approach for your team's improvement initiatives?

REFERENCES

Bjerke, M. B., & Renger, R. (2017). Being smart about writing SMART objectives. *Evaluation and Program Planning, 61*, 125–127. https://doi.org/10.1016/j.evalprogplan.2016.12.009

Carter, E. J., Usseglio, J., Pahlevan-Ibrekic, C., Vose, C., Rivera, R. R., & Larson, E. L. (2021). Differentiating research and quality improvement activities: A scoping review and implications for clinical scholarship. *Journal of Clinical Nursing, 30*(17–18), 2480–2488. https://doi.org/10.1111/jocn.15668

Centers for Disease Control and Prevention. (2021, April 1). *National Healthcare Safety Network*. https://www.cdc.gov/nhsn/index.html

Centers for Disease Control and Prevention. (2023, February 24). *Help your brain stay sharp*. https://www.cdc.gov/nccdphp/dnpao/features/physical-activity-brain-health/index.html

Granger, B. B. (2008). Practical steps for evidence-based practice: Putting one foot in front of the other. *AACN Advanced Critical Care, 19*(3), 314–324. https://doi.org/01256961-200807000-00011

Granger, B. B. (2020). Six simple steps to sustainability: A checklist for ongoing monitoring of clinical practice improvements. *AACN Advanced Critical Care, 31*(2), 203–209. https://doi.org/10.4037/aacnacc2020667

Institute for Healthcare Improvement. (n.d.). *History of Institute for Healthcare Improvement.* Retrieved May 15, 2023, from https://www.ihi.org:443/about/Pages/History.aspx

Institute for Healthcare Improvement. (2016, September 6). *Priority matrix: An overlooked gardening tool* [Video]. YouTube. https://www.youtube.com/watch?v=PtEMrYVGGgI

Institute for Healthcare Improvement. (2018). *How to improve with the model for improvement.* https://www.ihi.org:443/education/IHIOpenSchool/resources/Pages/QI-102-How-to-Improve-with-the-Model-for-Improvement.aspx

Laird, K. T., Vergeer, I., Hennelly, S. E., & Siddarth, P. (2021). Conscious dance: Perceived benefits and psychological well-being of participants. *Complementary Therapies in Clinical Practice, 44*, Article 101440. https://doi.org/10.1016/j.ctcp.2021.101440

Lawal, A. K., Rotter, T., Kinsman, L., Sari, N., Harrison, L., Jeffery, C., Kutz, M., Khan, M. F., & Flynn, R. (2014). Lean management in health care: Definition, concepts, methodology and effects reported (systematic review protocol). *Systematic Reviews, 3*, 103. https://doi.org/10.1186/2046-4053-3-103

Melnyk, B. M., & Fineout-Overholt, E. (2022). *Evidence-based practice in nursing & healthcare: A guide to best practice.* Lippincott Williams & Wilkins.

Montalvo, I. (2007). The National Database of Nursing Quality Indicators (NDNQI). *Online Journal of Issues in Nursing, 12*(3). https://doi.org/10.3912/OJIN.Vol12No03Man02

National Academies of Sciences, Engineering, and Medicine, Health and Medicine Division, Board on Health Care Services, Board on Global Health, & Committee on Improving the Quality of Health Care Globally. (2018). *Crossing the global quality chasm: Improving health care worldwide.* National Academies Press.

Nightingale, F. (1863). *Notes on hospitals* (3rd ed.). Longman, Roberts, and Green.

Predovan, D., Julien, A., Esmail, A., & Bherer, L. (2019). Effects of dancing on cognition in healthy older adults: A systematic review. *Journal of Cognitive Enhancement, 3*(2), 161–167. https://doi.org/10.1007/s41465-018-0103-2

Provost, L. P., & Murray, S. K. (2011). *The health care data guide: Learning from data for improvement.* Jossey-Bass.

Reynolds, S. S., & Granger, B. B. (2023). Implementation science toolkit for clinicians: Improving adoption of evidence in practice. *Dimensions of Critical Care Nursing, 42*(1), 33–41. https://doi.org/10.1097/DCC.0000000000000556

Roe-Prior, P. (2022). Questioning the answers, answering the questions: Evidence-based practice, quality improvement, and research. *Journal for Nurses in Professional Development, 38*(2), 114. https://doi.org/10.1097/NND.0000000000000861

Shankar, R. (2009). *Process improvement using Six Sigma: A DMAIC guide.* Quality Press.

Verghese, J., Lipton, R. B., Katz, M. J., Hall, C. B., Derby, C. A., Kuslansky, G., Ambrose, A. F., Sliwinski, M., & Buschke, H. (2003). Leisure activities and the risk of dementia in the elderly. *New England Journal of Medicine, 348*(25), 2508–2516. https://doi.org/10.1056/NEJMoa022252

Waldrop, J. & Dunlap, J.J. (2024). The Mountain Model for Evidence-Based Practice Quality Improvement Initiatives, *American Journal of Nursing,* In Press

IMAGE CREDITS

Fig. 9.1: Source: https://www.phf.org/resourcestools/Documents/PICK_Chart.pdf.
Fig. 9.3: Source: Adapted from https://www.ihi.org/resources/Pages/HowtoImprove/default.aspx.

CHAPTER 10

The Nurse's Role in Implementation of EBPQI Initiatives

Julee Briscoe Waldrop and Jayne Jennings Dunlap

KEY CONCEPTS

Implementation
Human subjects protection
Stakeholders
Buy-in
Facilitators
Barriers

LEARNING OBJECTIVES

1. Identify the implementation process for EBPQI initiatives.
2. Discover the importance of human subjects protection.
3. Explore purpose statements and multidisciplinary team formation.
4. Discuss integration and sustainability of practice changes.

> Positive progress towards excellence—that's what we want. If you stand still and settle for the status quo, that's exactly what you will have.
>
> —Hazel Johnson-Brown

Introduction

Ready, set, go! If you have read this far, you have likely observed a problem in healthcare as a patient, family member, or student nurse that you would like to improve. Problems or issues can be identified by anyone who is part of the healthcare experience. You know that identifying the problem is the first step in improvement, so you are on your way! Remember your

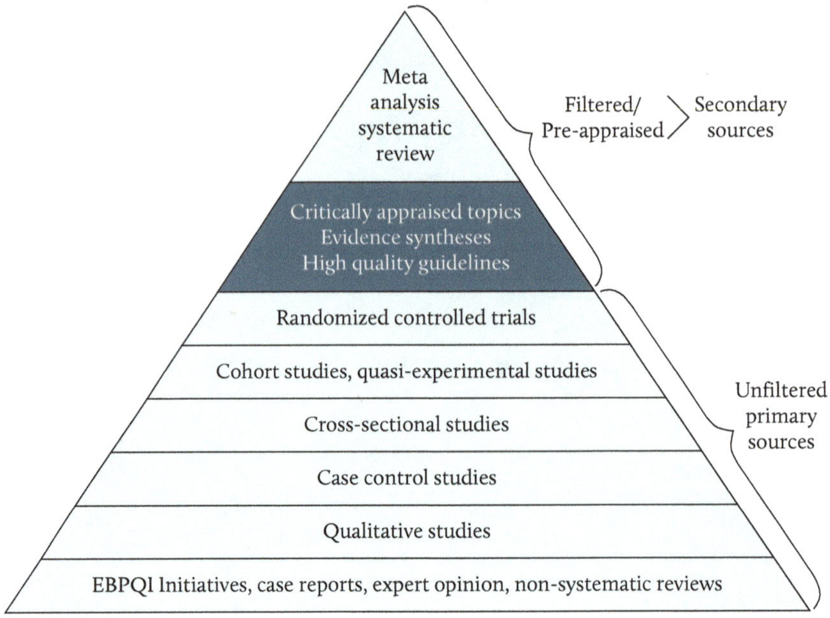

FIGURE 10.1 Hierarchy of Evidence Pyramid

power pose from Chapter 1? Embrace the opportunity to pose again because you are ready to make a change. This chapter focuses on the actual **implementation** of your EBPQI initiative—on the specifics of *doing* the initiative—so prepare to mobilize support for your practice change. We are approaching the top of the mountain model; this framework provides guidance for all EBPQI initiatives and can be used in conjunction with other detailed EBP or QI models during implementation of practice changes.

The Iowa model-revised (Cullen et al., 2022) is the most frequently used EBP process tool in magnet facilities (Speroni et al., 2020) and provides a roadmap for addressing all types of issues in healthcare. We will use the Iowa model in this chapter as a guide to the EBPQI process.

The Trigger

The *trigger* is simply the problem or issue in practice that you have identified and want to address. As we described in Chapter 2, identifying a trigger upon which to act is a key point of this textbook. Healthcare is not perfect; nurses' input is needed to address problematic issues to improve the system so that the quality and safety of patient care is optimized.

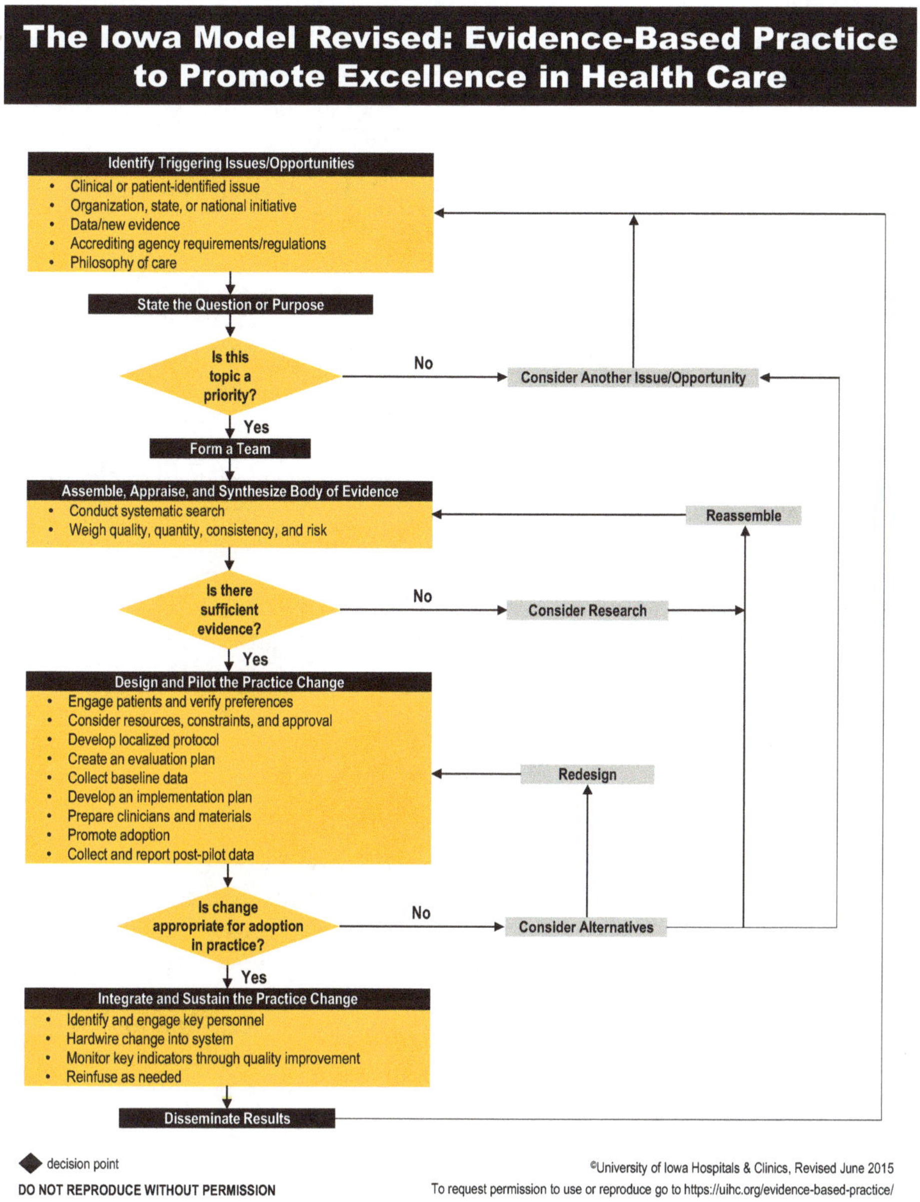

FIGURE 10.2 Updated Iowa Model

State the Question or Purpose

In Chapter 4, you learned how to write various types of questions to guide your search for evidence. Use one of those options (e.g., PPCO) that works for you to get started. You have also learned how to write purpose statements and SMART aims as you begin the process. Specifying the desired outcome of your EBPQI initiative will help you to communicate successfully with stakeholders (such as leaders in your organization) and facilitate their understanding of the benefits of supporting your initiative.

Determine Organizational Support: Is It a Priority?

If your organization does not support your initiative or has valid reasons (e.g., insufficient resources, anticipated personnel changes) to delay implementation of your recommended practice change, don't give up! Consider asking your leaders to share their concerns or outline the issues that they would like to see addressed before approving implementation. If you agree with their points, consider whether you can work on solutions. If organizational solutions are already in the planning stage, you can seek an opportunity to join the team. Of course, if your organization agrees with your recommended process change, you can pat yourself on the back and move ahead to form a team. Otherwise, consider what you have learned from this experience and be on the lookout for the next problem to solve. Every experience in your nursing career will make you wiser and more prepared as a problem solver and patient advocate.

Form a Team

Before you form a team, you must thoughtfully identify any people, environments, processes, or products likely to be affected by your proposed practice change. What behaviors, situations, or settings will be impacted when the innovation is implemented? As you determine who might make a good team member, remember that a successful solution takes into account multiple viewpoints; try not to overlook any persons or roles involved in your solution. Your first undertaking as a team will be to gather evidence on the problem in general and in your local context specifically; this effort can benefit from team members' diverse experiences and input.

Conduct a Systematic Search of the Evidence (the Literature)

A systematic search of the evidence is the hallmark of EBP (and thus a primary focus of this book). It forms the foundation in the mountain model (Waldrop & Dunlap, 2024) because research or practice change will be unfounded and potentially dangerous without it. However, in order to answer the essential question of whether sufficient evidence exists to change practice, you must use your clinical question to search the literature as well as your critical appraisal skills to judge the literature (Chapters 5–7). You will undoubtedly feel disappointed if you determine that the answer to this critical question is "no," but occasional disappointment is to be expected when working with evidence. In fact, you will find that a lack of or gap in evidence often presents an opportunity to engage in research and the production of a more solid foundation of new knowledge to support problem solving in the future.

Consider Research

You are familiar with basic characteristics of research studies, such as design, sample, measurement tools, and statistical analysis of results; however, because you care about the health of people, most of the research studies you have read likely included human beings. The most important part of a research study is its participants (sometimes called *subjects*). Always value them. Ask yourself, "What are their rights?" and "What are the responsibilities of the organizations who fund the research or for whom the participants work?" Most important of all, you and your team must determine and commit to doing whatever is needed to ensure your subjects' safety, privacy, and dignity.

As an example, let's suppose that in an RCT of a new drug for cancer, participants with cancer will be randomly assigned to receive either the experimental drug or a placebo. You might find yourself wondering, "What if this drug works yet only some receive it?" or "What if it provides no benefit to participants who could have taken a more beneficial drug instead?" You may even worry, "What if the experimental drug causes harm?" All researchers must consider the potential risks and benefits of the research process as well as ensure human subject protection, so you may be wondering how it is possible to do this and still answer research questions. Rest assured that you have explicit guidance to follow in this respect! Fortunately, national governing bodies exist that regulate research conducted with humans with the primary purpose of protecting them from harm. Historically, this has not always been the case.

History of Human Subjects Protection

One of the first research disasters regarding **human subjects protection** occurred in 1929–1930, when a researcher trying to prevent tuberculosis gave newborns the oral bacillus Calmette-Guerin vaccine. Of the infants in the study, 72 died within their first year of life, 135 became ill but recovered, and 44 stayed well and became resistant to further tuberculosis infection. The parents were never informed of the risks of the vaccine. This tragedy led to official guidelines in 1931 on human experimentation, addressing such issues as therapeutic intent, informed consent, and nonmaleficence; however, these guidelines did not prevent World War II atrocities committed by the Nazi and Japanese regimes on prisoners in concentration camps in the name of research. As a result of the crimes and named after the trials of physicians who had participated in unethical and harmful research, the

Nuremberg Code was written with the expectation that it would apply to human experimentation whenever and wherever conducted (Katz, 1996). As the code did not address the needs of children or other special populations, these moral, ethical, and legal concepts informed the World Medical Association's Declaration of Helsinki in 1964, which still guides research practice today (World Medical Association, n.d.). Unfortunately, the declaration's development did not prevent some research ethics violations from occurring (White, 2020).

You may have heard of the 40-year-long Tuskegee Study of Untreated Syphilis in the Negro Male. Begun in 1932, this infamous study's purpose was to observe the natural course of the infection, if left untreated, over many years. Researchers enrolled Black men (299 with syphilis and 201 without) who lived in poverty in rural Alabama. The participants were promised free medical care in return for participation but were given placebos, and when an effective cure (penicillin) became available, they were left uninformed and untreated so that the study could continue. When researchers' conduct was discovered and reported in 1969, their shocking experiment triggered Congress to pass the National Research Service Award Act of 1974, of which Title II created the National Commission for the Protection of Human Subjects of Biomedical and Behavioral Research (Centers for Disease Control and Prevention, 2022).

Although the commission issued several reports, the *Belmont Report* (National Commission for the Protection of Human Subjects of Biomedical and Behavioral Research,1979) had the largest influence on the conduct of human subjects research (Office of Human Research Protections [OHRP], 2010). This report established what is known as the "common rule" that any activity comprising an element of medical research (i.e., research that tests a theory, as opposed to medical practice, which has a known and expected result) should undergo review for the protection of human subjects. Currently, research with human subjects in the United States is clarified, guided, regulated, and overseen by the Office of Human Research Protections (OHRP) as part of the U.S. Department of Health and Human Services (https://www.hhs.gov/ohrp/index.html). Four ethical principles guide the protection of human subjects in research: respect of persons, beneficence, justice, and nonmaleficence.

The principle of *respect for persons* is grounded in the ethical conviction that individuals should be treated as autonomous agents able to choose or not choose (i.e., volunteer) whether to participate in research and, additionally, that persons with diminished autonomy (e.g., those with developmental disabilities, incarcerated persons) are entitled to protection (OHRP, 2010).

The principle of *beneficence* refers to the moral obligation to treat participants in an ethical manner, respect their decisions, protect them from harm, and make efforts to secure and maximize possible benefits for them. The benefits and risks of a research study must always be fully explained to potential participants as part of the process of obtaining their "informed consent."

Justice refers to fairness, equity, and appropriateness in the distribution of the benefits and possible burdens of research. Each eligible participant in research should have an equal opportunity for selection. No person should feel undue coercion or influence to participate in research.

In 1978, the National Commission for the Protection of Human Subjects completed a companion report stating that institutional review boards (IRBs) were the primary mechanism for ensuring that the rights of human subjects are protected. There are many federal requirements for the composition of individual IRBs and their function. The U.S. Department of Health and Human Services has regularly updated the regulations for protection of human subjects (45 C.F.R. 46 and 21 C.F.R. 50), most recently in 2018 (OHRP, 2018).

Many healthcare institutions where research is conducted have IRBs charged with protecting humans who are involved in research at their institution. These boards are composed of local members of the organization and representatives of the public. If your research involves human subjects, you must seek the appropriate IRB approval to determine whether and how you can proceed.

Human Participation in EBPQI Initiatives

EBPQI initiatives often do not meet the criteria of human subject research (HSR). Suppose you have strong evidence that can be translated into a practice change; in such a case, you are simply using existing research as an impetus to make changes that can benefit patients, providers, or the organization. However, this can get a little tricky because in EBPQI, the change to your customary practice with patients (or humans in other roles) generates internal data that is used to determine whether your change resulted in the improvement you intended. Whether the change in practice is considered HSR or not may depend not only on what you measure but on how you measure it: For example, did your actions or their consequences affect or change human behavior?

The Federal Policy for the Protection of Human Subjects, known as the Common Rule (OHRP, 2017), governs the use of human subjects for research by any institution receiving federal funding, and almost all university-associated IRBs abide by its regulations as well. IRBs apply different levels of review and oversight based on the following critical questions to evaluate (a) whether EBPQI initiatives and other types of research might be HSR and (b) the amount of oversight needed to ensure that humans are protected:

- Question 1: Is the activity a systematic investigation designed to develop or contribute to generalizable knowledge?

If the answer to this is question is "no" (and it generally will be), it will likely be the only question you will need to answer to obtain an IRB determination of non-human subject research (NHSR) for your EBPQI initiative. EBPQI initiatives are performed in a systematic way, but their purpose is to solve a problem for your local unit or organization only. The outcomes may be transferable but not generalizable (see Chapter 1 for a review of this concept).

- Question 2. Will you collect any identifiable information from living people?

Identifiable information refers to personal details (e.g., name, birthdate, address, age, etc.). There is generally no reason for you to collect this type of information

Full Board	- Studies are more than "minimal risk." - Studies are reviewed once a month. - Example: Interventions that involve physical or emotional discomfort & studies with deception of participants.
Expedited Review	- Studies are not greater than "minimal risk." - Studies fit under one of nine categories defined by the federal regulations (45CFR-46). - Example: Studies that collect identifiable information through surveys, interviews, and so on.
Exempt Review	- Studies not greater than "minimal risk." - Studies fit under one of six categories defined by the federal regulations (45CFR-46). - Example: Research with de-identified records & anonymous surveys.
Not Human Subjects Research	- Research that is not generalizable. - Research that does not collect identifiable information or biospecimens from living individuals. - Example: Program reviews & oral histories.

FIGURE 10.3 Levels of Human Subjects Protection

from the people involved in your EBPQI initiative; if you are not collecting this information, you can answer "no" to this question.

The level of oversight for protection of human subjects increases according to the potential for risks to humans or participants, as outlined in Figure 10.3.

- NHSR: does not meet the criteria for HSR.
- Exempt or expedited: HSR with no more than minimal risk (beyond that of daily living).
- Exempt: exempt from specific regulations and requirements.
- Expedited: must follow specific regulations and requirements (e.g., informed consent).
- Full board review: HSR that involves greater than minimal risk or vulnerable subjects and requires full board review by the IRB.

As a nurse, you are well-trained and positioned to engage in health-related research using your many skills: You have learned how to communicate responsibly and accurately with patients; you can administer protocols for treatments and drugs; you know how to document your interactions and interventions with patients/participants as well as their responses. In the Foreword section of this textbook, the contributors each provided a brief story about their decision to become a nurse. Julee Briscoe Waldrop's story describes her interactions with members of a nurse research team when she was a subject in a study; these nurses inspired her to become a nurse. Similarly, in Chapter 13, author Jennifer Wilson describes her role as a research nurse at the National Cancer Institute (see pages 230–31). Can you see yourself in this role?

Let's return to our earlier essential question, "Is there sufficient evidence to change practice?" This time, suppose that the answer is "yes." You are now ready to initiate a change in your practice, unit, or organization based on your review of the evidence. You will accomplish this by using evidence from the field of implementation science.

Implementation science is the scientific study of methods to promote the systematic uptake of research findings and other evidence-based practices to improve the quality and effectiveness of health services and care (Eccles & Mittman, 2006). In other words, by making something easier to do than not do, you make doing it relatively advantageous! Implementation science describes how you can encourage people/systems to accept or make a change, and QI describes how you can support them by facilitating their effort to make a change. This field developed when it became evident that simple linear EBP and QI models were not as effective as had been hoped in improving health and healthcare.

The study of implementation has demonstrated that implementing change is not usually as linear a process as following a step-by-step model (e.g., IHI PDSA cycles) (IHI, n.d.) . Systems are dynamic, people are diverse, and cultures may be deeply entrenched and resistant to change. You should be ready for unpredictable factors and adaptable to continued change in your plans (Braithwaite et al., 2018). Adaptability and iterative changes are the hallmark of effective improvement, and implementation science offers strategies that you can use to increase the success of your endeavors because multiple strategies are generally required (Leeman et al., 2021). The Expert Recommendations for Implementing Change was a project whose purpose was to develop common nomenclature for discrete implementation strategies. This project identified nonthematic clusters and 73 discrete implementation strategies (Kirchner et al., 2020; see Table 10.1).

TABLE 10.1 Implementation Stretegies

Strategies	Examples
Use evaluative and iterative strategies.	Assess for readiness. Identify barriers and facilitators. Audit and provide feedback.
Provide interactive assistance.	Provide clinical supervision. Leaders engage locally in facilitation.
Adapt and tailor to content.	Promote adaptability. Tailor strategies.
Develop stakeholder interrelationships.	Identify and prepare champions. Identify early adopters. Recruit, designate, and train for leadership.
Train and educate stakeholders.	Conduct educational meetings. Create a learning collaborative.
Support clinicians.	Create new clinical teams. Revise professional roles.
Engage consumers.	Prepare patients/consumers to be active participants. Intervene with patients/consumers to enhance uptake and adherence.

(Continued)

TABLE 10.1 *(Continued)*

Strategies	Examples
Utilize financial strategies.	Fund and contract for the clinical innovation. Develop disincentives.
Change infrastructure.	Change record systems. Mandate change.

Adapted from Kirchner et al. (2020)

Engage Stakeholders

Once you have articulated your initiative aims (Chapters 3 and 9), you can design and pilot your proposed practice change. The first step in this process involves engaging **stakeholders** (persons with related interests or concerns). Stakeholder input should be incorporated early in the design and piloting phases of EBP (Laures & Fowler, 2020), with key involvement from healthcare end users. Ideally, you will have asked key stakeholders to be on your EBPQI team, perhaps as healthcare co-designers, which will involve forming equal partnerships among (a) people who work within the system, (b) consumers within the system, and (c) healthcare change designers (Ward et al., 2018). Incorporating the perspectives of patients, families, and clinicians is vital to achieving effective practice change design (Kildea et al., 2019). Stakeholder engagement is ranked as the most significant facilitator of implementing change in healthcare; similarly, lack of stakeholder engagement is the most significant barrier to successful implementation of change (Alatawi et al., 2020).

You will recall the importance of appraising evidence (covered in Chapters 5–7). Now is the time to use your appraisal skills on data specific to your proposed change to identify stakeholders who should be contacted regarding your initiative. Special interest groups and advisory boards can provide stakeholder connections. Representation from the impacted population is important because failure to consider patient perspectives reduces the likelihood that practice change will be adopted (Mathieson et al., 2019). There are many ways to engage target individuals, including conversation, focus groups, individual interviews, and patient surveys (Cullen et al., 2022). You can then use the stakeholder input you have gathered to verify local practice change preferences.

Organizational Assessment and Identifying Facilitators and Barriers

You must now engage in real-time critical reflection on the resources you will need, personally and professionally, to ensure that your practice change can be well-executed. You should think deeply about potential resources, anticipated barriers to change, and needed approval pathways. Some nurses may abandon the initiative at this point due to multiple constraints or failure to see a clear path forward for change. Throughout this textbook, however, we have been introducing you to evidence-in-action strategies for personal application. Lean on those supports as you prepare to fully appraise what you will need to obtain from your workplace to implement positive change for the patients you serve.

Here was some examples of items and materials specific to your proposed change that you might consider:

- Time: How much time is needed and over what span? How can you make a solid case for your organization to provide the time needed for the initiative? Remember that behavior change may take substantial time to realize.
- Assistance: Who is needed? Remember that no EBPQI effort is completed solo. Does your organization have an EBP or QI department with access to supportive resources? Are training and technical assistance available? Would the research department render aid to an EBPQI initiative? If not, could neighboring organizations provide support? Consider both materials and statistical expertise as supportive resources. Specialized help from a statistician can reduce your workload tremendously.
- Leadership: Regular communication with local (and possibly system) leadership facilitates essential resources negotiation. Leaders can help jump-start and maintain change momentum.
- Approval: Where does initiative approval begin and end within your organization? Follow the organizational policy approval path closely, and as previously warned, do not begin the practice change until project designation is determined by the IRB and permission has been granted.

One way to identify **facilitators** and **barriers** is to complete an environmental assessment or scan of factors within and outside of your organization that may impact the practice change. This can be accomplished in several ways: a SWOT (strength, weakness, opportunities, threats) analysis provides a visual map of the existing organizational context to increase awareness of factors that will play into the proposed practice change (see Table 10.2).

TABLE 10.2 Example: SWOT—EBPQI Initiative to Improve Falls Rate

Internal	Strengths	Weaknesses
	Hospital administration is supportive, as they desire to improve this public benchmark. You have a good team dedicated to the initiative. You have a strong EBP mentor.	There are some nurses who are resistant to any new idea. The unit manager is worried about the possibility of overtime.
External	**Opportunities**	**Threats**
	If your initiative is successful on this unit, it might be considered as a practice change across the entire organization. Once completed, you can present the results at a conference or as a publication.	Nursing shortage has impacted your unit. Travel nurses are often on staff.

TABLE 10.3 Example: SOAR—EBPQI Initiative to Improve Falls Rate

Current	Strengths	Aspirations
	Hospital administration is supportive, as they desire to improve this public benchmark. You have a good team dedicated to the initiative. You have a strong EBP mentor.	The hospital will reach or exceed the national fall rate. The team will continue to work together on other problems. You may become an EBP mentor one day.
Future	**Opportunities**	**Results**
	If your initiative is successful on this unit, it might be considered as a practice change across the entire organization. Once completed, you can present the results at a conference or as a publication.	A successful EBPQI initiative can increase job satisfaction. Professional development opportunities also increase satisfaction in the workplace. Both will help the organization retain employees.

A SOAR (strengths, opportunities, aspirations, results) analysis is another method of identifying barriers and facilitators. SWOT describes the organization's current status, but SOAR's advantage is that it focuses more on the future—on what you want to make happen and the results that will ideally be achieved. We recommend listing each barrier you identify and creating a proactive path to address it (see Table 10.3).

Initiatives have an increased likelihood of failure when implementation is not integrated by all stakeholders (Sibbald et al., 2021), so be sure to create awareness and interest among those who will be involved in your EBPQI change. To successfully adopt an EBPQI change, nurses must identify and engage key personnel in practical ways and build upon sustained engagement early and often. Change agents can help you to leverage comparisons between the local practice and EBP in order to develop meaningful motivation to depart from the status quo. For example, in a clinic-based EBPQI initiative, you will want to continually involve influential healthcare workers with topical expertise across organizational levels as well as patients and community leaders who will help keep the change momentum going. Positive peers with intimate EBPQI involvement can improve learning and provide the team with messages to reduce cultural barriers and make practice change stick.

What is meant by "a specific change in practice"? A majority of clinical practice recommendations are broadly written and may not fit some specific patient populations or practice settings. This is why EBP change must be adapted to specific patient populations in the local environment as part of the QI process. Develop an organization-specific protocol that addresses the practice change; this may include EBPQI procedures and practice statements (see the mountain model). You will use the identified EBPQI recommendations (i.e., the "what" or innovations/interventions/changes) to create a new localized protocol with your stakeholders (see Box 12.2, page 217). As you use evidence to co-design the local practice change protocol, consider the complexities of the recommended change and try to simplify recommendations as appropriate and if feasible to reduce cognitive load (Cullen et al., 2022).

As your initiative will incorporate QI principles along with the EBP change, it is important that you use QI tools to further assess change within your environment (many of these tools were presented in Chapter 9). You will need to compile EBP information and package change recommendations within the local practice context.

In Chapter 3, you were provided with the example of a fall rate on your unit that was higher (6 per 1,000 patient days) than the benchmark (3.2 per 1,000 patient days). You developed a PPCO question and identified evidence to support a bundle of practice changes that had demonstrated improvement in fall rates in research and other EBPQI initiatives. From this external evidence and the internal evidence on the unit fall rate, you decide to develop SMART aims for a project (so you will know whether what you are doing makes a difference). The three types of aims are outcomes, process, and balancing (see Chapters 3 and 9 for more on aims). You should consider developing the process measure first for a couple of reasons: (a) because in almost every case, processes must change before you can expect outcomes to change and (b) because you can usually monitor process change immediately after implementation without waiting to see its impact on outcomes.

- Process: Nurses will document fall risk assessment 95% of the time at 3 months after implementing training on the falls bundle.
- Outcome: Fall rate will decrease to 5 per 1,000 patient days within the first 3 months after implementing the falls bundle.
- Balancing aim: Overtime on the unit will remain stable in the 3 months after implementing the falls bundle.

Your team decides to include the following evidence-based practices to implement as the "intervention bundle or falls bundle" on your unit:

- A comprehensive assessment of fall risk: This includes a comprehensive evaluation of fall risk factors, including patient history, physical assessment, medication use, and environmental assessment. It is important to identify any existing risk factors and take steps to reduce them.
- Education of staff and family: This includes educating staff and family members about the importance of fall prevention and how to help prevent falls.
- Documentation and evaluation: This includes full documentation of all falls and near-falls as well as ongoing evaluation of the effectiveness of the falls prevention bundle (more on this in Chapter 11).

Do you see how the aims you wrote are relevant to the practice changes you have included in your bundle? Now is a good time to get specific about how each "who, what, when, where, and how" aspect of this bundle will be carried out.

You may begin your initiative with a broad timeline, but once you are ready to implement change, you can develop a more specific timeline. Timelines in

EBPQI are not written in stone and may need to be adapted depending on how smoothly the implementation progresses.

Clinicians and materials should be thoroughly prepared for the practice change prior to initiation. This can be accomplished through training and educating stakeholders according to local needs, using strategies such as simulations, formal presentations, unit or clinic in-services, required continuing education modules, or lunch-and-learn sessions. We recommend additional preparation activities including but not limited to the following:

- Use evidence-based active learning to engage stakeholders when possible.
- Link the practice change to organizational goals and values.
- Share reliable evidence with practice recommendations early and often.
- Select change champions to lead locally.
- Ensure any needed supplies are accessible where locally needed.
- Make supportive resource materials available, including pocket guides, checklists, and algorithms.
- De-implement materials no longer in use or needed. (Cullen et al., 2022)

TABLE 10.4 Specifics of Intervention Bundle

What (intervention)	Who	When	Where	Why (evidence should provide the answers)	How (implementation strategy)
Falls risk assessment	Nurse	On admission	In patient room	Although all patients may be at some risk of a fall, some patients will be at higher risk. An individualized plan decreases fall rate.	Change infrastructure. Change record systems. Use evidence-based risk assessment tool embedded into admissions template in EHR.
Education of staff/family	Nurse	Within first 4 hours after admission	Patient room for patient Possibly other places or via phone or video call for family	When the patient and family understand the risks of falling and can work with the healthcare team to reduce falls, patient engagement and self-management increase (see Chapter 8).	Engage consumers, patients, and family as active participants.
Evaluation of compliance with interventions and outcome (fall rate)	EBPQI team members	Weekly for risk assessment and education Monthly for fall rate	Sample of charts Review data from quality department	All those involved in the EBPQI initiative want to feel that what they are doing is making a difference. Frequent and regular feedback improves motivation and willingness to continue with the change.	Evaluative and iterative strategies Audit and feedback

De-implementation describes the "stopping" of practices that are no longer "best" or representative of the "standard of care." There are frameworks and models to guide you in the de-implementation process (Walsh-Bailey et al., 2021). De-implementing old practices in order to implement new best practices and gold standards is essential but often easier said than done, particularly when nurses and other healthcare personnel have been engaging in practices that need to be stopped for a long time. Your evidence search might even lead you to de-implementing a practice as the practice improvement! For example, although auscultation of feeding tubes is a low-value practice, nurses are more likely to follow this tradition if they witness colleagues completing this action (Leeman et al., 2021). Remember to let the evidence guide your team's determination of practices, or elements of practice, which should be de-implemented and unlearned in order to update practice policy, procedures, and workflow. When electronic resources are available at the bedside, chairside, or tableside, we recommend digitally embedding reminders to increase frontline adoption with end users. You should complete these steps prior to your scheduled pilot start date.

The Iowa model and the model of change emphasize the importance of pilot testing before implementing practice change and encourage nurses to consider organizational context prior to the pilot (Cullen et al., 2022; Langley et al., 2009). In our practice change example, a pilot for 1 week might involve just one nurse on each shift performing risk assessment and patient education, then documenting and providing feedback on the process to the team. After this 1-week pilot, let's suppose that the feedback from the nurses has been positive, yet they are finding it time consuming to round up family members for patient education sessions. Your team brainstorms ways to improve this part of the process. One of the nurses involved in the pilot notes that as there is almost always at least one family member or significant person present with a patient on admission, it is an ideal time to provide family education. She suggests that the primary person who is with the patient can be charged with teaching other family and friends about fall prevention, thereby decreasing nursing time spent on repetitive family education and engaging the support person in an important responsibility related to patient care. The nurse will still be responsible for this aspect of patient care but can follow up with family and visitors over the course of the patient's hospital stay. Your team changes the "when" component of patient and family education from "within the first 4 hours of admission" to "on admission." This change is communicated to all involved, and the pilot proceeds accordingly.

Despite detailed planning, unexpected issues are likely to arise because that is simply the nature of working with people and organizations! We are confident that by this point, you understand that your localized EBPQI change must be tailored appropriately to the needs of your local setting and patient population. As the pilot progresses, engage the team in troubleshooting problems as they appear and develop responses/modifications/adaptations as indicated (Cullen et al., 2022).

Once the pilot is stable, it is time to include the rest of the unit. How you evaluate the unit-wide implementation will be based on your aims. The EBPQI team members will be responsible for collecting data on compliance with the falls bundle as well as on the fall rate and communicating it with all who need or want to know (as per Table 10.4). We will move on to the evaluation component of EBPQI in the next chapter.

WRAPPING UP

You have now been introduced to the basics of implementing an EBPQI initiative. When you have let the evidence guide your best-practice decision and you have proceeded through your organizational process and obtained approval from leadership, be sure to implement your practice change thoughtfully. Remember that implementing an EBPQI initiative is a team-based activity to which your skills as a patient care expert are critical.

Persistence and curiosity are key features of successful engagement in the practice change process. Should you encounter barriers to implementing your change, discuss and address their causes with your team and leadership in a timely manner. Implementation and sustainability require continuous monitoring, so you will learn how to evaluate and set up regular monitoring of your practice change next. First, though, let's pause and take some deep breaths.

WELLNESS IN ACTION: BREATHING

Breathing is the most important physiological process in our body (okay—we might be biased). It seems so simple; we do it without even thinking, yet it is under our control if we want it to be. Perhaps someone who has seen you upset or anxious has said, "Take a deep breath." This is always great advice! It has been known for thousands of years that focusing on breathing deeply and slowly calms the nervous system. Breathing is also one of the eight limbs of yoga practice (Satchidananda, 2012). Modern science has provided evidence of yoga and breathwork benefits (Journal & McCall, 2007). Adding a focused thought or mantra to your breathing can be especially helpful. The next time you are feeling overwhelmed, anxious, or angry (maybe right now), try this simple breathing exercise, wherever you happen to be.

1. Close your eyes.
2. Close your mouth and breathe in slowly through your nose as you think, "In 1, 2, 3, 4."
3. Focus on how the air feels as it comes in through your nose, travels down into your lungs, and fills them completely.
4. At the top of the inhale, hold your breath for a second, then breathe out through your nose as you think, "Out 1, 2, 3, 4."
5. Focus on how the air feels as it rises back up from your lungs and exits through your nose.
6. Pause for a second at the end of the exhale.
7. Repeat 3–10 times.

If you want to add a focused thought as you breathe in and out rather than counting, you might try this one: As you inhale, think, "I am strong," and as you exhale, think, "I am calm."

If you have just participated in this breathing practice, how do you feel? Both research evidence and our own consistent experience support that this practice is effective, and we hope it helps you!

REFLECTION QUESTIONS

1. What areas of strength and vulnerability did you identify related to a future EBPQI initiative of interest?
2. What strategies could you use to overcome a potential barrier to your best practice change?
3. Design a potential practice change for pilot purposes.

REFERENCES

Alatawi, M., Aljuhani, E., Alsufiany, F., Aleid, K., Rawah, R., Aljanabi, S., & Banakhar, M. (2020). Barriers of implementing evidence-based practice in nursing profession: A literature review. *American Journal of Nursing Science, 9*(1), 35. https://doi.org/10.11648/j.ajns.20200901.16

Braithwaite, J., Churruca, K., Long, J. C., Ellis, L. A., & Herkes, J. (2018). When complexity science meets implementation science: A theoretical and empirical analysis of systems change. *BMC Medicine, 16*(1), 63. https://doi.org/10.1186/s12916-018-1057-z

Centers for Disease Control and Prevention. (2022, December) *Tuskegee Study—timeline.* https://www.cdc.gov/tuskegee/timeline.htm

Cullen, L., Hanrahan, K., Farrington, M., Tucker, S., & Edmonds, S. (2022). *Evidence-based practice in action*. Sigma Theta Tau International.

Eccles, M. P., & Mittman, B. S. (2006). Welcome to implementation science. *Implementation Science, 1*(1), 1. https://doi.org/10.1186/1748-5908-1-1

Institute for Healthcare Improvement. (n.d.). *Quality improvement essentials toolkit* Retrieved December 18, 2022, from https://www.ihi.org/resources/Pages/Tools/Quality-Improvement-Essentials-Toolkit.aspx

Journal, Y., & McCall, T. (2007). *Yoga as medicine: The yogic prescription for health and healing.* Bantam.

Katz, J. (1996). The Nuremberg Code and the Nuremberg Trial: A reappraisal. *JAMA, 276*(20), 1662–1666. https://doi.org/10.1001/jama.1996.03540200048030

Kildea, J., Battista, J., Cabral, B., Hendren, L., Herrera, D., Hijal, T., & Joseph, A. (2019). Design and development of a person-centered patient portal using participatory stakeholder co-design. *Journal of Medical Internet Research, 21*(2), Article e11371. https://doi.org/10.2196/11371

Kirchner, J. E., Smith, J. L., Powell, B. J., Waltz, T. J., & Proctor, E. K. (2020). Getting a clinical innovation into practice: An introduction to implementation strategies. *Psychiatry Research, 283*, Article 112467. https://doi.org/10.1016/j.psychres.2019.06.042

Langley, G. J., Moen, R. D., Nolan, K. M., Nolan, T. W., Norman, C. L., & Provost, L. P. (2009). *The improvement guide: A practical approach to enhancing organizational performance* (2nd ed.). Jossey-Bass.

Laures, E., & Fowler, C. (2020). The power of the pilot. *Journal of PeriAnesthesia Nursing, 35*(5), 543–547. https://doi.org/10.1016/j.jopan.2020.02.009

Leeman, J., Rohweder, C., Lee, M., Brenner, A., Dwyer, A., Ko, L. K., O'Leary, M. C., Ryan, G., Vu, T., & Ramanadhan, S. (2021). Aligning implementation science with improvement practice: A call to action. *Implementation Science Communications, 2*(1), 99. https://doi.org/10.1186/s43058-021-00201-1

Mathieson, A., Grande, G., & Luker, K. (2019). Strategies, facilitators and barriers to implementation of evidence-based practice in community nursing: A systematic mixed-studies review and qualitative synthesis. *Primary Health Care Research & Development, 20*, Article e6. https://doi.org/10.1017/S1463423618000488

National Commission for the Protection of Human Subjects of Biomedical and Behavioral Research. (1979). *The Belmont Report: Ethical principles and guidelines for the protection of human subjects of research*. U.S. Department of Health and Human Services. https://www.hhs.gov/ohrp/regulations-and-policy/belmont-report/index.html

Office of Human Research Protections. (2010, January 28). *The Belmont Report*. https://www.hhs.gov/ohrp/regulations-and-policy/belmont-report/index.html

Office of Human Research Protections (2018). *45 CFR 46*. https://www.hhs.gov/ohrp/regulations-and-policy/regulations/45-cfr-46/revised-common-rule-regulatory-text/index.html

Office of Human Research Protections. (2017, October 11). *What regulations protect research participants?*. https://www.hhs.gov/ohrp/education-and-outreach/about-research-participation/protecting-research-volunteers/principal-regulations/index.html

Satchidananda, S. S. (2012). *The yoga sutras of patanjali* (Rev. ed.). Integral Yoga.

Sibbald, S. L., Van Asseldonk, R., Cao, P. L., & Law, B. (2021). Lessons learned from inadequate implementation planning of team-based chronic disease management: Implementation evaluation. *BMC Health Services Research, 21*(1), Article 134. https://doi.org/10.1186/s12913-021-06100-4

Speroni, K. G., McLaughlin, M. K., & Friesen, M. A. (2020). Use of Evidence-based Practice Models and Research Findings in Magnet-Designated Hospitals Across the United States: National Survey Results. *Worldviews on Evidence-Based Nursing, 17*(2), 98–107. https://doi.org/10.1111/wvn.12428

Waldrop, J. & Jennings Dunlap, J. (2024). The Mountain Model for evidence-based practice quality improvement. *The American Journal of Nursing*, May.

Walsh-Bailey, C., Tsai, E., Tabak, R. G., Morshed, A. B., Norton, W. E., McKay, V. R., Brownson, R. C., & Gifford, S. (2021). A scoping review of de-implementation frameworks and models. *Implementation Science, 16*(1), Article 100. https://doi.org/10.1186/s13012-021-01173-5

Ward, M. E., De Brún, A., Beirne, D., Conway, C., Cunningham, U., English, A., Fitzsimons, J., Furlong, E., Kane, Y., Kelly, A., McDonnell, S., McGinley, S., Monaghan, B., Myler, A., Nolan, E., O'Donovan, R., O'Shea, M., Shuhaiber, A., & McAuliffe, E. (2018). Using co-design to develop a collective leadership intervention for healthcare teams to improve safety culture. *International Journal of Environmental Research and Public Health, 15*(6), 1182. https://doi.org/10.3390/ijerph15061182

White, M. G. (2020). Why human subjects research protection is important. *The Ochsner Journal, 20*(1), 16–33. https://doi.org/10.31486/toj.20.5012

World Medical Association. (n.d.). *WMA Declaration of Helsinki—Ethical principles for medical research involving human subjects*. Retrieved August 23, 2023, from https://www.wma.net/policies-post/wma-declaration-of-helsinki-ethical-principles-for-medical-research-involving-human-subjects/

IMAGE CREDITS

Fig. 10.2: University of Iowa Hospitals & Clinics, "Updated Iowa Model," https://uiowa.qualtrics.com/CP/File.php?F=F_3lxS6fsUbWlBfKK. Copyright © 2015 by University of Iowa Hospitals & Clinics. Reprinted with permission.

CHAPTER 11

Evaluating the Impact of Evidence-Based Practice and Quality Improvement

Julee Briscoe Waldrop

KEY CONCEPTS

Outcome measures
Evaluation strategies
Electronic health record EHR

LEARNING OBJECTIVES

1. Identify the steps of the evaluation process.
2. Compare and contrast evaluation types.
3. Discuss the interpretation of statistics.
4. Explore basic strategies for evaluation.

> Education is the passport to the future, for tomorrow belongs to those who prepare for it today.
>
> —Malcolm X

Introduction

Finally! You are about to find out whether what you have planned, developed, implemented, and supported up to this point in your EBPQI journey has made a difference! You followed the process—from identifying a problem to implementation—and now you can evaluate the effectiveness of your EBPQI initiative.

The Evaluation Process

Evaluation is a systematic and objective assessment of your EBPQI initiative to determine its efficacy (success in producing the intended result) and areas for improvement. It usually involves data collection and analysis. The outcomes of the data analysis will inform the decision to adopt or reject the practice change. You can perform an evaluation at any stage of the process: (a) before implementation (formative) to evaluate baseline data; (b) during the implementation (process) to assess whether the change you intended is happening; and (c) after implementation (summative) to assess the results.

Let's Explore the Typical Steps Involved in the Evaluation Process

1. Designate a purpose. Evaluation should have a purpose. In EBPQI, the purpose is usually to determine whether the practice changes that were implemented resulted in improvements. Evaluations are often used to make future decisions. Because healthcare is a broad and diverse field, it comprises numerous areas and aspects on which healthcare improvements can be focused.
2. Adopt measurable aims. In Chapter 3, you were introduced to SMART (specific, measurable, achievable, relevant, and timely) aims (Table 3.5), so you know that your aims are already SMART. In Chapter 9, we added three specific types of aims that are used in quality improvement: process measures, **outcome measures**, and balancing measures. You will use these aims to guide your evaluation.
3. Determine the methods and tools you will use, based on your aims, to collect data. There are various methods from which to choose (see Table 11.1).
4. Collect the data. The data collection process should be systematic and reliable to ensure the accuracy and validity of the evaluation findings as well as ethical to protect participant privacy and confidentiality (as discussed in Chapter 10). Your data must be credible, valid, and reliable in order for your results to be considered trustworthy enough to support continuing and sustaining the change.
5. Analyze the data. The collected data should be analyzed in a way that addresses your evaluation objectives. Depending on the nature of the data, you can choose descriptive or statistical analysis, thematic analysis, or other methods, but the results should be presented in a useful and accessible manner.
6. Disseminate the findings. The final step is to communicate your evaluation results in a clear and comprehensive report that is shared with other people or organizations. The report should include an overview of the evaluation process, a presentation of the findings, and recommendations for future action(s) based on the findings. As you will see in Chapter 12, dissemination can take many forms.

Importance of Ongoing Evaluation

The outcomes of EBPQI initiatives must be evaluated on an ongoing regular basis to ensure the safety, satisfaction, and health of patients. It is crucial to know whether your practice changes are producing their intended results, ideally without increasing costs or workload. Once practices have been changed, evaluation supports their sustainability and holds those involved accountable for upholding the new standard of care; it also fosters a culture of inquiry and encourages continuous improvement. Evaluation can often determine whether regulatory standards or benchmarks are being met, an important point discussed in Chapters 2 and 9. Regular evaluation enables you to measure the impact of your interventions and verify whether they continue to deliver the expected results.

Remember that best practice may need to change again! Regular evaluation of practices will inform decision-making and strategic planning as new evidence or technologies become available. Sometimes initiatives can backslide; factors unrelated to the practice change become a priority, and the initiative can lose ground. Additional areas for improvement may be identified. This is part of the continuous improvement process. It is important to know when changes occur so that decisions can be made, based on current data, to adopt and sustain the best practices for our patients.

Evaluation Strategies

Evaluation strategies are the "how" of evaluation (see Table 11.1 for examples with descriptions). They should be familiar to you because many use the same methodologies that are used in research. Each has its strengths and limitations, and the choice of method depends on your specific evaluation objectives, available resources, and the nature of the EBP, QI, or EBPQI initiative being evaluated. Selecting appropriate and meaningful measures can be challenging. As you choose your measurement tools, be sure to consider any issues related to their reliability and validity or their ability to collect accurate and complete data (Silver et al., 2016).

TABLE 11.1 Evaluation Strategies and Descriptions

Evaluation strategy	Description
Surveys/questionnaires	Used to gather data from patients, healthcare providers, or other stakeholders. They can assess knowledge, attitudes, behaviors, or satisfaction levels. These tools can be administered before and after implementation to evaluate changes over time.
Observation	Direct observation of healthcare practices can provide insights into adherence to EBP guidelines, practice or system changes, the nature of patient-provider interactions, or the processes involved in care delivery.

(Continued)

TABLE 11.1 (*Continued*)

Evaluation strategy	Description
Patient record review	Involves systematically reviewing patient records to assess adherence to EBP guidelines, patient outcomes, and other quality indicators, as well as patient-oriented outcomes like blood pressure reduction or laboratory results.
Audits	Clinical audits compare current practices against established standards or guidelines to identify gaps and areas for improvement. Audits can be particularly useful for evaluating adherence to EBP and its impact on the quality of care. Results of audits are often used as feedback to inform participants in the EBPQI about compliance with a practice change.
Feedback	Feedback from patients, healthcare providers, and other stakeholders can be collected through various methods, including interviews, focus groups, and feedback forms. Feedback can provide valuable insights into the perceived effectiveness and acceptability of EBPQI initiatives.
Clinical outcomes	Involves tracking specific outcomes related to the EBPQI initiative, such as rates of hospital-acquired infections, patient readmissions, or mortality rates. The selection of appropriate outcome measures is crucial for an accurate evaluation.
Statistical process control (SPC) charts	Used to monitor and control processes in QI. They help identify variations in a process that may be due to specific causes and require intervention (see Chapter 9).
Benchmarking	Involves comparing an organization's performance or processes against industry standards or best practices. Benchmarking can help identify areas where an organization falls short and needs improvement (see Chapter 9).

Let's return to the intervention to address the patient falls example that you began in Chapter 3. Suppose that, at this point, you have started a unit-wide implementation to improve your unit's fall rate, and the plan for the EBPQI team is to collect evaluation data. Your aims were the following:

- Aim 1. Process: Nurses will document falls risk assessment 95% of the time at 3 months after implementing training on the falls bundle.
- Aim 2. Outcome: Falls rate will decrease to 5 per 1,000 patient days in the first 3 months after implementing falls bundle.
- Aim 3. Balancing aim: Overtime on the unit will remain stable for 3 months after implementing the falls bundle.

How will you measure these three aims?

Aim 1. This aim may prove difficult to monitor, but it is important. Consider the commonly used adage "If it is not documented, it was not done." Accordingly, if a practice change is not documented and thus "was not done," then an intended outcome cannot be found to have occurred. To measure Aim 1, you can immediately start reviewing patient records in the EHR and collecting data on compliance with the falls bundle. You will look for answers to the following two questions in nurses' documentation:

- Did the nurse complete a falls risk assessment on admission? (Yes/No)
- Did the nurse provide patient and family education on falls risks and prevention? (Yes/No)

You can use a simple chart or Excel spreadsheet to keep track of this information.

Now, let's say that your unit admits an average of 10 patients per day, and the average census is 20 patients. Do you need to review every single patient's record? Thankfully, no. You can perform this audit, or review a sample of charts, in increments of your choosing. First, you and your team must choose a method of determining which and how many records to review. Some possibilities would be to review all patients admitted every seventh day or the first or last patient admitted over the past 7 days. See Table 11.2. for one example of a first week of data collection.

TABLE 11.2 Documentation Compliance Audit: Patient Falls Bundle

Patient (Do not collect any PHI! Assign patient identification numbers to track how many records you have reviewed.)	Admission date	Falls risk assessment completed?		Education completed?	
		Yes	No	Yes	No
1.		X		X	
2.			X	X	
3.		X			X
4.			X	X	
5.		X			X
6.		X			X
7.		X		X	
8.			X	X	
9.		X			X
10.		X			X
Total Week 1		7	3	X	
Percent compliance		70%		50%	

This data from this pilot can be visualized using a bar or pie chart (see Figure 11.1). As you continue collecting this data, you can plot the weekly percent compliance on a run and then a control chart (see Figure 11.2).

Is Aim 1 being met? If not, what can you do about this problem?

The great thing about EBPQI is that you can continuously evaluate and make changes when needed. In this case, ask the nurses charged with changing their practice whether they encountered barriers to following the falls bundle; if they say that they are following it, ask whether something has kept them from documenting. Avoid accusation or reproach; just ask a sampling of nurses to explain and consider the information you receive. You might learn that a problem unrelated to the practice change or falls bundle affected nurses' behaviors. Perhaps the unit was short-staffed and used float pool nurses who were unaware of the new practice change. Perhaps the falls risk assessment documentation is too lengthy, and you and your team must discuss whether and how to shorten it to improve compliance. Regardless of the reasons for noncompliance, it is the EBPQI team's job to work with all involved to figure out how to successfully implement change and reach your improvement goal.

Aim 2. Lucky you! Your hospital already tracks patient falls, and you automatically get a report each month on the fall rate for your unit. However, let's suppose that your organization does not have a dedicated unit that collects and monitors falls and other safety concerns; where might you find information on patient falls? Remember the incident reports from Chapter 2? Every time a patient falls, an incident report must be completed. These reports will be stored in a file or database to which you can request access to complete your tracking on a regular (and preferably frequent) basis. People involved in practice change generally want to know whether what they are doing is making a difference, so the more frequently you can provide feedback, the better. You will need to balance how frequently what you are monitoring occurs with the time it takes to collect and analyze the data. For example, if your baseline fall rate is 6 per 1,000 patient days, you will probably not have any data to report on this aim after the first week of the pilot, but you will as the weeks progress (see Figure 11.2).

Aim 3. This is your balancing measure. Because staff overtime costs impact the unit's budget, the unit manager or another supervisor likely receives reports on overtime. To obtain this information, you must (a) find out who is responsible for the budget; (b) learn how frequently this information is reported and to whom; and (c) request access to the total number of overtime hours only (not information about individuals' work hours). This data can be plotted on a run chart and, as your initiative continues, on a control chart. Many organizations do a biweekly payroll, so you can plot this information on a run chart every other week, but as with Aim 2, you may not have any information to assess in Week 1 of the pilot.

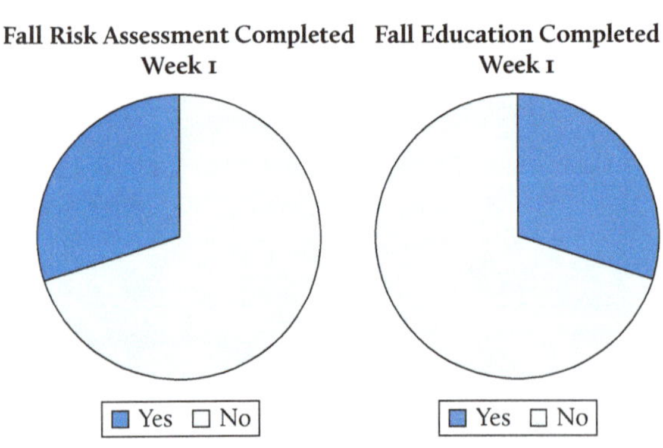

FIGURE 11.1 Compliance Charts

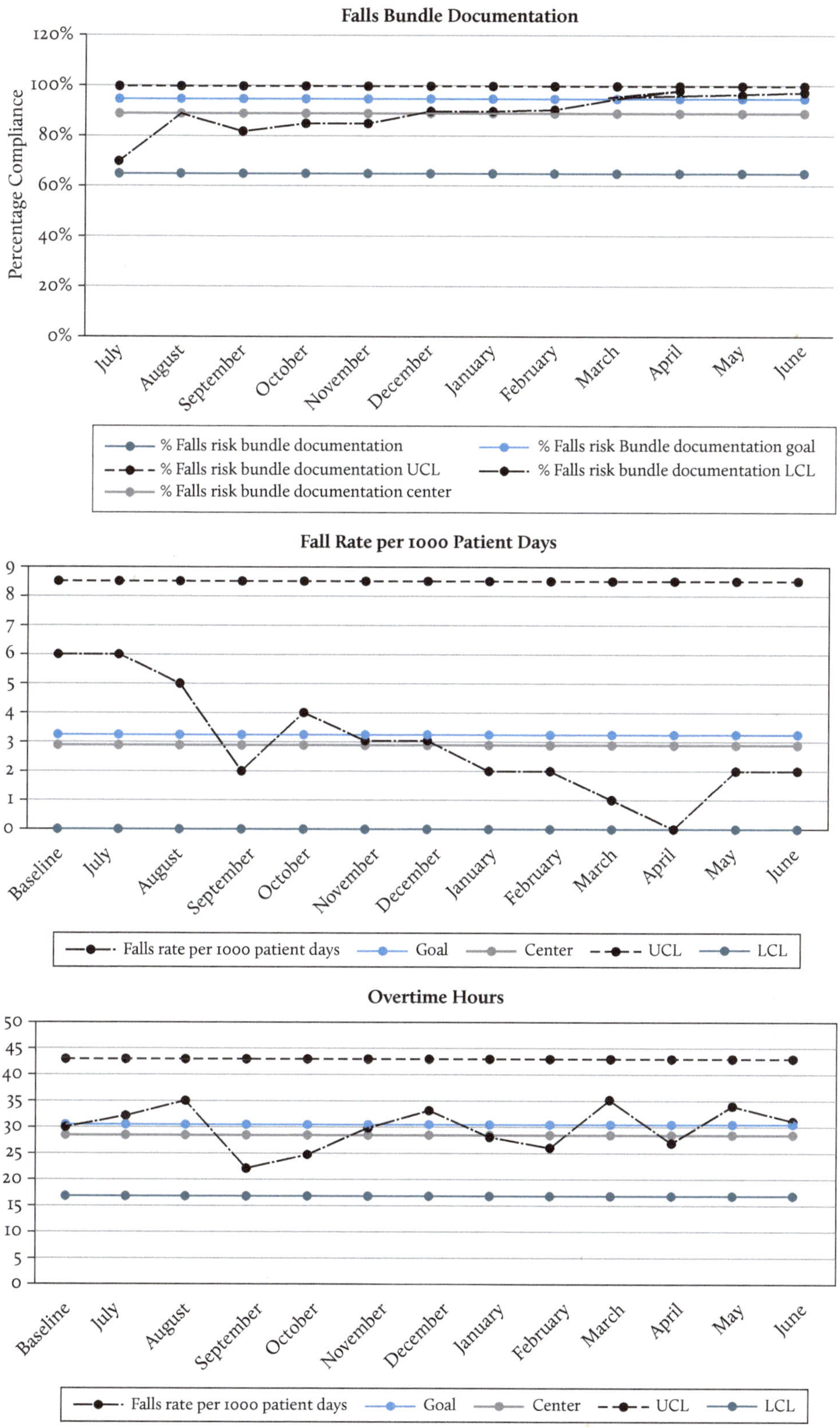

FIGURE 11.2 Family of Measures for 12 months

As you collect and analyze your data over the weeks and months of the project, you will develop a family of measures (see Chapter 9). Be sure to share this information regularly with all who are impacted by the initiative.

Figure 11.2 displays your family of measures for the first 12 months on SPC charts. Did you meet your goal? As you can see on the first chart, staff documentation of the falls bundle has steadily improved and, in the last 4 months, has met or exceeded the 95% goal. The second chart demonstrates that the fall rate has decreased as well: For the past 6 months, it has been below the national benchmark of 3.2! In addition, the last chart shows that overtime hours have remained constant at around 30 hours per pay period—all great news!

Analysis: Evaluating the Impact of an EBPQI Initiative

In addition to your family of measures, other evaluation strategies might help you and your stakeholders to understand the impact of your EBPQI initiative. These quantitative (numbers) and qualitative (stories) methods are the same ones you learned about in Chapters 5 and 6. Table 11.3 provides quantitative methods and their potential use for evaluation, and Table 11.4 does the same for qualitative methods.

TABLE 11.3 Quantitative Evaluation Methods

Method	How	Example
Surveys/questionnaires	Closed questions (e.g., multiple choice) can be scored numerically.	Patient satisfaction surveys Answers scored on a scale from 1 (*disagree strongly*) to 4 (*agree strongly*)
Clinical outcome measures	Tracks specific numeric outcomes related to the practice change	Patient readmission rates or infection rates
Benchmarking	Compares numerical data with industry standards	Patient fall rate compared with rates nationwide or in similar organizations
Return on investment	Compares the cost of the practice improvement with its effects OR a value of importance to the organization	Traditionally, a monetary value is assigned. Alternatively, although not quantifiable monetarily, another metric could determine the value (e.g., patient satisfaction).

Data you collect as numbers can be analyzed using statistics (see Chapter 5) and/or statistical process controls (see Chapter 9).

TABLE 11.4 Qualitative Evaluation Methods

Method	How	Example
Interviews	Asking questions verbally can provide more in-depth insight into participants' experiences, perspectives, and reasons for their attitudes or behaviors.	Interviews may be informal (e.g., in Chapter 7, during the pilot) or more formal with conversations recorded and transcribed.
Focus groups	Interviews with a group of people can generate information about shared experiences, beliefs in a community, or norms of behavior.	A group of nurses discuss a practice change (either formally or informally).
Case studies	A detailed investigation of a single instance or event (a case) can provide an in-depth understanding of the complexity of an issue.	Information can be collected from multiple sources, people, and documents to provide a full description of an adverse event (i.e., what happened before, during, and after the event from multiple perspectives).
Observation	Direct observation of activities or behaviors	Subject to the Hawthorne effect (see Chapter 4) but a valid method for determining whether an action is (or is not) being performed
Records review	Using text or documents to understand the context, processes, or impacts of the practice change or quality improvement processes	Evaluating nurses' notes or other documentation in the patient record

Data acquired through qualitative measures are analyzed differently than quantitative data, although descriptive (numerical) analysis can be done for some aspects of qualitative data (Sandelowski, 2000). For example, you might use descriptive statistics to describe the sample of nurses participating in your focus group (see Box 11.1 below). Most commonly, however, a thematic analysis is performed (see Chapter 6).

BOX 11.1: SAMPLE OF PARTICIPANTS IN A FOCUS GROUP EXAMPLE

Ten nurses, ranging in age from 25–55 years, participated in the two focus groups. They fell into the following three groups according to their years of experience: (a) four nurses had < 2 years; (b) five nurses had 2–10 years; and (c) one nurse had > 10 years. Of the nurses, 70% reported their ethnicity as non-Hispanic White and 30% as other ethnicities. Five nurses expressed a positive attitude about the new practices to prevent falls; the others expressed having neither positive nor negative attitudes about the practice change, although all reported that compliance added no extra time to their workday.

The most suitable method will depend on your specific evaluation objectives, the nature of the intervention, and the resources available. Using quantitative and qualitative methods (a mixed methods approach) can provide a more comprehensive understanding of the impact of evaluations by combining the "hard numbers" of quantitative data with the "rich stories" of qualitative data.

Challenges in Evaluating the Impact of EBPQI

Implementing a change in practice can present challenges, and evaluating whether that change is making a difference can prove challenging as well. Healthcare environments are complex and multifaceted, with various factors (e.g., patient characteristics, coexisting treatments, organizational culture) potentially influencing outcomes. Isolating the effects of a specific EBP can take time, effort, and patience. Assessing the impact of EBP may often require substantial resources, including personnel for data collection and analysis, technology to support these processes, and training to ensure that staff understand and can effectively contribute to evaluation efforts (Warren et al., 2016).

If the EBP is not applied consistently, it can be difficult to assess its true impact. Factors such as varying levels of staff training, resistance to change, or lack of support can lead to inconsistencies in EBP application. Clinicians often operate under significant time pressures, which may limit their ability to participate fully in EBP evaluations. Some staff might resist evaluation efforts due to fear of criticism, increased workload, or skepticism about the value of EBP or the evaluation process itself (Crawford et al., 2023).

Data collection and analysis for evaluation can be time-consuming. It is possible that EBP changes might not show immediate results. Effects could become evident only over a longer period, thus requiring long-term follow-up assessments that could be logistically and financially challenging. Confidentiality and privacy must also be maintained when collecting and analyzing patient data.

To overcome these challenges, it is essential that you cultivate a supportive culture for EBP and evaluation, allocate sufficient resources, provide necessary training, and ensure transparent and effective communication about the evaluation process and findings (Barnsteiner et al., 2023).

Role of Electronic Health Records in EBP and QI

You have learned that an organization's **electronic health record** (**EHR**) can be a valuable tool for evaluating EBPQI. EHRs provide a vast amount of patient data, including demographics, diagnoses, treatments, outcomes, and follow-ups. These data can be used to evaluate the impact of EBPQI initiatives, monitor trends over time, and identify areas for improvement. If you determine that there is currently not enough evidence to support a practice change, consider the EHR a rich source of data for research that can contribute to the evidence base for future practice. Table 11.5 presents some examples of how data from EHRs can be used.

TABLE 11.5 Examples of Information That Can Be Collected From Electronic Health Records

Quality metrics	EHRs may have built-in capabilities to track key quality metrics, such as readmission rates, medication errors, or adherence to preventive care guidelines.	These metrics can be used to evaluate the effectiveness of EBP and QI initiatives and to benchmark performance against external standards.
Audits	EHRs can be used to conduct audits to evaluate adherence to EBP guidelines.	For instance, you can check whether appropriate tests were ordered or evidence-based interventions were implemented consistently.
Clinical decision support	EHRs often include clinical decision support tools that guide providers and nurses in applying EBP.	These tools can also track compliance with such guidelines, offering insights for evaluation.
Patient outcomes	EHRs enable the tracking of patient outcomes, such as disease control measures (e.g., blood pressure or blood glucose levels) or complication rates.	These outcomes can be used to evaluate the impact of EBP or QI initiatives.
Population health management	EHRs can help identify patterns in large populations of patients, such as the prevalence of certain conditions or the effectiveness of interventions across different patient subgroups.	This information can be used to target and evaluate EBP and QI initiatives more effectively.

EHRs can offer many advantages for EBP and QI evaluation, but you should be aware of potential challenges, including data quality and integrity issues, privacy and confidentiality concerns, and the need for skill in extracting and analyzing EHR data. Moreover, EHRs capture data from routine clinical practice, which may not always align neatly with the data requirements for EBP or QI evaluations. A combination of EHR data and other data sources or collection methods is often needed for comprehensive evaluations (Agency for Healthcare Research and Quality, 2015).

The Role of Feedback in EBP and QI

Feedback is a continuous process that plays a critical role in EBPQI initiatives by providing information about performance and outcomes, helping to identify areas for improvement, and facilitating ongoing learning and development. Feedback is used to assess performance. For example, for Aim 1, did the nurse perform a falls risk assessment and provide the patient/family education? Feedback can motivate changes in behavior or practice, particularly when it highlights gaps between current and desired performance. By monitoring performance, you can identify areas that are working well and those that need improvement. Constructive feedback aids in learning and professional development, offering guidance on how to improve and sustain effective practices.

Regular feedback engages all stakeholders in continuous improvement, creating a sense of ownership and accountability. Ongoing feedback contributes to a culture of continuous improvement in which EBP and QI are considered integral parts of everyday practice rather than one-off initiatives.

BOX 11.2: FEEDBACK EXAMPLE

Let's suppose that a hospital is implementing an EBPQI project to reduce patient readmission rates by improving discharge planning and post discharge follow-up. To evaluate the effect of the improvements, the EBPQI team regularly collects data on (a) readmission rates, (b) adherence to the new discharge process, and (c) patient and staff experiences. They provide feedback to all involved staff every month. This feedback might include data on changes in readmission rates, insights into the reasons for readmissions, and examples of successful discharges without readmission. It might also include qualitative patient feedback about their experiences with the discharge process and their ability to manage their conditions at home.

As the EBPQI team discusses the feedback with the staff, they praise successes, identify challenges, and brainstorm solutions for identified issues. For instance, if the feedback indicates that some patients are unclear about their medication regimens post discharge, the team might decide to introduce a new step into the discharge process to ensure a more thorough medication reconciliation and education. This process not only informs the team about the progress of their QI initiative but also drives ongoing learning and improvement, contributing to the goal of reducing readmissions.

Integrating and Sustaining the Practice Change

For a change to stick, it must be hardwired into the system through such means as permanent policy or protocol revisions. Revisions can be integrated into new employee orientation, annual training, competency evaluations, or required learning modules or skills fairs that provide ongoing mechanisms to support the practice change. Educational resources with clear guidance should remain available to all stakeholders.

WRAPPING UP

In this chapter, you collected the data you needed to determine whether your initiative met your aims. You used your pilot data to adapt the practice change to fit your setting and continued to collect data. After 6 months, you began to see that the practice change was being implemented more consistently and making a difference in the fall rate without increasing costs (overtime hours). Congratulations!

You have one more step to climb to reach the top of the EBPQI mountain summit: disseminating your results! It is time to share the journey you have completed with others. This last step will determine the internal and external impact of your EBPQI work more than any other part of the process. In Chapter 12, you will be introduced to the importance of sharing information widely and learn about traditional and nontraditional methods of making target audiences aware of your results. Before moving on, let's take a well-earned moment to consider intentional engagement in active (scheduled) rest so that you can sustain the longevity of momentum.

WELLNESS IN ACTION: RESTORATIVE REST

Habits are powerful. In Chapter 3, we learned about the importance of getting adequate sleep, but it is also vital to practice some rest when we are awake. Participating in a pattern of planned relaxation according to your lifestyle and values can keep you energized and engaged. A scheduled rhythm of active (intentional) resting can increase your productivity, lifespan, and life quality while reducing stress and burnout. In one study, a group that practiced a weekly sabbath (rest for 1 day out of every 7) consistently lived 10 years longer than the average American (Buxton, 2014).

Interestingly, if a person rests for 1 day out of every 7, that adds up to approximately 10 years over a normal lifespan. Think of that! Active rest may look like relaxation or an hour, a day, a week, or more every month or year. Humans need time off from the daily grind to slow down, and by taking time to refresh and rejuvenate, we reap wellness benefits. Consider the value of practicing active rest in your life rhythm through the following steps:

1. Be intentional about setting aside time to rest in a way that works for your particular season of life. This can occur in various ways. Perhaps you can plan a vacation (or even a few hours) without access to screens to enjoy resting your mind rather than producing or processing information.
2. Plan a time to depart from labor and relax. For example, use a time cluster (e.g., a full or partial day) for rest, such as a half-day on Fridays to begin your weekend with restoration.
3. Redeem your workplace benefits of "time off" or vacation days before they expire. Don't lose this precious rest time: https://www.ustravel.org/toolkit/time-and-vacation-usage
4. Allow your mind to wander and relax during rest rather than occupying yourself with mindless activities. For example, instead of scrolling on your phone, read an interesting book for pleasure or take a walk in a beautiful landscape.

REFLECTION QUESTIONS

1. What are the benefits of conducting a pilot of your EBPQI practice change?
2. Explain the elements on one or all of the family of measures charts.
3. Using the example in Box 11.2 (feedback for a hospital that implements an EBPQI project to reduce patient readmission rates by improving discharge planning and post discharge follow-up), write one or more aims and develop strategies for collecting data to determine whether the aims were met.

REFERENCES

Agency for Healthcare Research and Quality. (2015, September). *Optimizing electronic health records (EHRs) for quality improvement (QI)*. https://www.ahrq.gov/evidencenow/tools/facilitation/qi-ehrs.html

Barnsteiner, J., Beebe, S., Dicker, R., Halm, M., Hirsch, M., Taulbee, R., & Troy, D. (2023). Facilitating a culture of evidence-based practice and quality improvement excellence: Streamlining processes to improve care. *Journal for Nurses in Professional Development*, *39*(4), 207–213. https://doi.org/10.1097/NND.0000000000000995

Buxton, R. (2014, July). *What Seventh-Day Adventists Get Right That Lengthens Their Life Expectancy.* https://www.huffpost.com/entry/seventh-day-adventists-life-expectancy_n_5638098

Crawford, C. L., Rondinelli, J., Zuniga, S., Valdez, R. M., Tze-Polo, L., & Titler, M. G. (2023). Barriers and facilitators influencing EBP readiness: Building organizational and nurse capacity. *Worldviews on Evidence-Based Nursing*, *20*(1), 27–36. https://doi.org/10.1111/wvn.12618

Sandelowski, M. (2000). Whatever happened to qualitative description? *Research in Nursing & Health*, *23*(4), 334–340. https://doi.org/10.1002/1098-240x(200008)23:4<334::aid-nur9>3.0.co;2-g

Silver, S. A., McQuillan, R., Harel, Z., Weizman, A. V., Thomas, A., Nesrallah, G., Bell, C. M., Chan, C. T., & Chertow, G. M. (2016). How to sustain change and support continuous quality improvement. *Clinical Journal of the American Society of Nephrology*, *11*(5), 916–924. https://doi.org/10.2215/CJN.11501015

Warren, J. I., McLaughlin, M., Bardsley, J., Eich, J., Esche, C. A., Kropkowski, L., & Risch, S. (2016). The strengths and challenges of implementing EBP in healthcare systems. *Worldviews on Evidence-Based Nursing*, *13*(1), 15–24. https://doi.org/10.1111/wvn.12149

CHAPTER 12

The Nurse's Responsibility to Ensure Dissemination

Jayne Jennings Dunlap, Tracy McManaman-Bridges, and Rosalie Mainous

KEY CONCEPTS

Dissemination
Plagiarism
Publication
Authorship
Presentations

LEARNING OBJECTIVES

1. Describe various approaches to EBPQI dissemination.
2. Compare and contrast the different types of dissemination.
3. Identify strategies for internal and external dissemination.
4. Discuss ways to include essential components of EBPQI initiatives in dissemination reports.

> If you have knowledge, let others light their candles in it.
>
> —Margret Fuller

Introduction

You have arrived at the top of the mountain! Take a breath and look around—after your climb, this pinnacle is an exhilarating place to be!

Throughout this final chapter, our focus will be on dissemination, the culminating step of the EBPQI process. Dissemination can be as simple as presenting evidence-based practice improvements to your patient populations and coworkers or as far-reaching as educating members of our profession (or allied professions) at the regional, state, national, or even international level. Although all EBPQI process components are equally essential, if your EBPQI initiative has proved successful, you should share it. The optimal impact of EBPQI initiatives occurs when others learn of your accomplishment and understand how to transfer and adapt your improvement to their own organization or setting. You will recall from Chapter 1 that transferability is the goal of EBPQI. As you leave school behind for a professional role, embrace the goal of disseminating knowledge about improvement opportunities and successes. Any project or initiative you embark upon in the future must have a sharing mechanism so that others can benefit from your completed work. Dissemination is critically important to advancing the field of nursing and enabling nurses to promote optimal health and healthcare.

Dissemination Approaches

What does the word "dissemination" mean to you? It has been our experience that many nursing students and practicing nurses do not fully understand what dissemination entails and the benefits of engaging in this professional mainstay. **Dissemination** is the spreading of ideas (often widely) to individuals and/or groups; in the context of healthcare, dissemination involves the purposeful distribution of information or materials to a specific audience. The goal of disseminating EBPQI work is to increase evidence-based interventions and/or actions that lead to sustained health improvements. Engaging in dissemination can be a fun and exciting process, if done effectively.

Before we discuss various types of dissemination, you should be aware of some essential components of information sharing. Imagine this scenario: You attend a conference at which another person or team presents your disseminated work, taking credit for your accomplishment. This is a prime example of plagiarism. **Plagiarism** means claiming someone else's work or ideas as your own. It is critical to avoid plagiarism under any circumstance, but researchers sometimes plagiarize inadvertently. A common cause of plagiarism is citing research or information without providing the proper reference. Suppose you copy and paste supportive information from a published study into your written work but forget to add a citation to the original source(s) along with a corresponding entry in your reference list. This oversight constitutes plagiarism! Accurate citation is a courtesy to fellow evidence seekers in that it guides them to the material on which your work is based as well as related research; however, providing appropriate credit is more than a mere courtesy! Ideas and accomplishments function as currency in the professional world, often contributing to a professional's career advancement or funding for future research, so plagiarism is considered a form of theft. Information source(s), whether paraphrased or directly quoted, must always be clearly credited. Additionally, you must enclose directly quoted material in quotation marks to indicate that you are crediting not only someone's work but their wording as well. Consequences for plagiarism are varied and can be very serious, including discreditation. Publishing your article in more than one journal constitutes self-plagiarism (reuse of your work from previously published text) and must be avoided. We want you to be empowered as a future nurse, so please heed our warning that participation in any form of plagiarism is disempowering and unethical.

You must also credit funding sources (budgetary resources) when your work is disseminated. Funding sources include any monetary support received for the project or initiative. For example, grants (internal or external) or donations should be credited appropriately when your work is shared. Name your funding source(s) in a visible location and fully comply with your institution's policy or the guidelines of the journal to which you are submitting your work for **publication**.

Authorship is a form of creating; it implies the production and organization of new material. The word "author" is derived from the Latin word *auctor*, meaning one who "originates or creates something" (Merriam-Webster, n.d.). Everyone listed as an author of the work should have substantially contributed to its completion. "Substantial" is the keyword here. For example, a person who shares ideas and helps to write the work is an author; conversely, a person who only reviews the finished work and provides feedback is not a contributing author to its completion. Remember that personal and professional rewards, as well as a great responsibility for the work, accompanies authorship (Oermann & Hays, 2019). For this reason, the order of authorship is important and should be determined honestly and respectfully from the start of dissemination. The first-listed (or primary) author is typically the initiative's leader and has contributed most substantially. Those who have contributed to the writing or presentation should be listed in order of contribution (work completed); for example, some expected contributions include conceptualization or writing/editing the content of drafts (works in progress). Make certain that the order of authorship truly reflects the standards of the International Committee of Medical Journal Editors (https://www.icmje.org/recommendations/browse/roles-and-responsibilities/defining-the-role-of-authors-and-contributors.html).

Conflicts of interest occur when your personal interests have the potential to compromise your professional judgment as a nurse. Any financial or competing interest that could cast doubt upon your fairness or judgment is a conflict of interest. For example, if you own a business that might impact or benefit from your EBPQI initiative, you must inform your audiences of this. Conflicts of interest or monetary relationships that are not disclosed for transparency may cause your disseminated work to be viewed skeptically if they are later discovered. Disclosure enables your audience to respect the accuracy and value of your disseminated information with complete confidence in your integrity as a researcher.

Identify Your Audience

Now that we have covered basic points about funding sources, authorship, and conflicts of interest, it is time to take the first step toward effective dissemination—identifying your target audience. When you imagine your intended audience, who comes to mind? What group of people or professionals might be interested in using your improvement initiative or components of your work in their settings? This is an important consideration, so take time to critically reflect on it. Relevant internal (e.g., local clinicians, clinical partners) and external (e.g., professional organizations, policymakers, community partners beyond your home organization) audiences will differ depending on your topic or initiative focus.

Typically, patients and clinical teams, including providers, nurses, ancillary and leadership staff, academic organizations, policymakers, and community partners, are interested in EBPQI work on local and systems levels. Nurses may not realize that if a positive change occurs through an EBPQI, the initiative may well be transferable to other departments or institutions on a broader scale. The only way to accomplish this is through dissemination!

An important point to remember:

- Dissemination of the same information may differ based on the audience. Asking yourself, "To whom do I want to provide this information?" will help you determine how best to target your impact. Think about the audience you want to reach before crafting your messaging strategy.

Dissemination Types

Passive dissemination involves one-way communication with targeted audiences. Passive dissemination is often a top-down approach to information sharing, generally taking the form of posted or published communications. *Active dissemination*, on the other hand, involves bidirectional interaction with target audiences, thus allowing you to impart key messages related to your work and entertain a back-and-forth exchange of ideas and questions in real time.

Which method will most effectively showcase your practice change to the right people? As you devise plans to share your work, consider incorporating elements of both passive and active dissemination. To reach internal audiences, for example, you could present a "brown bag" webinar, display a poster within the unit, or round routinely to thank involved stakeholders and staff for their contributions to the new EBPQI success. To reach external audiences, you could present a poster at a professional conference (e.g., sponsored by your local or state nursing association) or interface with decision-makers from other healthcare systems to offer inspiration and advice on developing a new practice at their organizations.

Dissemination may feel daunting, especially as you are learning to navigate the process, but keep in mind that you do not need to disseminate alone. You can elicit help from your teammates and/or trusted colleagues who may have specific strengths and experiential wisdom to share. For example, suppose you are a confident speaker and have a colleague who enjoys summarizing the initiative in written format but does not like to speak publicly. The two of you could form a solid partnership based on your complementary skills and preferences. Similarly, you may accept a smaller role on a larger team among whom dissemination tasks are divided. To increase your chances of successful dissemination, you should be willing to (a) recognize your strengths and challenges, (b) seek help from others who possess useful skill sets and a shared passion for tackling the problem your work addresses, and (c) communicate roles and responsibilities in a direct and reasonable manner.

Dissemination Methods

Traditional Methods

Oral Presentations

The key to a successful presentation is a clearly articulated, accurate, and meaningful message. **Presentations** can serve as an exciting way to distribute your EBPQI initiatives. If you are uncomfortable speaking in front of groups, we encourage you to stretch beyond your comfort zone, if possible. Try to put yourself in the place of fellow nurses from different units or organizations who want to know how this problem can be addressed successfully; by presenting your work, you are helping your peers and colleagues. Remember that your involvement in an EBPQI initiative has given you some mastery over this research topic, and sharing your expertise about your work is often much easier than speaking about yourself. You can start on a small scale by presenting evidence-based information to patients, perhaps by teaching an evidence-based class on childbirth, healthy activities, meditation—any topic about which you have some knowledge and passion! Similarly, you can start by presenting at a staff meeting with daily coworkers who will be supportive as you gain confidence in your presentation skills. Next, consider presenting your work at a conference attended by peers who share your interest in and devotion to improving healthcare and patient outcomes. Your fellow professionals will want to know what you have accomplished, just as you will want to learn from them. You may even come away from this exhilarating and helpful environment with ideas for future projects based on suggestions from your audience. This has been our repeated experience throughout our nursing careers.

Presentations can be either invited or peer-reviewed. Your presentation is "invited" if the conference/event leaders or organizers asked you to present on a topic related to an area of your known expertise. If your presentation is peer-reviewed, you likely followed the following process to have it considered:

1. You submitted an abstract (abbreviated content to be covered within the presentation) to a committee (often in response to a publicized call for presenters).
2. A group of peers reviewed the content and likely scored its strength on a rubric.
3. Your peer-reviewed abstract was accepted for presentation at the conference.

Presentations can be accepted or rejected. Seek feedback, if available, on rejected presentation abstracts so that you can work toward strengthening your messaging in the future. We recommend having a seasoned presenter review your abstract and presentation to offer suggestions to strengthen them. Remember, feedback should not be taken personally but considered objectively. Remember, too, that conference sessions have time frames, so organizers often must reject many good submissions; they may choose certain papers because their topics or approaches are complementary.

An important cautionary note:

- Verify the legitimacy of any conference before agreeing to present. Predatory conferences (or publications) claim to be scholarly but are typically organized entities focused on financial gain rather than quality scholarship. These conferences often seek out presenters and sometimes ask for payment to present. If you are suspicious, ask a trusted colleague with experience presenting at conferences for advice. Be alert for these red flags!

Preparing an Oral Presentation

Oral presentations at all levels (local, state, regional, national, and international) provide an excellent opportunity to share your EBPQI work. A common mistake seen at presentations, especially among novices, is placing too much material on slides. Oral presentations are of various types and lengths. You may present on a panel of researchers whose presentations touch on a common theme. Often, three similar presentations are scheduled within a blocked time frame (e.g., 1 hour). As with poster presentations, you must follow guidelines for oral presentations explicitly. We have the following suggestions:

- Think about the time allotted for your presentation when crafting your abstract and learning objectives/outcomes.
- Start and end with something meaningful, funny, or inspirational.
- Ensure the presented material is easy to read and engaging.
- Create visually appealing electronic slideshow presentations with minimal words.
- Let slideshows guide your presentation but not comprise the presentation.
- Avoid reading directly from your presentation materials.
- Practice your presentation until you can almost give it without your slides.
- Bring your enthusiasm for the work.
- Adhere to your time presentation allotment.
- Allow some time for questions and answers, if possible.
- Arrive early and ensure that your presentation is appropriately accessible.
- Ensure audio-visual equipment is functioning before the presentation.
- Have a backup plan in case of audio or visual equipment failure.

Poster Presentations

A poster is a visual representation of your EBPQI initiative. Poster presentations can serve as an entry point to dissemination at the start of your nursing career. Many professional meetings and settings will accept a poster about your work in progress. A key advantage of poster presentations is that they allow for one-on-one exchanges of information in a fairly private setting versus open discussions with an audience during a timed oral presentation in a room scheduled for successive activities. Be sure to follow the instructions for poster presentations completely and pay careful attention to details; if you do not adhere to the guidelines or format in the abstract submission, it is unlikely that your poster will be selected for presentation. EBPQI poster presentations often include the following:

- Poster title and listing of the author(s)
- Statement of the clinical problem/significance
- Display of the searchable question (e.g., PICO, PPCO)
- Details of the search process (e.g., dates of literature search, databases used, number of articles retrieved)
- Summary of the critical appraisal process, including tools used and synthesis of the evidence
- Data gathered from internal evidence
- Statement of initiative purpose and aims
- Description of the evidence-based practice change
- Methods used to implement the change (e.g., lean, Six Sigma, PDSA)
- Evaluation of outcomes

Include visual representations of your work as appropriate (e.g., evidence synthesis table, run chart) to increase readability/understanding; perhaps sketch out your ideas digitally or on paper as a poster mock-up to organize preparation efforts. Remember that many conferences offer peer evaluations and give awards (e.g., first place, second place, honorable mention). At the conference, try to remain near your poster so you can interface with conference attendees whenever possible. Aim high to elevate your work! The most recent trend in poster presentations is to place a visible QR code on your poster for scanning so that people reviewing your work may keep a copy of your abstract, poster, or material related to your initiative, such as a complete protocol or additional related information you wish to share.

Often, the organization you represent (at which you conducted your EBPQI initiative) will have a poster template and rules for presenting work publicly. The conference at which you are presenting may also have a required template. Templates provide a professional structure for displaying the content of your work. Although it may seem tempting to display your creativity without their guidance, templates ensure your presentation is complete and understandable.

Writing a Manuscript for Peer-Reviewed Publication

In nursing, as in all disciplines, peer review is a process that upholds integrity and validity in dissemination. It is an integral component of scholarship to have the scholarly quality of one's work systematically assessed and judged by peers. You certainly want your work measured against the highest standards of professional nursing practice (George & Haag-Heitman, 2011). In Chapters 5– 7, you learned about the critical appraisal of external evidence (i.e., peer-reviewed sources) to support EBPQI initiatives. Typically, *peer reviewers* are experts on a particular topic (e.g., cardiovascular nursing care) who volunteer to evaluate work as an unpaid service to the profession; they critique other scholars' work through constructive feedback in preparation for dissemination (Dougherty et al., 2011). Such reviews help to ensure legitimacy in the field. The peer-review process is the quality assurance system for the nursing discipline's body of knowledge. Readers depend on peer review to ensure the relevance, readability, and quality of articles (Morton, 2013).

There are various types of peer review. The type most commonly used by nursing journals is the *double-blind peer review*, in which reviewers do not know (are "blind" to) the identity of the authors whose manuscript they are reviewing and the authors are similarly "blind" to the identity of the peers who are reviewing their work (Waldrop & Likis, 2022). There is a trend in other disciplines to increase transparency in peer review by allowing the identity of the authors and/or reviewers to be known. Reputable journals should have accessible and transparent author guidelines that inform potential authors of how their peer-review process is conducted.

By sharing your EBPQI initiatives through **publication**, you contribute to the literature base so that others can potentially transfer/adapt your initiative to their local setting. Two examples of journals that publish peer-reviewed articles on a variety of nursing and healthcare topics monthly, thus reaching a wide audience of nurses and nursing leaders, are *American Nurse* (https://www.nursingworld.org/membership/ana-periodicals/americannurse/), a society journal of the American Nursing Association, and the *American Journal of Nursing* (https://www.wolterskluwer.com/en/solutions/ovid/ajn-the-american-journal-of-nursing-393).

Nurses can use a presentation to create a manuscript as well as to disseminate completed work. Depending on the topic and focus, you generally should present your content to a live audience before publishing a written version. After you have completed a live presentation, however, please commit to developing a manuscript and submitting it to a peer-reviewed journal. You can also write the manuscript first and build your presentation materials from your paper. Nurses are busy, so setting soft deadlines and asking for accountability from trusted colleagues will prove helpful. Set a goal for completion, such as 60 or 90 days, while the topic is still fresh and on your mind. Remember that production time (the amount of time it takes from submission to publication) varies, and you will want your manuscript to be made available digitally and/or in print as soon as possible. Stay focused on getting your message out so that others can benefit and learn from your work.

As you consider writing up your work in manuscript format, explore potential peer-reviewed journals that might have an interest in publishing it. You can access the International Academy of Nurse Editors' Nursing Journal Directory (https://airtable.com/shrjqveaKHtS9xku8/tblNXTxmTr18CC1If) for a current listing of vetted journals. The journals on this list are authenticated by nurse editor leaders. Use caution when selecting a target journal (a journal to which you intend to submit), as predatory publications often use names similar to those of legitimate peer-reviewed journals. Sadly, nurses have engaged in predatory publication erroneously, thus compromising and invalidating their work. Watch out for red flags! Predatory journals often offer a rapid path to publication and may ask for payment to publish your work. If in doubt, always consult a trusted colleague before submitting your work to a journal.

After identifying a target journal, read its mission or purpose statement (usually found in the "About" section on the journal website) to ensure that your topic is a good fit for that specific journal given its focus (e.g., pediatrics, hematology, diabetes care). Next, check the author guidelines (found under "Information for Authors") to discover which types of manuscripts the journal accepts. For example, if you wish to submit an EBPQI initiative, it would likely be nonproductive to submit it to a journal that accepts only research studies, clinical features, and case studies. Read the author guidelines in their entirety. Once you have selected a target journal that might be a good fit and verified its legitimacy, consider emailing a query to the editor to gauge interest in your topic or ask whether they would be interested in an EBPQI manuscript. It is essential to first familiarize yourself with the journal (in print or online) by reading its previously published articles in recent issues. Follow the directions on the journal's website for author queries and be clear and succinct in your messaging about your manuscript's topic and why you believe the article would be a good fit for the journal's readership.

Occasionally, some journals will announce a call for manuscripts on specific topics of interest, usually on the journal's homepage. As with presentations, you must follow the journal's author guidelines closely to increase your chances of receiving a peer review rather than a desk rejection. A *desk rejection* occurs when an editor rejects the manuscript without sending it for peer review because the journal guidelines were not followed or the article was not deemed a good fit for that journal.

We strongly suggest that you ask a trusted colleague to review your article before you submit it for publication. Make this a systematic part of your writing and dissemination process! Remember that articles are often accepted conditionally pending successful revisions (changes requested by peer reviewers and editors), so soliciting advice before submission may help you to anticipate reviewer concerns. If you are invited to revise and resubmit your manuscript, rejoice! This means that the editor believes that your manuscript is publishable if improved based on the reviewers' feedback. Follow the suggestions for revision and resubmit your revised manuscript within the allotted time frame. If you need an extension to complete a significant revision, proactively correspond with the editor and request this. The purpose of peer-review feedback is to strengthen the article, so accommodate all the suggestions that you can; if a reviewer's request seems unfeasible to you, politely explain why. Clearly itemize your author response to each of the individual changes suggested by the reviewer(s) or editor; we recommend organizing these itemized responses in a table format (see Table 12.1 for an abbreviated example). You can adapt a similar table by copying/pasting each reviewer comment, listing how the item was addressed (or why you felt the particular request could not be accommodated), and noting where the change is located in your revised manuscript (or pasting in a copy of the revised wording).

The publishing world is smaller than it seems, and you may be associating with the same colleagues in various capacities throughout your career: at conferences, on presentation panels, on committees, or as a reviewer or author. Remember that peer review is a voluntary professional service provided by your colleagues, and it is important to respect others' time and effort throughout the submission process. Always be polite and professional in your dealings with editors and reviewers, even if you disagree with a decision or comment. If you decide not to resubmit following a peer review, communicate your decision with the editor so they won't be expecting your revised manuscript.

TABLE 12.1 Sample Author Response Table

Thank you for your thoughtful support and comments to strengthen our paper. Please see the author response table addressing each item below.		
Reviewer/editor comments	**Author response**	**Location of revisions**
Reviewer 1		
I found the Introduction and the Background to be confusing at times and lacking a flow of ideas. I am not sure the contents included in both of these sections are totally relevant.	Introduction and Background sections rewritten. Additionally, author use of print materials was removed to increase clarity.	Page 2, paragraphs 1–4
The first sentence in the last paragraph doesn't seem to reflect the remainder of that paragraph. I think it could simply be deleted and start the first paragraph with the second sentence. This article is timely, and I suggest adding more content.	First sentence deleted.	Page 6, paragraph 1
Reviewer 2		
Thank you for the opportunity to review this manuscript. I suggest omitting the Introduction. Overall, I found this work to be interesting, but more content is needed.	Key points from the Introduction were included in the rewrite of the background article.	Page 2, paragraphs 1–4
Editor		
Both reviewers suggested additional content for the paper. In addition, you need more references. I am recommending you add content with more details to this paper so it is an original manuscript, not a department (because of the word limits).	Format changed from department to original feature manuscript	Throughout

Nontraditional Dissemination

In addition to traditional dissemination methods as appropriate for your work, you can use nontraditional outlets to increase its reach to your intended audience. We recommend that formal dissemination methods, such as peer-reviewed publications, be augmented with nontraditional methods to reach the broadest audiences. Institutional repositories as a form of open access have been used successfully to disseminate practice scholarship and are held by librarians in an oversight role. Institutional, governmental, and discipline-specific repositories maximize digital dissemination (Kesten & Hoover, 2022). One of the best examples is the Sigma Theta Tau International Honor Society of Nursing's Sigma Repository (https://www.sigmarepository.org/).

State nursing associations, boards of nursing, chapters of Sigma Theta Tau, local and state chapters of the National Black Nurses Association, and the National Association of Hispanic Nurses have newsletters and various publications from formal journals down to very brief communiques. Most health/hospital systems have newsletters and various publications offered to the public on topics of interest and best health practices. Some are peer-reviewed, and some are not. Some require references; some publish opinion pieces. Policy work can often be shared in these modalities, and they are a great place to publish some work that may be a bit controversial. All you need do is query the editor with your idea to ensure a good fit and, of course, follow the publication guidelines.

Practice-oriented projects are well-suited for lay publications, and the public is hungry for evidence-based guidelines for promoting health or managing symptoms, screening guidelines, and anticipatory guidance for pediatric populations. There are many places to publish the results of the scholarship of nursing practice. Have you considered the audiences (readership) of common lay publications, such as *Reader's Digest*, *Family Circle*, *Women's Health*, *Men's Health*, and *Cosmopolitan*? These are among the most popular magazines in the country; each is a niche publication that would benefit from timely articles steeped in evidence to support decision-making related to health practices. In addition, there are publications in most clinics and healthcare provider's offices, which are purposeful in reaching the audience of their waiting room.

Blogs are another means to disseminate your work. *Blogs* are updated websites/pages that are very informal but informational. In general, blogs associated with organizations or businesses require access and often a fee. Personal blogs are more likely to be free. Typically, a blog would not be a good method to offer a single piece of work; instead, it could represent a series or a broad topic area. Pick your topic and then seek a blogging platform (web content home). Long and short articles, updates, and breaking news are all acceptable. Many bloggers try to develop their blog to support a revenue stream through advertising, but such an endeavor is generally labor intensive, possibly costly, and requires a lot of content. For some, however, it can be a dedicated way to build a professional presence.

Podcasts began as an alternative format to the written word and broadcast radio. *Podcasts* present information to share with listeners for entertainment and education in a prerecorded audio format. They can have many purposes, and there are many health-focused podcasts available to the public. Podcasts have increased in popularity over the past decade (Gotting, 2023) and can be an excellent venue for dissemination. However, a challenge to developing a successful podcast is securing an audience. How will potential listeners know about your podcast? Podcasts need to be marketed, and individuals must feel compelled to subscribe to listen; therefore, developing a podcast requires financial resources. Generally, we approve use of this means to reach a professional audience, and many nurses have done so. If you search "nurse" on Apple or other podcast sites, you will find a variety of podcasts on nursing topics to listen to.

Brief Methods of Dissemination

Elevator Speech

All professionals who wish to bring attention to their work should have at the ready an elevator speech, so titled because you can give the entire speech on the elevator as you move from one floor to another. Elevator speeches may serve as a means of introduction, advocacy, or the dissemination of your work's key findings. This speech should be crafted to a specific audience, so you may need several versions. Start by writing a draft with a clear opening, solid message, and closure. Practice speaking it within an approximately 3-minute time frame. Share your speech with a trusted colleague and ask for feedback on your delivery and messaging. Elevator speeches have the potential for indelibly imprinting your message on your target audience.

Executive Summary

Another succinct way to communicate the key points of your EBPQI initiative is with an executive summary. An *executive summary* is usually a 1- to 2-page document that serves as a cover sheet for a comprehensive report. You may have seen one attached to a business case, white paper, market analysis, or the findings from a task force or large collaborative. Like an abstract, the executive summary should be written last, as it summarizes the more extensive report. It usually has sections including an introduction, the key points of the report with the findings, and conclusions; however, it must be able to stand on its own merit. Your executive summary should be formal and exact yet sufficiently interesting to engage an audience to read the full report.

Social Media

Social media has introduced novel ways to enable rapid information sharing locally and globally. Some journals and many professional nursing organizations have social media channels. Nursing journals use social media to promote their content and increase engagement with their readers (Dunlap & Waldrop, 2022). Twitter (X) is the most used social media channel among nursing journals, followed by Facebook. Other types of social media used to promote nursing journal content include Pinterest, YouTube, and Instagram (Waldrop & Dunlap, 2021). If a journal posts about your article, share and comment on the post. Use hashtags to loop in others who may be involved in disseminating your work. Many nursing journals and PubMed Central have social media plugins to enable one-click sharing (Waldrop et al., 2022).

BOX 12.1: AMPLIFY YOUR NURSING VOICE

- Follow nursing and healthcare peer-reviewed journals on your social media channels.
- Share relevant articles with your personal and professional networks.
- Include appropriate hashtags for related topics or audiences and/or organizations who may be interested in your posted content.

(*Waldrop et al., 2022*)

Speaking to the Media

Nurses should give thoughtful consideration to sharing information with the media through lay outlets. Although this is one way to make the public aware of best practices, speaking to the media can be challenging, even for the most experienced nurses or administrators. If you are approached by the media to showcase your work or provide commentary on a hot topic, proceed very cautiously. First, we recommend notifying the communications and marketing department in your institution for guidelines on media interviews. You may need to obtain formal approval to speak with the media. Often, the communications department can help you produce a statement consistent with the institution's philosophy that highlights your accomplishments or critique. Second, recognize that an interview with the press for a television or radio segment will likely be edited down to short sound bites that make the most impact; thus, it may not contain parts of your message. Third, ask whether the news agency will allow you to preview and edit the piece before it appears in print. If so, always take advantage of this opportunity to review the accuracy of the final piece and make any necessary changes. Fourth, listen carefully to what you are being asked and do not respond until the interviewer has finished asking their question. If you do not understand the question or if you do not have a full and clear sense of what is being asked, request that the question be repeated or rephrased. It is possible that the interviewer has a hidden agenda or is seeking to support a view their sponsor wants to represent. If you cannot provide an informed answer, do not hesitate to admit this, and offer to get back to the interviewer as soon as possible, or refer them to someone else.

BOX 12.2: DISSEMINATION IN ACTION

A new nurse approached me (Tracy) in the labor and delivery unit and stated that she wanted to decrease the C-section rate on our unit. She had noticed that the unit's C-section rates did not meet the organization's goal of less than 20%. As her assigned preceptor and mentor, I encouraged her to explore the research/evidence on this topic. The evidence-based interventions she initially uncovered were interventions that would require implementation by our physician and provider partners, such as postponing inductions until later gestation and adding cervical ripening to the induction procedure. We discussed the nurse's role at the bedside and refocused her search on nursing interventions. She used the PPCO framework to develop a question to guide her search.

Element	Description	Example
Problem (P)	What is the problem in general (external evidence) and specifically in the local context (internal evidence)?	Cesarean birth rate above benchmark
Population (P)	Whom does the problem impact?	Women and newborns
Change (C)	What has been recommended or done to address the problem (practice or process changes)?	Changes in nursing practice or processes
Outcomes (O)	How are outcomes reported (measured)? (This may be the same as the problem originally noted or its components.)	Reduction in cesarean rate

Waldrop and Dunlap 2024a (in press)

The new nurse let the literature guide her to a potential nursing invention supported by evidence. Many laboring patients receive epidural anesthesia (the medication is administered continuously into the epidural space in the spinal cord) and thus have limited mobility during labor. The new nurse found research evidence on the use of a "peanut ball" for position changes during labor. This noninvasive nurse-led practice was associated with decreased C-section rates. Through the systematic appraisal of the evidence, she found that when the laboring patient hugged the peanut ball, it provided a dual benefit: (a) It changed the angle of the pelvis, allowing labor to progress more quickly; and (b) the patient was actively involved in her care (Caughey et al., 2014; Mercier & Kwan, 2018; Roth et al., 2016). The nurse pitched her evidence-based recommendation for a change in practice to reduce the C-section rate to the unit manager.

- SMART aim: On the labor and delivery unit, introducing the peanut ball as a labor aid will result in a 2% reduction in the C-section rate after 1 month of use.

The unit manager was convinced and purchased four peanut balls to support the EBPQI initiative. After being educated on its use, the healthcare team offered the peanut ball to all laboring patients. As a process measure, the nurse asked questions of the healthcare team members about participation; as a balancing measure, she asked questions about comfort and satisfaction. A decrease in the C-section rate was noted within the first month for mothers using the ball during labor, and a notable difference in how involved the patients felt in their care was evidenced through data collection. After the successful pilot, the nurse created a unit policy for the use, cleaning, and storage of peanut balls. She also disseminated her findings via poster presentation at a state-wide women's health conference. Four years later, the peanut ball continues to be a staple in every delivery room across our unit, symbolizing a unit-wide EBPQI change led by a new RN that is directly benefiting patients. By following the steps of EBPQI to realize practice improvement (Waldrop & Dunlap, 2024b), working with the healthcare team to ensure that the change was sustained internally as well as disseminated externally, and targeting transferability, this nurse surpassed her initial EBPQI goal. Her work may decrease C-section rates beyond her unit (the initial goal), help mothers feel more involved in their labor, and save valuable healthcare dollars—a contribution to be proud of indeed!

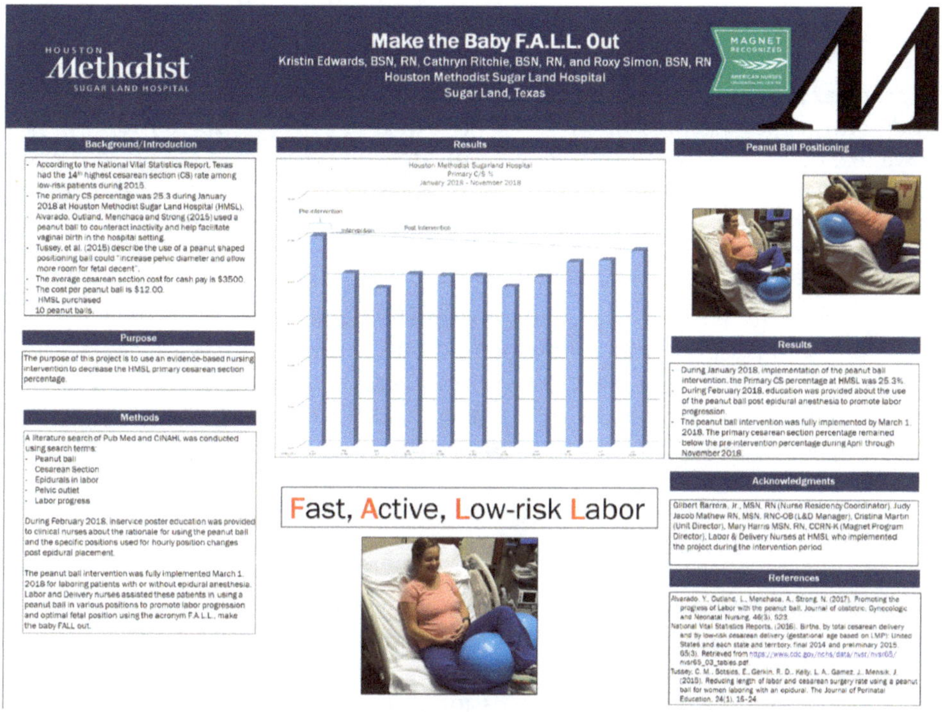
HOUSTON Methodist SUGAR LAND HOSPITAL
Make the Baby F.A.L.L. Out
Kristin Edwards, BSN, RN, Cathryn Ritchie, BSN, RN, and Roxy Simon, BSN, RN
Houston Methodist Sugar Land Hospital
Sugar Land, Texas
MAGNET RECOGNIZED
Background/Introduction
- According to the National Vital Statistics Report, Texas had the 14th highest cesarean section (CS) rate among low-risk patients during 2015.
- The primary CS percentage was 25.3 during January 2018 at Houston Methodist Sugar Land Hospital (HMSL).
- Alvarado, Outland, Menchaca and Strong (2015) used a peanut ball to counteract inactivity and help facilitate vaginal birth in the hospital setting.
- Tussey, et al. (2015) describe the use of a peanut shaped positioning ball could "increase pelvic diameter and allow more room for fetal decent".
- The average cesarean section cost for cash pay is $3500.
- The cost per peanut ball is $12.00.
- HMSL purchased 10 peanut balls.
Purpose
The purpose of this project is to use an evidence-based nursing intervention to decrease the HMSL primary cesarean section percentage.
Methods
A literature search of Pub Med and CINAHL was conducted using search terms:
- Peanut ball
- Cesarean Section
- Epidurals in labor
- Pelvic outlet
- Labor progress
During February 2018, inservice poster education was provided to clinical nurses about the rationale for using the peanut ball and the specific positions used for hourly position changes post epidural placement.
The peanut ball intervention was fully implemented March 1, 2018 for laboring patients with or without epidural anesthesia. Labor and Delivery nurses assisted these patients in using a peanut ball in various positions to promote labor progression and optimal fetal position using the acronym F.A.L.L., make the baby FALL out.
Results
Houston Methodist Sugarland Hospital
Primary C/S %
January 2018 - November 2018
Pre intervention
Post intervention
Fast, Active, Low-risk Labor
Peanut Ball Positioning
Results
- During January 2018, implementation of the peanut ball intervention, the Primary CS percentage at HMSL was 25.3%.
- During February 2018, education was provided about the use of the peanut ball post epidural anesthesia to promote labor progression.
- The peanut ball intervention was fully implemented by March 1, 2018. The primary cesarean section percentage remained below the pre-intervention percentage during April through November 2018.
Acknowledgments
Gilbert Barrera, Jr., MSN, RN (Nurse Residency Coordinator), Judy Jacob Mathew RN, MSN, RNC-OB (L&D Manager), Cristina Martin (Unit Director), Mary Harris MSN, RN, CCRN-K (Magnet Program Director), Labor & Delivery Nurses at HMSL who implemented the project during the intervention period.
References
Alvarado, Y., Outland, L., Menchaca, A., Strong, N. (2017). Promoting the progress of Labor with the peanut ball. Journal of obstetric, Gynecologic and Neonatal Nursing, 46(3), S23.
National Vital Statistics Reports. (2016). Births, by total cesarean delivery and by low-risk cesarean delivery (gestational age based on LMP): United States and each state and territory, final 2014 and preliminary 2015. 65(3). Retrieved from https://www.cdc.gov/nchs/data/nvsr/nvsr65/nvsr65_03_tables.pdf
Tussey, C. M., Botsios, E., Gerkin, R. D., Kelly, L. A., Gamez, J., Mensik, J. (2015). Reducing length of labor and cesarean surgery rate using a peanut ball for women laboring with an epidural. The Journal of Perinatal Education, 24(1), 16-24.

FIGURE 12.1 Poster Presentation

WELLNESS IN ACTION: GRATITUDE

Gratitude helps us relish good experiences, feel positive emotions, improve health, deal with adversity, and strengthen relationships. Higher levels of gratitude have been associated with increased life satisfaction. As you continue your lifelong exploration of evidence-based wellness practices, consider trying these two simple gratitude actions:

1. Write a thank-you note to someone who has helped you (you can deliver the letter or not).
2. At the end of the day, journal about a circumstance or event for which you are grateful.

Notice how these reflective actions shift your mental focus away from possessions and pressing undertakings and guide it toward people you appreciate and your gratitude for the ways in which they have helped you. These straightforward practices can provide short-term gratitude boosts, train our brains to notice the positive people around us and meaningful events in which we are involved, spotlight the personal strengths we leverage to create supportive relationships, and remind us of the resources available to us as we move through life (Bolier et al., 2013; Proyer et al., 2015).

WRAPPING UP

Remember that EBP is the recommended practice. You do your coworkers, patients, and community a professional service by sharing EBPQI information. As you have learned, practice is often heavily influenced by steeped tradition ("what we have always done") and resistance to change, yet this does not mean that the current practice is necessarily the best possible practice. As a newer nurse, you can establish an essential role in your work setting by partnering in EBPQI initiatives with seasoned nurses and other healthcare professionals. Be open to exploring opportunities for positive improvements, and follow such journeys through from conception to dissemination. Stay focused on sharing information throughout this process and garner support from your leadership team. Internal and external dissemination typically reflect well on the organization and, ultimately, benefit patients, populations, communities, and you!

REFLECTION QUESTIONS

1. What barriers may keep you from sharing your work with target audiences? If you can push past these challenges, who will benefit?
2. What forms of dissemination seem most realistic to you?
3. Who do you have in your professional support matrix to help you achieve EBPQI dissemination?
4. How can you take a simple step toward amplifying the work of others?

REFERENCES

Bolier, L., Haverman, M., Westerhof, G. J. Riper, H., Smit, F., & Bohlmeijer, E. (2013). Positive psychology interventions: A meta-analysis of randomized controlled studies. *BMC Public Health, 13*, Article 119. https://doi.org/10.1186/1471-2458-13-119

Caughey, A., Cahill, A., Guise, J., & Rouse, D. (2014). Safe prevention of the primary cesarean delivery. *American Journal of Obstetrics and Gynecology, 210*(3), 179–193. https://doi.org/10.1016/j.ajog.2014.01.026

Dougherty, M. C., Freda, M. C., Kearney, M. H., Baggs, J. G. & Broome, M. (2011). Online survey of nursing journal peer reviewers: Indicators of quality in manuscripts. *Western Journal of Nursing Research, 33*(4), 506–521. https://doi.org/10.1177/0193945910385715

Dunlap, J. J., & Waldrop, J. (2022). An exploratory study of social media use and management by nursing journals. *Advances in Nursing Science, 45*(3), 218–226. https://doi.org/10.1097/ANS.0000000000000403

George, V., & Haag-Heitman, B. (2011). Nursing peer review: the manager's role. *Journal of Nursing Management, 19*(2), 254–259. https://doi.org/10.1111/j.1365-2834.2011.01225.x

Gotting, M. C. (2023). *U.S. podcasting industry—statistics & facts*. Statista. https://www.statista.com/topics/3170/podcasting/ #topicHeader_wrapper

Kesten, K. S., & Hoover, S. N. (2022). Doctor of nursing practice dissemination through an open access repository. *Journal of Professional Nursing, 41*, 19–25.

Mercier, R. J., & Kwan, M. (2018). Impact of peanut ball device on the duration of active labor: A randomized control trial. *American Journal of Perinatology, 35*, 1006–1011. https://doi.org/10.1055/s-0038-1636531

Merriam-Webster. (n.d.). Author. In *Merriam-Webster.com dictionary*. Retrieved May 23, 2023, from https://www.merriam-webster.com/dictionary/author

Morton, P. G. (2013). Insights about the manuscript review process. *Nurse Author & Editor, 23*(3), 1–4. https://doi.org/10.1111/j.1750-4910.2013.tb00158.x

Oermann, M. H, Hays. J. (2019). *Writing for publication in nursing* (4th ed.). Springer.

Proyer R. T., Gander, F., Wellenzohn, S., & Ruch, R. (2015). Strengths-based positive psychology interventions: A randomized placebo-controlled online trial on long-term effects for signature strengths-vs. a lesser strengths-intervention, *Frontiers in Psychology, 6*. https://doi.org/10.3389/fpsyg.2015.00456

Roth, C., Dent, S. A., Parfitt, S. E., Hering, S. L. & Bay, R. C. (2016). Randomized controlled trial of use of the peanut ball during labor. *Maternal Child Nursing, 41*, 140–146. https://doi.org/10.1097/NMC.0000000000000232

Waldrop, J., & Dunlap, J. J. (2021). Analysis of Tweeting on journal usage and identification of nursing journals using social media. *Computers, Informatics, Nursing, 39*(6), 291–295. https://doi.org/10.1097/CIN.0000000000000774

Waldrop, J., & Dunlap, J. J. (in press). *American Journal of Nursing*.

Waldrop, J & Dunlap, J.J. (2024a). An Evidence-Searching Question for Nurses, *American Journal of Nursing*, In Press

Waldrop, J. & Dunlap, J.J. (2024b). The Mountain Model for Evidence-Based Practice Quality Improvement Initiatives, *American Journal of Nursing*, In Press

Waldrop, J. B., Dunlap, J. J., & Kennedy, M. S. (2022). Social media and journals: Suggested best practices for nursing editors, authors, readers. *Nurse Author & Editor, 32*(1), 11–14. https://doi.org/10.1111/nae2.33

Waldrop, J., & Likis, F. (2022). Nurse editors' roles and practices. *Journal of Nursing Scholarship, 54*(4), 477–484. https://doi.org/10.1111/jnu.12745

Waldrop, Julee DNP, FNP-BC, PNP-BC, FAANP, FAAN; Jennings-Dunlap, Jayne DNP, FNP, CNE, EBP-C. CE: Beyond PICO—A New Question Simplifies the Search for Evidence. AJN, American Journal of Nursing 124(3):p 34–37, March 2024. | DOI: 10.1097/01.NAJ.0001007676.91191.dd

IMAGE CREDITS

Fig. 12.1: Copyright © by Kristin Edwards, Cathryn Ritchie, and Roxy Simon. Reprinted with permission.

CHAPTER 13

What Stories Will You Tell?

Lifelong Learning and Legacy Building in Nursing

Jennifer Wilson, Christiana Acho, and Jayne Jennings Dunlap

KEY CONCEPTS

Lifelong learning
Forethought
Intellectual curiosity
Intentional practice
Advocacy
Legacy
Mentorship

LEARNING OBJECTIVES

1. Connect EBPQI's importance to personal nursing practice.
2. Explore ways to promote lifelong learning engagement and patient advocacy.
3. Define intellectual curiosity and professional legacy building.
4. Identify the importance of professional mentorship.
5. Encourage engagement in creative outlets and activities.

Let us never consider ourselves finished nurses. We must be learning all of our lives.

—Florence Nightingale

Introduction

EBP and QI are valuable tools that allow clinicians to make intentional and sound evidence-based decisions in clinical practice (Melnyk & Fineout-Overholt, 2023; White et al., 2021). When we set out to write this book, we noticed that published information describing EBP and QI processes often concluded with dissemination, yet we know that these processes do not end with professional sharing; rather, they are tethered to **lifelong learning**. Join us as we conclude our journey with an important call for continued learning, advocacy, legacy building, and mentoring in nursing. Your lasting impact starts now.

Lifelong Learning

Throughout this book, you have accessed true stories illustrating the impact of EBPQI across several settings and populations. As you have read about these initiatives, have you noticed what they share?

- In each story, at least one person was impacted or benefited from a nurse's actions.
- Each story involved a nurse who understood the problem and decided to consider the evidence, then use that evidence to take action and refused to settle for less than best practice, even though doing the right thing was challenging or risked conflict or practice change.
- Each story involved some form of opposition that required a nurse to swim upstream, challenge the status quo, and take risks.
- The nurse knew *why* they were willing to advocate for best practices.
- The nurse was ultimately respected for their decision and action, even if the practice change was uncomfortable at the time.
- Each story demonstrated a learning opportunity.

Do you remember the first real case example (Box 1.3) from Chapter 1? In this situation, a surgical team defended outdated practices after family members shared current evidence and recommendations to proceed differently. Faced with a decision to maintain the status quo or consider adhering to the most current evidence, the surgical team chose the former. The patient was in a compromised condition that limited his ability to advocate for himself properly, and he ultimately trusted the opinion of the healthcare team because the nurse chose a passive role. In this real-life scenario, the nurse and team, like most healthcare workers, likely began their day with positive intentions to deliver sound care. The patient trusted all the members of his care team to provide the best possible care, just as our patients do day after day. Suppose the nurse or even one member of the health care team had made a conscious decision to listen with an open mind to information about a newer approach, find the confidence and skill to speak up, and base their practice on current evidence. Had that been the case, the patient's outcome might have been significantly different. Thankfully, the patient survived, but his preventable complications from a lack of EBP prematurely ended his remarkable career. Every clinical decision you make as a nurse leads to an outcome, so you must remember that we are responsible and accountable for our nursing judgments.

Forethought, Curiosity, and Thoughtfulness/ Intentional Practice

Intellectual curiosity and a spirit of inquiry enable nurses to question the status quo habitually and seek answers on a deeper level (Harper et al., 2019; Melnyk et al., 2017). **Forethought** entails thinking ahead, which allows nurses to anticipate (rather than react to) challenges or complications. Forethought sharpens the ability to assess and identify complications quickly or ideally to prevent them, rather than jumping in reactively when they occur (Wilson, 2012). Forethought often encompasses an intentional desire to do the right thing, which drives successful decision-making. When nursing students are asked in post conference to describe an example of an exemplary nurse they witnessed in clinical practice, their stories usually describe that nurse's **intellectual curiosity** (need to know), enthusiasm for learning, use of data to support their decisions, search for evidence on a topic before acting, and confidence in educating others to solve clinical problems. Nurses' curiosity and desire to understand on a deeper level are linked to improved patient care (Scala et al., 2019). Many students are surprised yet inspired when they see nurses confidently educating physicians, pharmacists, respiratory therapists, and other team members with respect for the unique perspective that each discipline brings to the clinical situation and allowing those team members to educate them in turn.

Students regularly share that on a certain unit, even the most seasoned and experienced nurses regularly search for evidence-based information on new medications, disease processes, and novel procedures as they prepare to offer excellent, well-informed care the next day. The nurse then asks a nursing student to pretend to be the parent of tomorrow's patient so that the nurse can practice explaining the new medication, procedure, or treatment; this practice not only helps the nurse to prepare but also engages the student in both a factual learning experience as a future nurse and an experience of receiving patient education as a family member. When students describe their experiences of working with or observing these nurses, they share that they were inspired by their intellectual curiosity, their "need to know" as a vital component of providing evidence-based care for patients, and their habitual desire to stay updated on the latest and best evidence and share it with the entire team.

The stories in this book embody thoughtfulness, or **intentional practice**. In the context of evidence-based nursing, *thoughtfulness* encompasses the habit of examining a situation or encounter from the perspective of the person with whom you are interacting, such as a patient, family member, fellow nurse, provider, nursing student, or interdisciplinary team member (Wilson, 2012). Clinical decision-making in nursing is complex, and nursing students regularly describe the most meaningful clinical days as those during which nurses involve them in clinical decision-making and patient care, take time to teach them, and ask their opinions. In clinical settings, nursing students will only understand the complexity of thinking that drives nurses' decisions if those nurses are willing to take time to explain their thought processes and include students in clinical decisions throughout the day (Caputi, 2016).

As you make clinical decisions throughout your career, you will have to choose when and how to exercise the courage to challenge the status quo and pursue EBPQI. All healthcare providers encounter similar situations and dilemmas. We hope that you will embrace these experiences as opportunities to become a better nurse. As painful as they may seem at the time, these experiences are our best teachers, and the lessons we learn from them motivate and prepare us to make better future choices (Wilson, 2012). The more we learn from our experiences, the stronger clinicians we become. This is precisely why reflecting on our stories and sharing them with others is so important. Storytelling is integral to professional nursing identity formation, empowerment, and lifelong learning (Attenborough & Abbott, 2020).

Can you think of a time when you witnessed a nurse make a "wrong" decision during a conflict because they were afraid of disappointing or angering someone else or unable to support their position with evidence? Many nurses struggle with such challenges, especially in their early career. A nurse loses fear, however, by becoming empowered to do the right thing through making evidence-supported decisions. With this empowerment, their clinical decision-making becomes sounder and more efficient, and their commitment to doing the right thing becomes easier to defend and sustain. It is essential to consider that as we gain new evidence, clinical practices will continue to change, and clinical conflict resolution will remain an integral component of our nursing role.

One of the most significant and rewarding aspects of nursing is that we learn new knowledge daily. Although it is well known that caring, curiosity, and critical thinking are essential to the nursing role, both the complex relationships between these concepts and the most effective strategies to cultivate curiosity remain less understood and warrant further research (Nadelson et al., 2022). As we gain new knowledge, we have a professional responsibility to share it with our colleagues so that it can be synthesized into the current body of evidence. It is impossible to become experts in all things, so each of us must be responsible for remaining teachable and allowing others to introduce new evidence; this is especially true during times of clinical conflict as we establish our own nursing stories.

What Stories Do You Already Have to Share About Your Experiences?

As a nursing student, you have likely accumulated stories of your own. Have you shared these stories with others or just thought, "I am a student, so my stories do not matter"? Not only do your stories matter but writing them down or telling them to others can provide numerous benefits. All humans, including nurses, become characters in stories, whether they intend to or not (Kouzes & Posner, 2006). What kinds of stories do you think the patients in your clinical experiences would tell about you? Would you be the character who advocated for others by standing up and doing the right thing? We recommend that as you approach each nursing interaction, you stay mindful of the stories you and others will potentially tell about the interaction and its impact. If you do this, you will likely become a more thoughtful and intentional person and nurse. Even as a nursing student, you cannot avoid being part of a story. The good news is that approaching your clinical experiences with intention and having clarity about the evidence-based factors that drive your decision-making can significantly influence the stories of which you are a part. When you share your stories, you educate others and lead by example.

EXPLORING ONGOING EBPQI ENGAGEMENT

As an RN, you will have many choices, including where and how you will practice. We hope you will consider enhancing your EBPQI knowledge and skills through the many current opportunities that exist for RNs, including continuing education opportunities. For no cost, several QI self-paced courses are available through the Institute for Healthcare Improvement (IHI) open school (https://www.ihi.org/education/ihi-open-school). You can pursue the new certification in evidence-based practice (EBP-C) as a new national standard; more information about this can be found online (https://fuld.nursing.osu.edu/ebp-certification). You can also become a certified professional in healthcare quality (CPHQ). Two years of professional nursing experience are recommended to qualify to sit for the certification in healthcare quality examination; more information can be found on the National Association for Healthcare Quality website (https://nahq.org/individuals/cphq-certification). These certifications will showcase your continued competence in EBP and QI knowledge and skills, enhance your credibility with your peers and leadership team, and, most important of all, directly impact your care of patients and the success of their outcomes. Pathways to reimbursement for certification costs may be available within your current or future healthcare system. Do not be afraid to seek out these unique opportunities to enhance your EBPQI knowledge throughout your nursing career! Many of us are pursuing additional EBPQI opportunities driven by our career-long commitment to learning.

Advocacy

As frontline providers and decision-makers, nurses are essentially the last line of defense for patients because our choices affect whether, when, and how medications are administered (Stimpfel et al., 2020), procedures are conducted, patients are discharged or transferred, staffing is determined, and policies are developed. **Advocacy** is a universally accepted primary nursing role. If you were to conduct an informal poll of nurses, most would likely say that they act as patient advocates every day and could provide plenty of examples. Professionals who initiate and propel positive change are guided by a vision of success, a certainty that others will benefit from change, clarity in their decision-making, and the ability to push past their fears. When responsible nurses encounter clinical situations that threaten the quality of patient care, they become motivated by empathetic curiosity to seek additional information and reflect more deeply on their practice; this process inevitably strengthens their critical thinking skills, resulting in better decision-making and an improved quality of care (Nadelson & Nadelson, 2019).

Nurses who base their daily practice on current evidence and have the confidence to apply that evidence to practice, knowing that their patients will benefit, ultimately make better clinical decisions. Nursing is the most trusted profession, a distinction/honor held by the nursing profession for over 2 decades, yet our 2022 confidence ratings lag 10% below those of 2020 for honesty and ethical standards (Brenan, 2023). This latest data should serve as a wake-up call to all nurses and healthcare leaders; it presents a reminder that we must strive to understand each person's perspective and take accountability at the individual level for our daily practice within an expansive and dynamic system.

To promote successful change and advance our profession, all nurses must accept advocacy as a core value that is equivalent in importance to caring, accountability, safety, and integrity. Nurses on the frontlines are often emotionally spent, overworked, and exhausted after providing care for patients in understaffed settings due to a global pandemic. As we adapt to sustained challenges introduced by COVID-19, nurses must recognize their responsibility to advocate for a better future through policy changes that foster wellness, improvement in public health infrastructure, safe and healthy working environments, health equity, diversity, and holistic health nursing practices (Hasmiller, 2022). Clarity about these values allows us to stay focused on "doing the right thing" despite personal or emotional influences that might otherwise cloud our judgment or affect clinical decision-making.

Nurses today have at their fingertips unlimited access to data, evidence, and resources. Quality care requires conscious decisions made by individual nurses to access information and allow the best available evidence to define their clinical practice and guide their decision-making. Because nurses operate primarily within a team, however, it is the shared responsibility of a system, its leadership, and various organizations to create a culture in which nurses feel supported and safe when reporting issues. The primary reasons for not reporting patient issues are fear of retaliation and a belief that reporting patient safety issues will not result in positive change (Cole et al., 2019). Quality and safety improvement requires investment by organizations in resources that support the well-being of nurses and other healthcare providers (Melnyk et al., 2021). However, it is equally important that nurses be willing to access resources, knowledge, and support in order to equip themselves with the skills and courage needed to apply evidence to practice effectively.

Legacy

This book provides a variety of examples of how EBPQI, used at the individual level, can impact patients, but the work of some influential people has a large-scale impact, and their legacy continues to provide benefits to others long after their death. The term **legacy** is open to interpretation but generally may describe (a) significant achievement(s) for which a notable person (e.g., Steve Jobs, Benjamin Franklin, Thomas Edison, Florence Nightingale, Mary Mahoney) is remembered; (b) the inheritance a person leaves their beneficiaries; (c) the ways in which a person has impacted others; or (d) the reasons for which others remember a person. We believe that legacy is primarily defined by the ways in which we choose to consistently fill our days with meaning. Each day, even when we may feel limited in our options, we make choices about how to make that day impactful for our patients through our decisions and actions.

AUTHOR'S LEGACY IN ACTION

I (Christiana) obtained an associate degree in nursing in Africa, after which I came to the United States and pursued a BSN while working as a nurse on an inpatient unit. At that time, my husband and I began taking medical mission trips to my home country of Nigeria every summer; we would educate people about health maintenance and screenings to help prevent urgent visits to the hospital. We invited friends to join us on these trips, yet even with extra hands to help, the need we encountered was far too great to address periodically.

I noticed that many people had very high blood pressure readings and signs and symptoms of diabetes but no useful resources or access to evidence-based care. This unmet health need and profound lack of EBP led me to return to school and become a family nurse practitioner capable of diagnosing and treating complex conditions. With the help of friends and colleagues, I transformed those periodic trips into a much larger operation, and the services we provided expanded to include general medical, general surgical, and specialty services.

The spark of hope that these free medical services lit in the eyes of my people became the impetus for the creation of the Living Hope Medical Center, a modern hospital with state-of-the-art facilities that rests on a large span of land and beckons all who are experiencing illness or disability to come to a place where they can receive medical services year-round, 24 hours per day, 7 days per week. My people no longer wait anxiously for summer medical visits from the American people; when needed, they receive timely care through the Living Hope Medical Center. For me, the American dream was actualized only when it was shared with others less fortunate.

Let us first explore this concept on a micro level. How many times a day do you tell yourself that you have to do something (e.g., go to work, pass a class, complete an assignment, get up at 4:30 a.m. to go to clinical, pay the bills, pick up a friend from the airport)? If you stop and think about it, you do not have to do any of these things. Each of your activities is a choice, although there may be consequences to doing or not doing them. You decided to go to nursing school and become a nurse, and you can always decide to pivot. All your daily tasks, especially the school-related ones, are optional. Viewing the activities in our lives as mandatory tasks can cause us to forget that education is a choice we made, even a privilege. During stressful times, all these "have to's" can feel overwhelming and make us forget the reason we decided to pursue our goals in the first place. At times like this, it's helpful to remember how hard you worked to earn acceptance into nursing school, how many people want to be in your shoes but can't be, how many opportunities your future will hold, and, most important, how many people will benefit because you completed the assignments and finished your program. We promise that you will look at "have to's" differently when you remind yourself daily of your "why." Every day when you wake up, remind yourself that the choice of what to do with your day—and with your life—is yours to make. This shift in thinking can be freeing and empowering; it will enable you to view your life and learning through a different lens, with purpose, intent, wonder, and awe.

Next, let us explore this concept on a macro level. What would you like your legacy to be at the end of your career? As a nurse, you will have countless opportunities to work in various roles and settings and encounter people from many different walks of life. Throughout your career, you will choose the work you engage in as well as the education options you take advantage of to achieve your goals. At the start of your career, you will have only a partial knowledge of where your journey will take you and all that will transpire along the way; nevertheless, if you think of your career as the groundwork of your legacy, its trajectory will be substantially affected. Florence Nightingale's legacy was transforming nursing into a respected profession. Her achievements as a researcher, a pioneer in epidemiology and public health, an advocate for populations, and an architect of modern hospitals collectively transformed our healthcare system (Tye, 2020). Nightingale's achievements began with a vision of what nursing and hospitals could be. She made a commitment to fight for what was right, then she turned to the evidence. A century later, our healthcare system continues to face new challenges, and Nightingale's example remains relevant. As one nursing researcher recently noted, "Any health care executive striving to improve clinical quality and patient satisfaction could do much worse than studying the way Florence Nightingale—in the face of strident opposition and severely limited resources—created a blueprint for the modern hospital" (Tye, 2020, p. 225).

FOCUS ON LEGACY BUILDING

Envisioning a legacy can feel daunting, but it begins with a few simple questions. Why did you decide to become a nurse? If you do not know where to start, review the authors' stories at the front of this book, then write down your own story of why you pursued nursing. Include why you are still in the program, the strengths and talents that led you here, and how you can use them in your profession.

As part of your story, think about what you consider an excellent clinical day that leaves you fulfilled and energized. What types of experiences draw or build upon your strengths, satisfy your personal interests, and create a sense of accomplishment? Consider, too, what you would like to accomplish to make the profession better. This exercise can provide valuable clarity both as you prepare to pursue nursing job opportunities as well as over the course of your career; for example, you might initially choose to pursue neonatal nursing and become a NICU nurse because you love babies, later realize that you feel more satisfied and fulfilled when interacting with older children, and eventually discover that you have become passionate about adolescent mental health and want to improve mental health services across populations. Legacy exploration facilitates a career that is an ever-evolving process, allowing you to pivot as you gain experience and evolve as a person and professional nurse.

AUTHOR'S LEGACY IN ACTION

I (Jennifer) began my career as a pediatric oncology nurse, which significantly shaped my life perspective. In this role, I frequently entered the scene on the worst days of my patients' lives: when a child was diagnosed with cancer or died prematurely. I determined every day to savor the precious time I had with my patients and their families. As I cared for these children, I watched in awe as they approached life with purpose, honesty, dignity, and bravery. At the very least, I realized, they deserved the same from others in return and to receive the best care possible, based on the evidence available (which was limited at the time). I recognized early on that in addition to caring for patients individually, I could advocate for them on a larger scale by gaining more education. I earned an MSN in oncology and began working as a clinical research nurse at NIH in the Pediatric Branch of the National Cancer Institute. My work and connections at NIH led to additional opportunities to advocate for children with cancer. In this setting, I came to deeply appreciate research and the critical role that evidence plays in clinical decision-making. At NIH, every policy that impacted patients, nurses, and other providers was based on data gathered by the entire staff. Research and data-driven decision-making were integral to the nursing culture and gave us the confidence to deliver exemplary care. I learned that evidence is required to garner support for the resources we need, whether for new drugs for patients or improved working conditions that allow nurses to perform our jobs in an exemplary fashion. Each day at work, I was reminded that the young children with whom I interacted had, in many ways, achieved more, touched more lives, and influenced my life more than most adults I knew. I decided that regardless of where my life and career took me, I would approach it with a daily awareness that if I committed to a vision of using my talents to benefit others with purpose, a legacy would naturally follow. My initial vision was imprecise: a desire, by the time I finished my career, to have improved the lives of children with cancer.

As an oncology clinical nurse specialist, my work focused on conducting research and empowering nurses through education and advocacy to use knowledge, skills, and resources to provide the best quality care. By actively seeking out mentors who possessed expertise, knowledge, or skills that I lacked, I was able to collaborate with other national experts to establish best practice standards based on the current body of evidence. Years later, as a clinical professor, I now teach and empower nursing students, regardless of their role or title, to engage in a process that both improves the lives of patients and elevates the profession. At every level of my career, in each role I have played, my scope of impact has multiplied simply because I have been willing to believe that I can make a positive change, one day at a time.

Mentorship

What is mentorship, and why is it valuable? **Mentorship** describes the powerful influence, direction, and guidance that an experienced person has on or gives to a less experienced person over months or years to achieve an expected outcome (in this case, quality care). Mentorship happens when one person commits to assisting another toward optimal growth, role development, and effectiveness (Hoover et al., 2020; Koon et al., 2020). Specific to our profession, mentors are usually seasoned nurses who share their knowledge, experience, and connections with junior nurses. Each of us has at least one mentor, a trusted teacher or coach who has helped us with EBP or some other endeavor, to thank for where we are today (Melnyk & Fineout-Overholt, 2023). True mentors serve as role models, offering essential advice and candid feedback while establishing and maintaining professional boundaries (Clark, 2015). New graduate nurses have been found to be more likely to follow role-model practices than recently learned evidence-based patient care methods (Breckenridge-Sproat et al., 2015). This finding magnifies the value of trusted mentors who are willing to share their extensive EBPQI knowledge and skills. EBP mentors have been implemented successfully to build EBP programs in healthcare and deliver a message of high day-to-day EBP organizational commitment. EBP mentors stimulate a culture of clinical inquiry through education among nurses and healthcare providers (Melnyk et al., 2017).

How Will You Mentor and Be Mentored Throughout Your Career?

As you navigate your next clinical day, pay careful attention to the culture of the unit or clinic. How would you describe it? How could one person positively influence that environmental culture? As you read this final chapter, ask yourself, "Whom have I mentored in my lifetime? How will I mentor others?" and then challenge yourself to find someone to mentor. To be a good mentor, you must continue to advance your career through continuing education so that you can offer the most current EBPQI knowledge and skills to your mentees.

PRACTICAL RECOMMENDATIONS FOR MENTOR SELECTION

1. Actively seek out mentors who are exemplary nurses (they are likely skillful with patients). Please do not wait for them to select you.
2. Choose a mentor who can be trusted to provide honest feedback and cares enough about you to tell you the truth.
3. Tell the potential mentor why they inspire you, and be clear about why you are requesting their mentorship specifically.
4. Share your professional successes in life with the mentors who have helped you to achieve them.
5. Remember that you are worthy of providing as well as receiving mentorship, and seek out new nurses to mentor.

WRAPPING UP

We hope that this book has provided you with a thorough introduction to the EBPQI process and convinced you to think critically and creatively about current healthcare issues. We hope you are thoughtfully considering how you will optimally impact our profession as future nurses. Our ultimate desire is that you will enter the nursing field prepared to engage patients and stakeholders fully in EBPQI codesign to enact positive healthcare transformation. We also hope that a spark has been kindled within you that will ignite an inextinguishable passion for learning, inspire others, and expand your scope of impact. We believe the concepts in this book, applied to your professional practice and other aspects of your life, will accelerate your growth and confidence, and allow you to thrive in your endeavors. In the process, we hope you will experience wonder every day that leaves you fulfilled and empowered. Above all, we want you to continue accumulating and sharing stories.

As seasoned nurses, we welcome you to the profession, and we are in awe of your possible future achievements. We want you to know that we believe in you enough to have invested in your career by sharing our expertise and knowledge through writing this textbook. We remain committed to lifelong learning, and the process of sharing our personal stories on these pages has served as a reminder that none of us are alone on this exciting and important journey. As nurses who have gone before you, we encourage you to keep questioning current practices. Learn and understand the up-to-date rationales for the care you provide. Take action to educate yourself so that you can educate your patients.

When we began this journey, the first question we asked was why you chose the nursing profession. We challenge you to now consider your legacy as you become the nurses of tomorrow who will have untold EBPQI opportunities of the future at your fingertips. If you commit to the EBPQI process early, as a curious lifelong learner and future mentor, we are certain that you will improve the health of patients, populations, and the nurses who will come after you. Remember the critical value of mentorship as you begin your nursing career.

As you close this book, we urge you to focus on the countless lives you will touch, often during moments of great need. Nourish and take good care of yourself to sustain the EBPQI mountain climbs ahead. Ensure that your patient is the most important person in every healthcare encounter; effective patient care hinges on expert patient advocacy, often the first and last defense from harm in healthcare. Connect with the outstanding nurses you want to emulate and learn from them. Together, you can keep the candle lit and blaze new EBPQI trails in healthcare. The world is ready for your legacies.

WELLNESS IN ACTION: CREATIVITY FOR DISCOVERING AWE AND WONDER

Creativity is contagious. Pass it on.

—Albert Einstein

Engaging in creative goals has been linked to increased positive affect and flourishing behaviors (Conner et al., 2018). What types of creative activities interest you? Recall a moment from your recent or distant past when you were awestruck. What were you doing? Compose a personal list of items or experiences that have inspired wonder within you. Consider how you can schedule a time into your regular (daily, weekly, monthly, or annual) routine to engage in creative opportunities, perhaps including a visit to a new or familiar place where you can experience or design a creative ritual. Be curious and open to creative goals that leave you inspired and rejuvenated. As a future nurse, creative engagement can help fuel your passion for caring for yourself and others in innovative ways. As we adapt to an ever-changing healthcare system, nurses must remain vigilant to preserve the awe and wonder that derives from engaging with and caring for others and inspire the values and elements essential to our beloved profession and heritage (Milton, 2022).

REFLECTION QUESTIONS

1. What is the most interesting or important lesson you have learned through engagement with this textbook?
2. How will you use the competencies gained through this EBPQI journey to impact your future practice?

REFERENCES

Attenbourough, J., & Abbott, S. (2020). Using storytelling in nurse education: The experiences and views of lecturers in a higher education institution in the United Kingdom. *Nurse Education in Practice, 40*,1–6.

Breckenridge-Sproat, S. T., Throop, M. D., Raju, D., Murphy, D. A., Loan, L. A., & Patrician, P. A. (2015). Building a unit-level mentored program to sustain a culture of inquiry for evidence-based practice. *Clinical Nurse Specialist, 29*(6), 329–337. https://doi.org/10.1097/NUR.0000000000000161

Brenan, M. (2023, January 10). *Nurses retain top ethics rating in U.S., but below 2020 high.* Gallup. https://news.gallup.com/poll/467804/nurses-retain-top-ethics-rating-below-2020-high.aspx

Caputi, L. (2016). *Building the future of nursing* (3rd ed.). Woltesr-Kluwer.

Clark, C. (2015). The power and potential of positive mentoring. *Nurse Educator, 40*(3), 109–110. https://doi.org/10.1097/NNE.0000000000000158

Cole, D., Bersick, E., Skarbek, A., Cummins, K., Dugan, K., & Grantoza, R. (2019). The courage to speak out: A study describing nurses' attitudes to report unsafe practices in patient care. *Journal of Nursing Management, 27*(6), 1176–1181.

Conner, T. S., DeYoung, C. G., & Silvia, P. J. (2018). Everyday creative activity as a path to flourishing. *The Journal of Positive Psychology, 13*(2), 181–189. https://doi.org/10.1080/17439760.2016.1257049

Harper, M., Warren, J., Bradley, D., Bindon, S., & Maloney, P. (2019) Nursing professional development's spirit of inquiry focus areas. *Journal for Nurses in Professional Development, 35*(3), 118–124. https://doi.org/10.1097/NND.0000000000000515

Hasmiller, S. B. (2022). How nurses can help to create a better post-pandemic world. *Policy, Politics, & Nursing Practice, 23*(1), 3–4. https://doi.org/10.1177/15271544221075201

Hoover J., Koon A. D., Rosser E. N., & Rao, K. D.(2020). Mentoring the working nurse: A scoping review. *Human Resources for Health, 18*, Article 52. https://doi.org/10.1186/s12960-020-00491-x

Kerley, L., & Toney-Butler, T. J. (2022). *Nursing advocacy.* StatPearls. https://www.ncbi.nlm.nih.gov/books/NBK499928/

Koon A. D., Hoover J., Sonthalia S., Rosser E., Gore A., & Rao K. D. (2020). In-service nurse mentoring in 2020, the year of the nurse and the midwife: Learning from Bihar, India. *Global Health Action, 13*(1), Article 1823101. https://doi.org/10.1080/16549716.2020.1823101

Kouzes, J. M., & Posner, B. Z. (2006). *A leader's legacy.* Jossey-Bass.

Melnyk, B. M., & Fineout-Overholt, E. (2023). *Evidence-based practice in nursing & healthcare: A guide to best practice* (5th ed.). Lippincott Williams & Wilkins.

Melnyk B. M., Gallagher-Ford L., & Fineout-Overholt E. (2017). *Implementing evidence-based practice competencies in healthcare: A practical guide for improving quality, safety, & outcomes.* Sigma Theta Tau.

Melnyk, B. M., Tan, A., Hsieh, A. P., Gawlik, K., Arslanian-Engoren, C., Braun, L. T., Dunbar, S., Jacob, J. D., Lewis, L. M., Millan, A., Orsolini, L., Robbins, L. B., Russell, C. L., Tucker, S., & Wilbur, J. (2021). Critical care nurses' physical and mental health, worksite wellness support, and medical errors. *American Journal of Critical Care*, *30*(3), 176–184. https://doi.org/10.4037/ajcc2021301

Milton, C. L. (2022). The future of nurse scholarship: The ethical challenge. *Nursing Science Quarterly*, *35*(1), 25–27. https://doi.org/10.1177/08943184211051335

Nadelson, S. G., & Nadelson, L. S. (2019). Connecting critical thinking, caring, and curiosity in nurse education: Exploring the beliefs and practices of nurse educators. *Journal of Nursing Education and Practice*, *9*(8), 1–10. https://doi.org/10.5430/jnep.v9n8p1

Nadelson, S., Reed, D., Massey, M., Lowder, T., & Yarberry, F. (2022). Faculty perceptions of curiosity in the education of nursing and health science students. *Journal of Modern Nursing Practice and Research*, *2*(1), 1–9. https://doi.org/10/53964/jmnpr.2022001

Scala, E., Patterson, B. Stavarski, D. H., & Mackay, P. (2019). Engagement in research: A clinical nurse profile and motivating factors. *Journal for Nurses in Professional Development*, *35*(3), 137–143. https://doi.org/10.1097/NND.0000000000000538

Stimpfel, A. W., Fatehi, F., & Kovner, C. (2020). Nurses' sleep, work hours, and patient care quality, and safety. *Sleep Health*, *6*(3), 314–320. https://doi.org/10.1016/j.sleh.2019.11.001

Tye, J. (2020. Florence Nightingale's lasting legacy for health care. *Nurse Leader*, *18*(3), 220–226. https://doi.org/10.1016/j.mnl.2020.03.023

White, K.M ., Dudley-Brown, S., & Terhaar, M. F. (2021). *Translation of evidence into nursing and healthcare* (3rd ed.). Springer.

Wilson, J. (2012). *The new graduate nurse's survival handbook: How to avoid being labeled as scary.* Infinity Publishing.

Appendix A: Competency Index

American Association of Colleges of Nursing: The Essentials: Core Competencies for Professional Nursing Education

Essential EBP-Related Competencies and Level 1 Sub-Competencies for the Professional Nurse Addressed by Chapter

The American Association of Colleges of Nursing's (AACN, 2021) core competencies for professional nursing education provide 10 domains of competence that constitute the expectations of the practicing nurse with integration of the concept of EBP throughout all domains and quality and safety with its own designated domain.

- Domain 1: Knowledge for Nursing Practice
- Domain 2: Person-Centered Care
- Domain 3: Population Health
- Domain 4: Scholarship for the Nursing Discipline
- Domain 5: Quality and Safety
- Domain 6: Interprofessional Partnerships
- Domain 7: Systems-Based Practice
- Domain 8: Informatics and Healthcare Technologies
- Domain 9: Professionalism
- Domain 10: Personal, Professional, and Leadership Development

This textbook will provide you with the knowledge and tools to demonstrate several AACN competencies and Level 1 sub-competencies related to EBPQI expected of the entry-level nurse. While you will learn much about EBPQI throughout this book, you are not expected to be an expert or lead these initiatives alone when you begin your nursing career. As discussed in Chapter 1, EBPQI is a collaborative effort best achieved through the expertise and participation of interdisciplinary teams.

CHAPTER 1 Setting the Stage for Clear Understanding of Research, Evidence-Based Practice, and Quality Improvement

Domain	Competency	Sub-Competency
1	1.1 Demonstrate an understanding of the discipline of nursing's distinct perspective and where shared perspectives exist in other disciplines.	1.1a Identify concepts derived from theories from nursing and other disciplines, which distinguish the practice of nursing. 1.1b Apply knowledge of nursing science that develops a foundation for nursing practice.
1	1.2 Apply theory and research-based knowledge from nursing, the arts, humanities, and other sciences.	1.2b Demonstrate intellectual curiosity. 1.2e Demonstrate ethical decision-making.
4	4.1 Advance the scholarship of nursing.	4.1c Apply theoretical framework(s)/models in practice. 4.1d Demonstrate an understanding of basic elements of the research process. 4.1e Participate in scholarly inquiry as a team member.
4	4.2 Integrate best evidence into nursing practice.	4.2c Use best evidence in practice.
9	9.1 Demonstrate an ethical comportment of one's practice reflective of nursing's mission to society.	9.1b Reflect on one's actions and their consequences.
9	9.5 Demonstrate the professional identify of nursing.	9.5a Describe nursing's professional identity and contributions to the healthcare team.
10	10.1 Demonstrate a commitment to personal health and well-being.	10.1a Demonstrate healthy, self-care behaviors that promote wellness and resiliency.

CHAPTER 2 Quality and Safety as Nursing Practice Mainstays

Domain	Competency	Sub-Competency
1	1.2 Apply theory and research-based knowledge from nursing, the arts, humanities, and other sciences.	1.2c Demonstrate social responsibility as a global citizen who fosters the attainment of health equity for all. 1.2d Examine influence of personal values in decision-making for nursing practice. 1.2e Demonstrate ethical decision-making.
1	Demonstrate clinical judgment founded on a broad knowledge base.	1.3a Demonstrate clinical reasoning. 1.3b Integrate nursing knowledge (theories, multiple ways of knowing, evidence) and knowledge from other disciplines and inquiry to inform clinical judgment. 1.3c Incorporate knowledge from nursing and other disciplines to support clinical judgment.

Domain	Competency	Sub-Competency
2	2.2 Communicate effectively with individuals.	2.2e Use evidence-based patient teaching materials, considering health literacy, vision, hearing, and cultural sensitivity.
2	Develop a plan of care.	2.5c Prioritize care based on best evidence. 2.5d Incorporate evidence-based intervention to improve outcomes and safety.
3	Manage population health.	3.1h Describe general principles and practices for the clinical management of populations across the age continuum. 3.1i Identify ethical principles to protect the health and safety of diverse populations.
4	4.1 Advance the scholarship of nursing.	4.1a Demonstrate an understanding of the different approaches to scholarly practice. 4.1e Participate in scholarly inquiry as a team member.
4	4.2 Integrate best evidence into nursing practice.	4.2c Use best evidence in practice.
4	4.3 Promote ethical conduct of scholarly activities.	4.3d Recognize the impact of equity issues in research.
5	5.1 Apply quality improvement principles in care delivery.	5.1a Recognize nursing's essential role in improving healthcare quality and safety. 5.1b Identify sources and applications of national safety and quality standards to guide nursing practice.
5	5.2 Contribute to a culture of patient safety.	5.2a Describe the factors that create a culture of safety. 5.2b Articulate the nurse's role within an interprofessional team in promoting safety and preventing errors and near misses. 5.2c Examine basic safety design principals to reduce the risk of harm. 5.2d Assume accountability for reporting unsafe conditions, near misses, and errors to reduce harm. 5.2e Describe processes used in understanding causes of error. 5.2f Use national patient safety resources, initiatives, and regulations at the point of care.
5	5.3 Contribute to a culture of provider and work environment safety.	5.3c Promote policies for prevention of violence and risk mitigation. 5.3d Recognize one's role in sustaining a just culture reflecting civility and respect.
6	6.4 Work with other professions to maintain a climate of mutual learning, respect, and shared values.	6.4a Demonstrate an awareness of one's own biases and how they may affect mutual respect and communication with team members. 6.4b Demonstrate respect for the perspectives and experiences of other professions.
7	7.1 Apply knowledge of systems to work effectively across the continuum of care.	7.1b Explain the relationships of macrosystems, mesosystems, and microsystems.

(Continued)

CHAPTER 2 *(Continued)*

Domain	Competency	Sub-Competency
9	9.1 Demonstrate an ethical comportment of one's practice reflective of nursing's mission to society.	9,1b Reflect on one's actions and their consequences. 9.1e Report unethical behaviors when observed.
9	9.3 Demonstrate accountability to the individual, society, and profession.	9.3a Engage in advocacy that promotes the best interest of the individual, community, and profession. 9.3b Demonstrate the moral courage to report concerns.
9	9.4 Comply with relevant laws, policies, and regulations.	9.4a Advocate for policies that promote health and prevent harm.

CHAPTER 3 Clinical Questions and Specific Aims

Domain	Competency	Sub-Competency
1	1.2 Apply theory and research-based knowledge from nursing, the arts, humanities, and other sciences.	1.2b Demonstrate intellectual curiosity.
2	2.5 Develop a plan of care.	2.5c Prioritize care based on best evidence.
3	3.1 Manage population health.	3.1c Assess the priorities of the community and/or affected clinical population. 3.1d Compare and contrast local, regional, national, and global benchmarks to identify health patterns across populations. 3.1f Develop an action plan to meet an identified need(s), including evaluation methods.
4	4.1 Advance the scholarship of nursing.	4.1e Participate in scholarly inquiry as a team member.
4	4.2 Integrate best evidence into nursing practice.	4.2a Evaluate clinical practice to generate questions to improve nursing care.
6	6.1 Communicate in a manner that facilitates a partnership approach to quality care delivery.	6.1a Communicate the nurse's roles and responsibilities clearly. 6.1c Elicit the perspectives of team members to inform person-centered decision-making.
6	6.4 Work with other professions to maintain a climate of mutual learning, respect, and shared values.	6.4d Collaborate with interprofessional team members to establish mutual healthcare goals for individuals, communities, and populations.
7	7.1 Apply knowledge of systems to work effectively across the continuum of care.	7.1a Describe organizational structure, mission vision, philosophy, and values.
10	10.2 Demonstrate a spirit of inquiry that fosters flexibility and professional maturity.	10.2d Expand personal knowledge to inform clinical judgment.

CHAPTER 4 The Nurse's Role in Searching for Evidence: A Foundation to Explore and Embrace Evidence

Domain	Competency	Sub-Competency
1	1.2 Apply theory and research-based knowledge from nursing, the arts, humanities, and other sciences.	1.2b Demonstrate intellectual curiosity.
1	1.3 Demonstrate clinical judgment founded on a broad knowledge base.	1.3b Integrate nursing knowledge (theories, multiple ways of knowing, evidence) and knowledge from other disciplines and inquiry to inform clinical judgment.
2	2.5 Develop a plan of care.	2.5c Prioritize care based on best evidence.
3	3.4 Advance equitable population health policy,	3.4c Identify the best evidence to support policy development.
4	4.1 Advance the scholarship of nursing.	4.1e Participate in scholarly inquiry as a team member.
4	4.2 Integrate best evidence into nursing practice.	4.2a Evaluate clinical practice to generate questions to improve nursing care. 4.2c Use best evidence in practice.
10	10.2 Demonstrate a spirit of inquiry that fosters flexibility and professional maturity.	10.2d Expand personal knowledge to inform clinical judgment.

CHAPTER 5 Critically Appraising Quantitative Evidence

Domain	Competency	Sub-Competency
1	1.2 Apply theory and research-based knowledge from nursing, the arts, humanities, and other sciences.	1.2d Examine the influence of personal values in decision-making for nursing practice.
4	4.1 Advance the scholarship of nursing.	4.1b Demonstrate application of different levels of evidence. 4.1d Demonstrate an understanding of basic elements of the research process. 4.1e Participate in scholarly inquiry as a team member. 4.1f Evaluate research.
4	4.2 Integrate best evidence into nursing practice.	4.2b Evaluate appropriateness and strength of the evidence. 4.2c Use best evidence in practice.
7	7.3 Optimize system effectiveness through application of innovation and evidence-based practice.	7.3a Demonstrate a systematic approach for decision-making.

CHAPTER 6 Critically Appraising Qualitative Evidence

Domain	Competency	Sub-Competency
1	1.2 Apply theory and research-based knowledge from nursing, the arts, humanities, and other sciences.	1.2d Examine the influence of personal values in decision-making for nursing practice.
4	4.1 Advance the scholarship of nursing.	4.1b Demonstrate application of different levels of evidence. 4.1d Demonstrate an understanding of basic elements of the research process. 4.1e Participate in scholarly inquiry as a team member. 4.1f Evaluate research.
4	4.2 Integrate best evidence into nursing practice.	4.2b Evaluate appropriateness and strength of the evidence. 4.2c Use best evidence in practice.
7	7.3 Optimize system effectiveness through application of innovation and evidence-based practice.	7.3a Demonstrate a systematic approach for decision-making.

CHAPTER 7 Appraising Other Types of Evidence to Inform Best Practices

Domain	Competency	Sub-Competency
1	1.3 Demonstrate clinical judgment founded on a broad knowledge base.	1.3b Integrate nursing knowledge (theories, multiple ways of knowing, evidence) and knowledge from other disciplines and inquiry to inform clinical judgment.
4	4.1 Advance the scholarship of nursing.	4.1b Demonstrate application of different levels of evidence. 4.1d Demonstrate an understanding of basic elements of the research process. 4.1e Participate in scholarly inquiry as a team member. 4.1f Evaluate research.
4	4.2 Integrate best evidence into nursing practice.	4.2b Evaluate appropriateness and strength of the evidence. 4.2c Use best evidence in practice.
7	7.3 Optimize system effectiveness through application of innovation and evidence-based practice.	7.3a Demonstrate a systematic approach for decision-making.

CHAPTER 8 Patient Preferences and Values

Domain	Competency	Sub-Competency
1	1.2 Apply theory and research-based knowledge from nursing the arts, humanities, and other sciences.	1.2b Demonstrate intellectual curiosity. 1.2c Demonstrate social responsibility as a global citizen who fosters the attainment of health equity for all. 1.2e Demonstrate ethical decision-making.
2	2.1 Engage with the individual in establishing a caring relationship.	2.1c Establish mutual respect with the individual and family.
2	2.5 Develop a plan of care.	2.5a Engage the individual and the team in plan development. 2.5b Organize care based on mutual care goals. 2.5c Prioritize care based on best evidence. 2.5d Incorporate evidence-based intervention to improve outcomes and safety. 2.5g Address individuals' perspectives in designing plans of care.
4	4.2 Integrate best evidence into nursing practice.	4.2c Use best evidence in practice.
9	9.1 Demonstrate an ethical comportment of one's practice reflective of nursing's mission to society.	9.1g Advocate to the individual's right to self-determination.
9	9.2 Employ participatory approach to nursing care.	9.2e Demonstrate cultural sensitivity and humility in practice.

CHAPTER 9 Fundamentals of Quality Improvement for Nurses

Domain	Competency	Sub-Competency
5	5.1 Apply quality improvement principles in care delivery.	5.1a Recognize nursing's essential role in improving healthcare quality and safety. 5.1b Identify sources and applications of national safety and quality standards to guide nursing practice. 5.1c Implement standardized evidence-based processes for care delivery. 5.1d Interpret benchmark and unit outcome data to inform individual and microsystem practice. 5.1e Compare quality improvement methods in the delivery of patient care. 5.1f Identify strategies to improve outcomes of patient care in practice. 5.1h Develop a plan for monitoring quality improvement change.

(Continued)

6	Perform effectively in different team roles, using principles and values of team dynamics.	6.2a Apply principles of team dynamics, including team roles, to facilitate effective team functioning. 6.2c Engage in the work of the team as appropriate to one's scope of practice and competency. 6.2e Apply principles of team leadership and management to improve quality and assure safety. 6.2f Evaluate performance of individual and team to improve quality and promote safety.
7	7.1 Apply knowledge of systems to work effectively across the continuum of care.	7.1d Recognize internal and external system processes that impact care coordination and transition of care.
7	7.3 Optimize system effectiveness through application of innovation and evidence-based practice.	7.3a Demonstrate a systematic approach for decision-making. 7.3b Use reported performance metrics to compare/monitor outcomes.

CHAPTER 10 The Nurse's Role in Implementation of EBPQI Initiatives

Domain	Competency	Sub-Competency
1	1.3 Demonstrate clinical judgment founded on a broad knowledge base.	1.3a Demonstrate clinical reasoning. 1.3b Integrate nursing knowledge (theories, multiple ways of knowing, evidence) and knowledge from other disciplines and inquiry to inform clinical judgment. 1.3c Incorporate knowledge from nursing and other disciplines to support clinical judgment.
2	2.6 Demonstrate accountability for care delivery.	2.6a Implement individualized plan of care using established protocols. 2.6d Monitor the implementation of the plan of care.
4	4.2 Integrate best evidence into nursing practice.	4.2c Use best evidence in practice. 4.2d Participate in the implementation of a practice change to improve nursing care.
4	4.3 Promote the ethical conduct of scholarly activities.	4.3a Explain the rationale for ethical research guidelines, including Institutional Review Board (IRB) guidelines. 4.3b Demonstrate ethical behaviors in scholarly projects, including quality improvement and EBP initiatives. 4.3c Advocate for the protection of participants in the conduct of scholarly activities. 4.3d Recognize the impact of equity issues in research.

5	5. Apply quality improvement principles in care delivery.	5.1c Implement standardized evidence-based processes for care delivery. 5.1g Participate in the implementation of a practice change.
6	Perform effectively in different team roles, using principles and values of team dynamics.	6.2a Apply principles of team dynamics, including team roles, to facilitate effective team functioning. 6.2c Engage in the work of the team as appropriate to one's scope of practice and competency.

CHAPTER 11 Evaluating the Impact of Evidence-Based Practice and Quality Improvement

Domain	Competency	Sub-Competency
2	2.6 Demonstrate accountability for plan of care.	2.6d Monitor the implementation of the plan of care.
2	2.7 Evaluate outcomes of care.	2.7a Reassess the individual to evaluate health outcomes/goals. 2.7b Modify plan of care as needed. 2.7c Recognize the need for modifications to standard practice.
3	3.4 Advance equitable population health policy.	3.4c Identify best evidence to support policy development. 3.4d Propose modifications to or development of policy based on population findings.
4	4.2 Integrate best evidence into nursing practice.	4.2d Participate in the evaluation of outcomes and their implications for practice.
5	5. Apply quality improvement principles in care delivery.	5.1d Interpret benchmark and unit outcome data to inform individual and microsystem practice. 5.1f Identify strategies to improve outcomes in patient care in practice.
6	6.2 Perform effectively in different team roles, using principles and values of team dynamics.	6.2f Evaluate performance of individual and team to improve quality and promote safety.
7	7.3 Optimize system effectiveness through application of innovation and evidence-based practice.	7.3b Use reported performance metrics to compare/monitor outcomes. 7.3c Participate in evaluating system effectiveness.

CHAPTER 12 The Nurse's Responsibility to Ensure Dissemination

Domain	Competency	Sub-Competency
2	2.2 Communicate effectively with individuals.	2.2c Use a variety of communication modes appropriate for the context. 2.2e Use evidence-based patient teaching materials, considering health literacy, vision, hearing, and cultural sensitivity.
3	3.4 Advance equitable population health policy.	3.4d Propose modifications to or development of policy based on population findings.
3	3.5 Demonstrate advocacy strategies.	3.5d Implement messaging strategies appropriate to audience and stakeholders.
4	4.1 Advance the scholarship of nursing.	4.1g Communicate scholarly findings.
8	8.4 Use information and communication technology to support documentation of care and communication among providers, patients, and all system levels.	8.4d Explain the impact of health information exchange, interoperability, and integration on healthcare.

CHAPTER 13 What Stories Will You Tell? Lifelong Learning and Legacy Building

Domain	Competency	Sub-Competency
9	9.5 Demonstrate the professional identity of nursing.	9.5a Describe nursing's professional identity and contributions to the healthcare team. 9.5b Demonstrate the core values of professional nursing identity. 9.5c Demonstrate emotional intelligence.
10	10.1 Demonstrate a commitment to personal health and well-being.	10.1a Demonstrate healthy, self-care behaviors that promote wellness and resiliency.
10	10.2 Demonstrate a spirit of inquiry that fosters flexibility and professional maturity.	10.2a Engage in guided and spontaneous reflection of one's practice. 10.2b Integrate comprehensive feedback to improve one's practice. 10.2c Commit to personal and professional development. 10.2d Expand personal knowledge to inform clinical practice. 10.2e Identify role models and mentors to support professional growth.

Appendix B: Evidence-Based Personal Improvement Plan (EBPIP)

Looking beyond engagement with the evidence-based wellness activities included at the end of each chapter, we encourage you to consider addressing challenging areas of your personal life by creating a customizable, evidence-based improvement plan of your own. As nurses and people, we can personalize evidence-based recommendations anecdotally and then track our progress toward health and wellness improvements. An evidence-based personal improvement plan (EBPIP) uses many but not all of the steps of EBP:

1. Identify the problem.
2. Search for evidence.
3. Develop a plan.
4. Implement.
5. Evaluate.

To help you identify the problem and search the evidence, we adapted the PPCO question (below). Rather than stand for population, the second "P" in PPCO stands for "person" when used for the purpose of EBPIP, and that person is a special individual and future nurse ... you!

Here we offer two of our own EBPIP examples in hopes that sharing them will help you on your own wellness journey.

Julee: Emotional Wellness

1. Person: Me (Julee)

   Problem: Feelings of anger and fear that were expressed in my relationships with a quick temper, hurtful outbursts, and arguing.

   My husband of 43 years was terminally ill and bedbound. I resented him leaving me with all the responsibilities of life, my jobs, our home, and our family and his expectation that because I was a nurse, being his primary caregiver shouldn't be a problem for me.
2. Search the evidence: For anger and fear (problem), what interventions (change) can impact emotional balance (outcome)? The top evidence-based practices that improve emotional balance were:

   a. Exercise
   b. Mindfulness
   c. Behavioral therapy (pet therapy)

I already went on a daily run with my German Shepherd (exercise and pet therapy), but I needed more. I had practiced yoga for 30 years, and right as my husband's illness worsened, I received an email from the yoga nurse, Annette Tersinghi, RN. Ten years ago I had participated in her course "The Yoga Nurse Essentials" and now she was offering a yoga nurse teacher training (https://yoganurse.mykajabi.com). As a certified yoga teacher, I just knew this was something I needed to do. I began to explore the evidence-based practices of yoga postures (asanas) and breathing (pranayama) that could support me in this phase of life (Pascoe et al., 2017; Zolotow, 2022).

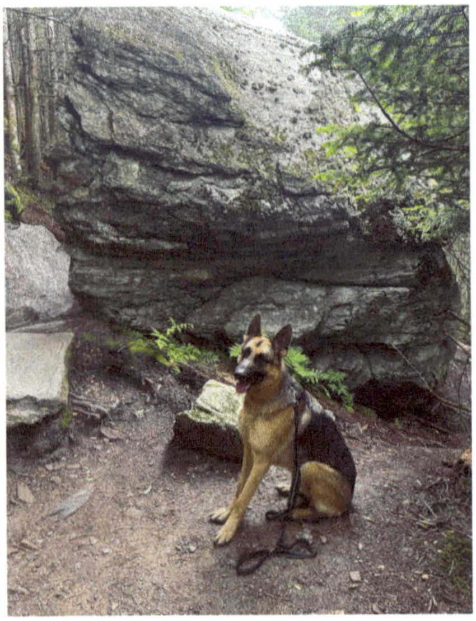

Image B.1

3. Plan: Daily intention of meditation with a mantra.
4. Implementation: I developed an intention every morning that I would return to throughout the day whenever feelings of resentment and anger threatened to overwhelm me.
5. Evaluate: It helped right away and continues to help decrease my hurtful outbursts and increase my feelings of acceptance, compassion, and patience for myself and others.

Jayne: Mental Fatigue and Stress

1. Person: Me (Jayne).

   Problem: Fatigue and feelings of overwhelm. I had increasingly started my day in a hurried manner (upon awakening). This was compounded by my life phase as a wife and mother of young children. I believed the compelling evidence endorsing getting enough sleep each night, and as my sleep decreased, my productivity and creativity began to drop. So, I often stayed up later than normal to complete my work after my family was asleep, which resulted in my oversleeping and then rushing and repeating this cycle. I also noticed that when I woke up later without any time for solitude, I had difficulty prioritizing my daily tasks to align with my values. I sought wise counsel about this problem and simultaneously searched the evidence for a potential solution(s).
2. Search the evidence: What interventions or changes were used to mitigate these issues?

   a. Sleep routine/consistency (Herzog-Krzywoszanska et al., 2021; Chaput et al., 2020)
   b. Meditation/intentionality (Davidson & Kennedy, 2004; Goyal et al., 2014)

3. Plan: (1) Consistent sleep routine and (2) daily meditation/prayer upon awakening each morning

4. Implementation: (1) Go to bed 1 hour earlier consistently and set an alarm to wake up 1 hour earlier before my children were awake; (2) upon awakening, for the first minutes I would breathe deeply while meditating/praying and set my intention for the day ahead.
5. Evaluate: Problem improvement was immediate and has been sustained for several months.

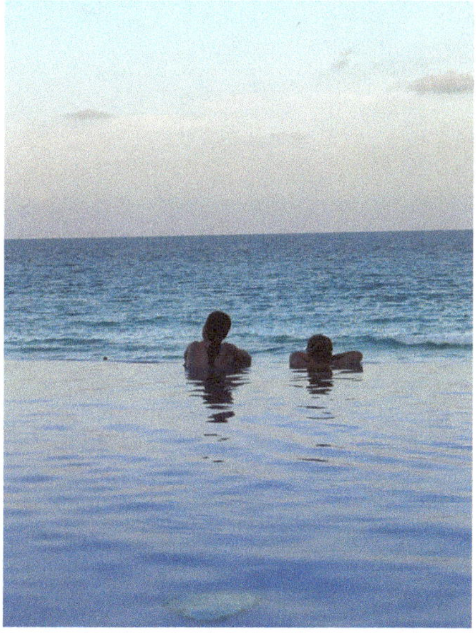

Image B.2

Through implementing this plan, I have learned that I require consistent, earlier sleep, and morning wakeups for quiet time before my children are awake to set my daily intention. If I am not intentional with these habits, I have trouble sustaining focused energy and productively throughout the day. These scheduled practices also help connect me to my purpose and values and enable me to tend to my family's needs at bedtime, often when the kids seek parental help from my husband and I as they process their own daily feelings and challenges. No matter what chaos and setbacks occur throughout the day, I have found that greater peace, calm, and emotional availability is experienced when I have been intentional about rest and those very first, powerful moments of the day. Here is a photo of my children watching a recent sunset. I was grateful to remain present in this moment with them—rested and refreshed after a full day.

REFERENCES

Chaput, J. P., Dutil, C., Featherstone, R., Ross, R., Giangregorio, L., Saunders, T. J., Janssen, I., Poitras, V. J., Kho, M. E., Ross-White, A., Zankar, S., & Carrier, J. (2020). Sleep timing, sleep consistency, and health in adults: A systematic review. *Applied Physiology, Nutrition, and Metabolism*, *45*(10 (Suppl. 2)), S232–S247. https://doi.org/10.1139/apnm-2020-0032

Davidson, R. J., & Kennedy, J. F. (2004). Alterations in brain and immune function produced by mindfulness meditation. *Psychosomatic Medicine, 66*(4), 564–570.

Goyal, M., Singh, S., Sibinga, E. M., Gould, N. F., Rowland-Seymour, A., Sharma, R., ... Haythornthwaite, J. A. (2014). Meditation programs for psychological stress and well-being: A systematic review and meta-analysis. *JAMA Internal Medicine, 174*(3), 357–368.

Herzog-Krzywoszanska, R., Jewula, B., & Krzywoszanski, L. (2021). Bedtime procrastination partially mediates the impact of personality characteristics on daytime fatigue resulting from sleep deficiency. *Frontiers in Neuroscience, 15*, Article 727440. https://doi.org/10.3389/fnins.2021.727440

Pascoe, M. C., Thompson, D. R., & Ski, C. F. (2017). Yoga, mindfulness-based reduction and stress-related physiological measures: A meta-analysis. *Pschoneuroendocrinology, 86*, 152–168.

Zolotow, N. (2022). *Yoga for times of change: Practices and meditations for moving through stress, anxiety, grief, and life's transitions*. Shambala.

Appendix C: Critical Appraisal Tools

As you learned throughout Chapters 5–7, critically appraising the evidence is a critical step in EBPQI. Remember that critical appraisal involves assessing the quality and strength of evidence. We use checklists because they enable us to do things in a systematic way and remind us to be diligent in all the critical aspects of the process. The information included in this appendix will provide you with a stepwise approach to guide you through examples of critically appraising three research studies and one quality improvement report. These tools are freely available to you, and you can access them on your own through the weblinks provided. We hope these examples facilitate your quest for competency as an EBPQI team member.

How to Use the Critical Appraisal Skills Programme (CASP) Checklist for Systematic Reviews (SR)

Step 1. Download a copy of the fillable document from the CASP website.

https://casp-uk.net/checklists/casp-systematic-review-checklist-fillable.pdf

Step 2. Have a copy of this article as the reference example we will use.

Chang, S. J., Lee, J., An, H., Hong, W., & Lee, J. Y. (2020). Animal-assisted therapy as an intervention for older adults: A systematic review and meta-analysis to guide evidence-based practice. *Worldviews on Evidence-Based Nursing*, *18*(1), 1–70. https://doi.org/10.1111/wvn.12484

Step 3. Read the article and answer the questions.

The CASP checklist includes 10 (sometimes multicomponent) questions to help you make sense of an SR. There are instructions within the checklist that this example will help you interpret.

The three big questions that you want to answer when critically appraising any piece of evidence are generally the same, and the questions in sections A, B, and C of the CASP checklist for SR help you answer them. Most of the questions (except 7, which asks about precision) are answered with a *Yes*, *Can't Tell*, or *No*, but the real appraisal information that will help you remember why you answered the way you did should be placed in the comments box. After reading the article, see if you agree with what we put in the boxes.

Section A

Are the results valid?

Validity is appraised based on the study designs and has to do with how the study was conducted.

Section B

What are the results?

Results are the actual outcomes of the study based on the data collected in this study.

Section C

Will the results help locally?

Only you can determine if the results be applied to the patients you care for in your setting.

Section A

Question 1—Answer: Yes

Comments:

This study was guided by the PICOS framework.

P - Older Adults

I - Animal Assisted Therapy

C - Other therapies

O - Health outcomes, including behavioral, psychosocial, cognitive, and physiological

Purpose: To 1) explore this literature on AAT as applied to older adults, 2) analyze the effects of ATT on health outcomes, including behavioral, psychosocial, cognitive, and physiological variables, and 3) provide evidence for future interventions.

Question 2—Answer: Yes

Comments:

Inclusion criteria:

People aged 60 and older

Interventions using animals for interventions

Other therapies

Behavioral, psychosocial, cognitive, physiological outcomes

The authors included only RCTs and high-quality quasi-experimental studies.

Question 3—Answer: Yes

Comments:

Yes, the authors used the PRISMA as a guide. They searched 7 databases. They began with 5,520 studies and removed duplicates and used inclusion / exclusion criteria to include 47 studies.

Question 4—Answer: Yes

Comments:

Joanna Briggs appraisal tools were used. An inter-rater reliability was also calculated at .95.

Based on the appraisal tools, the level of evidence could be considered moderate.

Question 5—Answer: Yes
Comments:

While the studies presented many diverse outcomes withing the "health outcome" categories, there were enough studies who reported on depression as an outcome to perform a meta-analysis of effect size.

Section B

Question 6—Answer: Yes
Comments:

The results demonstrated that AAT therapy, no matter the intervention dose, animal, or intensity, was associated with improved health outcomes.
The meta-statistic for effect size, the standardized mean differences (SMD) was -1.310 / CI [-1.900,-.721] $p < .001$

Question 7—Answer: Yes
Comments:

The CI is relatively narrow, indicating that all studies demonstrated an improvement in depression scores.

Section C

Question 8—Answer: Yes
Comments:

If the local population is persons older than 60 - yes!
It is recommended that trained therapy dogs be used for patient and animal safety.

Question 9—Answer: Can't Tell
Comments:

All the outcomes that were planned were considered.
An outcome that included harms would have been helpful to determine risk in clinical practice.
An outcome related to cost and resource use would also be helpful for those who might want to initiate an AAT program.

Question 10—Answer: Yes
Comments:

While no harms or costs were included in this review, it appears that the strong positive health outcomes would be worthwhile.

Note: This tool does not have a scoring system or a validated benchmark of what constitutes a poor, moderate, or high-quality report. But I think you can see from the fact that 9 of the 10 questions were answered with "met" that it is safe to say that this is a systematic review of solid quality and could be included in evidence to support an EBPQI that used animal-assisted therapy with older adults.

How to Use the Critical Appraisal Skills Programme (CASP) Checklist for Randomised Controlled Trials

Step 1. Download a copy of the fillable document from the CASP website.

https://casp-uk.net/checklists/casp-rct-randomised-controlled-trial-ch

Step 2. Have a copy of this article as the reference example we will use.

Yan, H., Du, Y. X., Wu, F. Q., Lu, X. Y., Chen, R. M., & Zhang, Y. (2022). Effects of nurse-led multidisciplinary team management on cardiovascular hospitalization and quality of life in patients with atrial fibrillation: Randomized controlled trial. *International Journal of Nursing Studies*, *127*, 104159. https://doi.org/10.1016/j.ijnurstu.2021.104159

Step 3. Read the article and answer the questions.

This CASP checklist includes 11 (sometimes multicomponent) questions to help you appraise an RCT. There are instructions within the checklist that this example will help you interpret.

The three big questions that you want to answer when critically appraising any piece of evidence are generally the same, and the questions in sections A, B, C, and D of the CASP checklist for RCT help you answer them. Most of the questions are answered with a *Yes*, *Can't Tell*, or *No*, but the real appraisal information that will help you remember why you answered the way you did should be placed somewhere in the answer box. After reading the article, see if you agree with what we put in the boxes.

Section A

Is the study valid?

Validity is appraised based on the study design and has to do with how the study was developed.

Section B

Was the study method sound?

The study method should always be guided by and appropriate for the research question.

Section C

What are the results?

Results are the actual outcomes of the study based on the data collected in this study.

Section D

Will the results help locally?

Only you can determine if the results be applied to the patients you care for in your setting.

Let's Go!

Section A

Question 1—Answer: Yes

Comments:

The population is patients hospitalized with atrial fibrillation.
The intervention is nurse-led interdisciplinary team.
The comparator is usual care.
The outcomes are cardiovascular hospitalizations, death, and quality of life.

Question 2—Answer: Yes

Comments:

Computer generated random sequence upon admission to either unit 1 or 2 by personnel who were not aware of the allocation nor took part in the study.

Question 3—Answer: Yes

Comments:

All participants were accounted for in the CONSORT diagram in Figure 1.
An intention to treat analysis was done on participants per assigned groups.
There were no compelling reasons to stop the study early (adverse events or treatment effects).

Section B

Question 4—Answer: No

Comments:

Two of three components in this question were not met. It is difficult to blind an intervention where there is significant interventionist contact. Participants would likely be able to determine which group they were in, if not early in the hospital, then during follow up. Similarly, it is virtually impossible to blind such an intervention from those who are involved in its delivery. Two independent researchers who were unaware of the allocation did collect and analyze the data.

Question 5—Answer: Yes
Comments:

Yes, in Table 1 baseline characteristics between the groups are presented with only one significant difference between groups. The control group had more persons with hypertension.

This could possibly affect the outcome of cardiovascular hospitalizations and death, and it was not discussed or presented as a limitation.

Question 6—Answer: Yes
Comments:

The components of the interdisciplinary intervention were clearly described, and follow up intervals were the same for each group at 1, 3, 6, and 12 months.

Section C

Question 7—Answer: Yes
Comments:

A power analysis was done. There were 110 patients in each group using a 2 tailed alpha of 0.05 and a power of 0.80. Absolute values N (%) were reported (e.g., hospitalized or died = yes/no). Results were reported for each outcome at each follow up and there was no missing or incomplete data used. There were no significant differences in drop out between groups.

Potential sources of bias were not being able to blind the intervention and having contamination between groups in the different units. In hindsight, it was felt a crossover design may have been better. Chi Square analysis was reported using p values (see Table 2).

Question 8—Answer: Yes
Comments:

Precision was reported with p values but not confidence intervals.

Question 9—Answer: No
Comments:

The intervention produced statistically significant results in the primary outcome of hospitalizations (but not deaths) and in the secondary outcome of QOL. No harms were reported, but COVID may have impacted the final study time period.

There was no cost-effectiveness analysis, and it was reported as a limitation.

Section D

Question 10—Answer: Only you can determine this based on the patients you care for.

Question 11—Answer: Only you can answer based on your organization setting.

Appraisal Summary:
This is a resource-intensive intervention despite that not being taken into consideration by the researchers. It may or may not be feasible depending on the type of healthcare delivery system in your country and your organization. However, it is important to know what does work and that nurses can be leaders of interdisciplinary teams to reduce costly rehospitalizations and improve quality of life for patients with AF.

Note: This tool does not have a scoring system or a validated benchmark of what constitutes a poor, moderate, or high-quality report. In this case, there were *No* answers to two of the nine questions without knowing your answer to questions 10 and 11. This RCT is probably of solid quality and could be included in a synthesis of evidence to support an EBPQI initiative that puts nurses as leaders of care teams.

How to Use the Critical Appraisal Skills Programme (CASP) Checklist for Qualitative Research

Step 1. Download a copy of the fillable document from the CASP website.

https://casp-uk.net/checklists/casp-qualitative-studies-checklist-fillable.pdf

Step 2. Have a copy of this article as the reference example we will use.

Holmes, T., Vifladt, A., & Ballangrud, R. (2019). A qualitative study of how inter-professional teamwork influences perioperative nursing. *Nursing Open*, 7(2), 571–580. https://doi.org/10.1002/nop2.422

Step 3. Read the article and answer the questions.

This CASP checklist includes 10 (sometimes multicomponent) questions to help you appraise a qualitative research study. There are instructions within the checklist that this example will help you interpret.

The three big questions that you want to answer when critically appraising any piece of evidence are generally the same, and the questions in sections A, B, and C of the CASP checklist for a qualitative study help you answer them. All but the last question are answered with a *Yes*, *Can't Tell*, or *No*, but the real appraisal information that will help you remember why you answered the way you did should be placed in the comments box. After reading the article, see if you agree with what we put in the boxes.

Section A

Are the results valid?

> Validity is appraised based on the study design and has to do with how the study was developed. In qualitative research if the design is not appropriate to address the purpose of the study, then it may not be worth continuing your appraisal.

Section B
What are the results?

Results are the actual outcomes of the study based on the data collected in this study.

Section C
Will the results help locally?

Only you can determine if the results be applied to the patients you care for in your setting.

Let's Go!

Section A

Question 1—Answer: Yes
Comments:

The aim of this study was to explore Norwegian OR nurses' perceptions of how team skills in the interprofessional OR team influence perioperative nursing in relation to patient safety.

Question 2—Answer: Yes
Comments:

Qualitative descriptive using interviews. The design is appropriate because there are mostly quantitative studies on the OR team and few focusing on OR nurses' team skills and their perception of teamwork in the OR.

Question 3—Answer: Yes
Comments:

Yes, to explore perceptions of OR nurses, interviewing them is appropriate.

Section B

Question 4—Answer: No
Comments:

A convenience sample of 10 OR nurses at one organization were recruited via an invitation letter distributed by email from their nurse managers.

Question 5—Answer: Yes
Comments:

Yes, it was collected via individual interviews with a semi-structured interview guide based on TeamSTEPPS framework.
The same person conducted all interviews. The interviews were audio-recorded, and field notes were made.
There was no discussion of saturation of data.
The interview guide was included as an Appendix to the article.

Question 6—Answer: No
Comments:

The researchers did not examine the potential bias their role or life experience might have on the conduct of the study or the interpretation of the results. They did note in the limitations that the sample recruitment process and the sample size may have introduced bias.

Section B

Question 7—Answer: Yes
Comments:

Yes, this study was approved by the ethics committee and informed consent occurred. Interviews were conducted in a private space and data was anonymized.

Question 8—Answer: Yes
Comments:

But not as rigorous as it could have been. Examples were given and a description of the analysis process. However, again, the researcher analyzing the data did not reflect on their own role and potential bias or influence this might have. The data was also coded by only one author.

Question 9—Answer: No
Comments:

Findings were developed into clear themes with subthemes which were clearly supported by example quotes. Discussion presented the results in the context of prior studies and identified areas for application and future research.

Section C

Question 10—Answer: Only you can determine this based on the patients you care for.

Note: This tool does not have a scoring system or a validated benchmark of what constitutes a poor, moderate, or high-quality report. In this case, there were *No* answers to two of the nine questions and the answer to question 10 is up to you. However, in general, this study describes findings that need further validation but that may contribute to practice now. For example, the low confidence operating room nurses have in leading the team can be bolstered with further education and skills. Depending on how similar your population and setting are, you may or may not decide to include this study as evidence that supports a proposed EBPQI initiative.

How to Use the Quality Improvement Minimum Quality Criteria Set (QI-MQCS)

Step 1. Download a copy of Appendix 1 (the QI-MQCS Form) from this reference.

https://doi.org/10.1136/bmjqs-2014-003151

Hempel, S., Shekelle, P. G., Liu, J. L., Sherwood Danz, M., Foy, R., Lim, Y. W., Motala, A., & Rubenstein, L. V. (2015). Development of the Quality Improvement Minimum Quality Criteria Set (QI-MQCS): A tool for critical appraisal of quality improvement intervention publications. *BMJ Quality & Safety*, *24*(12), 796–804. https://doi.org/10.1136/bmjqs-2014-003151

Step 2. Have a copy of this article as the reference example we will use.

Kulesa, J. T., Tyris, J. N., McQuiston-Lane, K., Herstek, J., & Rush, M. L. (2023). Increasing nurse-physician family-centered rounds communication: A quality improvement pilot project. *Journal of Nursing Care Quality*, *38*(4), 304–311. https://doi.org/10.1097/NCQ.0000000000000701

Step 3. Read the article and answer the questions.

The QI-MQCS includes 16 Domains to assess to determine the quality of a QI report. There are instructions within the checklist (and a 17-page guide) that this example will help you interpret.

All domains are appraised with a *Met* or *Not Met*. The domain AND a minimum standard are described, and I find it helpful to add notes to support the minimum standard. This will help you remember why you answered the way you did. You can place your comments in either box, keeping them visible for quick review if needed. After reading the article, see if you agree with what we put in the boxes.

Let's Go!

Top Section
Fill in the blanks if they are appropriate for the critical appraisal process you are using. It is helpful to always determine and document what the intervention is and what the outcomes are.

Intervention:
1. Senior residents determined rounding order with a pre-Family Centered Rounds (FCR) huddle and sent text messages to nurses via RoundAbout before their patient's FCR started.
2. Standardized FCR summary at the end of each patient's FCR.
3. Sent standardized FCR summary to nurses unable to attend FCR.

Outcome:
1. Increase nurses' perceived awareness of the three components of the shared mental model (medical problems, escalation parameters, and the plan of care for the day),
2. Increase nurse attendance at FCR,
3. Evaluate resident physicians' compliance with completing FCR summaries, and
4. Evaluate the average time spent per FCR encounter.

Domain 1—Answer: Met
Organizational Motivation: One motivating factor - nurses' attendance at FCRs was often declined.

Domain 2—Answer: Met
Intervention Rationale: Rationale - Nurses not being present impacts nurse-physician communication negatively (evidence reviewed in introduction).

Domain 3—Answer: Met
Intervention Description: At least one specific change is described with who executes it (in this case, it is the same as the interventions listed in the top section).

See PDSA cycle interventions:
1. Senior residents determined rounding order with a pre-Family Centered Rounds (FCR) huddle and sent text messages to nurses via RoundAbout before their patient's FCR started.
2. Senior Residents completed standardized FCR summary at the end of each patient's FCR.
3. Senior Residents sent standardized FCR summary to nurses unable to attend FCR.

Domain 4—Answer: Met
Organizational Characteristics: Examples of at least two organizational characteristics.
Academic urban freestanding children's hospital, three academic rounding teams (can be found in setting and stakeholders' section).

Domain 5—Answer: Met

Implementation: At least one approach is used.
Pilot testing and PDSA cycles, all stakeholders are involved.

Domain 6—Answer: Met

Study Design: Named as Pilot QI that used the IHI PDSA cycles.

Domain 7—Answer: Met

Comparator: Compared to at least one standard before the practice change.
Nurse attendance at FCR.

Domain 8—Answer: Met

Data Sources: Surveys of nurses were used to measure awareness (Aim 1) and a checklist for physicians to document time in FCR and nurse attendance (Aims 2 and 3).

Domain 9—Answer: Met

Timing: Of intervention, follow up, and evaluation.
Data was collected five times during two weeks for three separate teams and included test of change for three PDSA cycles.

Domain 10—Answer: Met

Adherence/Fidelity: Compliance to intervention. Process measure was the resident summaries completion and nurse attendance at FCR.

Domain 11—Answer: Not Met

Health Outcomes: This project focused on systems change and provider/nurse behaviors.

Domain 12—Answer: Met

Organizational Readiness: Reports organizational barrier or facilitator.
Reported three specific barriers to communication (see identifying communication problems section).

1. Residents not determining a rounding order
2. Residents not sending a notification to nurses about FCR
3. Nurses faced with conflicting patient care demands at time of FCR

Domain 13—Answer: Not Met

Penetration: Proportion of participation.
Three teams were a pilot but not reported what percentage this is of the total number of teams in the organization.

Domain 14—Answer: Met

Sustainability or Potential for Sustainability:
Any hospital with a text system and nursing alert systems integrated with the EMR. More evaluation is needed to determine impact on patient safety or outcomes.

Domain 15—Answer: Met

Spread: Reported potential for other hospitals with nursing alert systems to integrate with the EMR to adapt the practice change.

Domain 16—Answer: Met

Limitations: At least one related to design/evaluation.
Lack of access to RoundAbout usage information.

Note: This tool does not have a scoring system or a validated benchmark of what constitutes a poor, moderate, or high-quality report. But we think you can see from the fact that 14 of 16 of the domains are met that it is safe to say that this is a pilot EBPQI with solid quality and could be included in evidence to support improvement in nurse-physician communication.

Index

About the Editors

Jayne Jennings Dunlap, DNP, APRN, FNP-C, CNE, EBP-C

Texas Woman's University, Associate Clinical Professor and Interim DNP Program Director

Baylor Scott and White Health, Family Nurse Practitioner

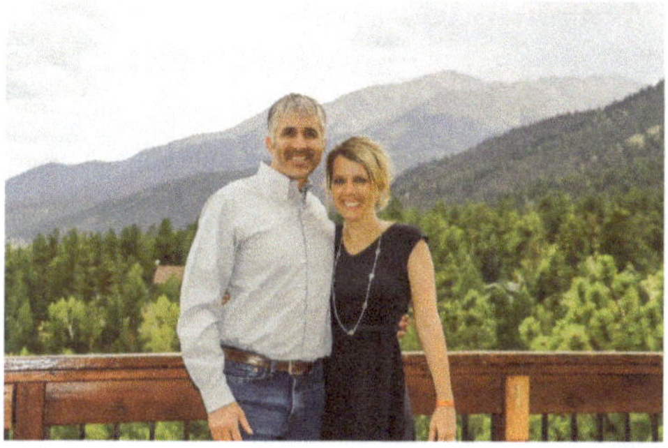

Image 0.1

My childhood dream was to become a singer. Healthcare careers seemed scary to me. I remember plugging my ears during situations I perceived as dangerous for others because I couldn't bear to hear suffering and not know how to respond. In high school, I became a certified lifeguard and discovered that I thrived on knowing how to help when someone needed to be rescued. I realized that my fear of physical suffering was really a fear of feeling helpless without the proper role or training. Once I'd figured this out, teaching swim lessons became meaningful work.

At my university, I was unsure whether I wanted to pursue a career in education or nursing, so I attended the freshman orientation at both colleges. My parents told me that I looked bored during the teaching orientation, but I appeared to come alive as the nursing instructors spoke. Nursing seemed dynamic to me then, and it still does. From my first nursing job in the neonatal intensive care unit to my current primary care nurse practitioner role, I have loved being on the frontline, serving patients and families. I live my calling by teaching tomorrow's nurses (like you) who represent our future.

Julee Briscoe Waldrop, DNP, PNP, FNP, CNE, EBP-C, FAANP, FAAN

Duke University, Professor and Assistant Dean, DNP Program

The Journal for Nurse Practitioners, Editor in Chief

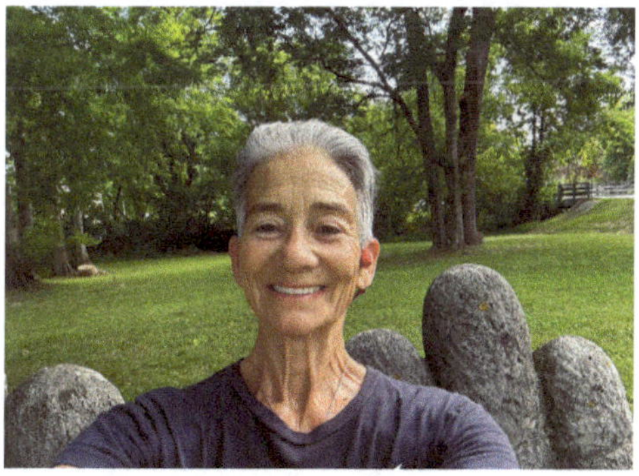

Image 0.2

I was an athlete in high school and college. I really did not consider any other possible career besides teacher and coach. These were the people who influenced me, so I earned my first degree in education with a physical education focus. Sadly, it was only during the final semester of the program, when I experienced student teaching, that I discovered how little teaching PE met my expectations and that it was not for me. After graduation, I embarked on a few years of discontent doing clerical and secretarial work, which did not pay very well. I was always looking for ways to make extra money. My husband had a fellowship at a major medical center, so the opportunity to be a subject in research studies for pay was often available. I gave blood, carried around 24-hour urine containers, and allowed tubes to be stuck in numerous places. It was through being a human research subject, however, that I met nurses for the first time, and they seemed to be really enjoying their work.

As a nurse, you never know when you are going to change someone's life, as those nurses did mine. Their great attitude motivated me to go back to school and earn my second undergraduate degree. This time, the fit was good, and with my Bachelor of Science in Nursing (BSN) in hand, I began my true career. I had my first child while in nursing school, which led me to specialize in the health of infants and mothers.

Image 0.1 Credit: Copyright © by Trail West Lodge, Young Life. Reprinted with permission.

About the Contributors

Christiana N. Acho, DNP, APRN, CNP, FNP-C

Assistant Clinical Professor & FNP Hybrid Track Coordinator, Texas Woman's University

Growing up in Africa, I had no opportunity to interact with nurses. People in my country of Nigeria believed you went to the hospital to die. There were no primary care clinics for minor ailments; most people sought treatment from herbalists. My father and an auntie were teachers, so my desire was to become a high school teacher. When I was a teenager, my older brother started medical school and interacted with nurses for the first time. He told me, "I think you will be a very good nurse because you're very caring," so I applied to a famous nursing school in my country. I was embarrassed during the interview because I knew nothing about nursing history. Oh, my goodness, I was asked about Florence Nightingale! I had overheard another candidate call her the "lady with the lamp," and that one fact was all I could offer as my answer. Given my interview, I was very surprised when I was admitted into the program with a full scholarship.

Knowledge cannot be taken from an individual. I have sought new learning opportunities throughout my nursing career. My childhood dream of becoming a teacher has been realized thanks to a profession I did not know existed when I was young. I have the joy of maintaining a clinical practice and teaching nurse practitioners who will light the way for patients in the future.

Francisco Javier Ayala, DNP, APRN, FNP-C

Assistant Clinical Professor, Texas Woman's University

I became a nurse by being exposed to nursing on a continual basis from a very young age. Suffering from a congenital heart disease, I was consistently in the hospital and had several surgical interventions as a child and adolescent. I interacted with many kind nurses, and one in particular who went above and beyond to make me feel comfortable and cared for inspired me and truly piqued my interest to pursue nursing as a career path.

Until I finished high school, the hospital always felt like my second home, so it was only natural that I felt comfortable and ended up pursuing the profession of nursing. Nursing has always been rewarding to me, and I have continued to advance in areas of interest. That is how I ended up in academia educating and exploring our profession further with our next generation of nurses.

Cynthia D. Beckett, PhD, RNC-OB, LCCE, LSS-BB, CHRC, EBP-C

Assistant Clinical Professor, The Ohio State University

Assistant Director–Academic Core, Helene Fuld Health Trust National Institute for Evidence-Based Practice in Nursing and Healthcare

When I was in high school, I wanted to be a physician. At 16, I became a nurse's aide and worked each summer at a critical access hospital in a small rural community until I started college. The nurses there were caring and compassionate; they knew that I wanted to pursue a career in healthcare, so they allowed me to accompany the charge nurse to the emergency room at night to "answer the bell." We would triage patients and determine which physician or surgeon needed to be called to address their needs. I was also allowed to go to the labor and delivery unit to help with deliveries and recoveries and to the postoperative recovery room to assist and learn.

I became aware of the many and varied roles that nurses play across a hospital and their profound impact on patient care and outcomes. Although I respected physicians and the importance of their role, I realized that nursing had caught my heart. Nursing is a career that offers role flexibility and opportunities across many specialties. I wanted to marry and have children, and nursing has allowed me to combine growth in my profession with being a wife and mother of three boys. It has been the best decision for me.

Tracy L. Brewer, DNP, RNC-OB, CLC, EBP-C

Clinical Professor & DNP Program Chair, University of Tennessee, Knoxville

I cannot remember a time when I did not want to be a nurse; it was my destiny! Every holiday, I would ask for the latest "nurse kit" on the market based on the best TV commercial evidence. I excelled in every advanced science course available in high school, although my performance in other academic subjects was average or below average. I grew up on a farm in a college town in rural Southwest Ohio, and I assumed I would attend the university in my hometown—until the dreaded ACT. I bombed the first time and did no better on my second try. My high school counselor told me that no college of nursing would ever accept me. I was attending a technical school for medical assisting when an instructor asked, "Why are you not going to college to become a nurse?" I explained, "I was told that I am not smart enough."

I am now a nurse with four college degrees, paying it forward to other students. I have faith that every one of them can succeed! My gratitude and respect for those who gave me a chance and pushed me to become the nurse and educator I am today is overwhelming. The moral of my story is clear: Never doubt that you can become and accomplish what you choose. No one else knows your destiny.

Niki Cobb, MSIS

Assistant Professor & Health Sciences Librarian, University of Tennessee, Knoxville

As a child, I was captivated by books. Their stories took root in my imagination and fostered a sense of discovery that has affected every aspect of my life. When I got older, I was determined to pursue my love of literature and learning on a professional level but could not decide whether to do so through teaching or librarianship. After exploring both pathways during my academic career, I can safely assert that librarianship chose me!

As a librarian, I am the type of educator I always wanted to be: a lifelong learner, teacher, navigator, and mentor. Information is everywhere, and being a librarian allows me to explore all the ways in which people can find, understand, and disseminate information as well as how interacting with it affects everyday lives. I connect people with the resources they need and with tools and services that they can use to conduct an informed search and locate information on their own. All the while, I'm learning from everything I do and everyone I encounter on my journey.

Kathleen Kistner Ellis, PhD, RN, CCRN-K, CNE

Nurse Scientist, Children's Health

As a child, I always wanted to be a teacher. I entered college as a music education major, intending to become a band director. While I loved my classes and made good grades, I began to feel that this wasn't the best fit for me. I'd grown up healthy, so my only images of nursing were brief interactions with my school nurse and images on television. The reasons that nursing appealed to me were similar to my interest in education—primarily working in a helping profession.

During college, I lost two friends to illness. This reinforced my need to do something meaningful and gave me new perspectives on health, illness, and loss. As I pursued nursing, I found the fit I'd been lacking. My desire to teach remained intact, just focused on another area. I resolved to be there for others in a way to honor my friends. Over the years, I've appreciated the sacred trust our profession holds: to support others, to be with them in times of immense joy and intense sadness, and to ensure that they receive evidence-based care.

Bradi B. Granger, PhD

Professor, Duke University School of Nursing, the Duke-Margolis Center for Health Policy

Director, Duke Heart Center Nursing Research Program

I became a nurse so I could work with patients and peers on scientific evidence to promote health and support new developments in health behaviors through nursing science. I began my nursing career in a cardiothoracic step-down unit in Charleston, West Virginia, in 1986 after graduating from the University of Tennessee. The following year I transferred to Duke University to attend graduate school and work as a critical care nurse, earning a master's degree from Duke in 1991 and a PhD from UNC–Chapel Hill in 2004. Currently, I serve as a clinical nurse specialist and director of the Heart Center Nursing Research program at Duke and core faculty at Duke Margolis Center for Health Policy.

Throughout my career, my passion to partner with patients and peers to advance nursing science has led me to grow the Heart Center Nursing Research program at Duke to serve and lead 23 staff nurse research studies and the International Study Buddies program, a program developed to mentor international nurses in developing research programs abroad. My career focus has been helping nurses think differently about their practice using a unit-based, team-centered model. My own research focuses on improving patients' health behaviors to reduce mortality and hospital readmissions and to implement strategies for safe care transitions across settings of care, from hospital to home and community-based settings. I feel fortunate to work with the patients and nurses who make each day worthwhile!

Melissa Marie Hessock, DNP, APRN, FNP-C, EBP(CH)

Clinical Assistant Professor, University of Tennessee, Knoxville

I was not called to nursing; rather, I was gently pushed toward it. Other than a short-lived interest in becoming a navy pilot the year I turned 16 (thanks to the movie *Top Gun*), I spent my youth wanting to become a veterinarian. My first year of college was hard. I was a pre-veterinary science major, 800 miles from home, and unready to commit to 8 more years of education.

I left the program and returned home, feeling a little lost and unsure of my future path. My mother suggested that I consider the nursing program at our local community college. Nursing presented good job opportunities and aligned with my interest in science and helping people. Without a better plan, I agreed, but I wasn't sure how I felt about taking care of humans!

On my first clinical day, I thought I had made the wrong career choice, but shortly afterwards, I observed a birth. As I watched the nurses seamlessly provide skilled care, quell fear, educate, and share the joy of new life, I realized the tremendous importance of their role. I understood what a privilege it is to be part of the best (and sometimes worst) days of a person's life. Many years, nursing degrees, and roles later, I continue to be humbled by the honor of providing exceptional evidence-based care to those who entrust me with their health.

Rosalie O. Mainous, PhD, APRN, FNAP, FAANP, FAAN

Dean and Warwick Professor, University of Kentucky

I was a 17-year-old who graduated from high school a year early and applied that December to attend Eastern Kentucky University in January. I had no major, no advising, and it was the last day of registration. I walked into the registration area, which was in the university gym, and was contemplating where to start when a woman approached me and said, "Honey, how would you like to be a nurse? I normally take 100 students into the class, and this is the last day of registration, and I have two slots left. I will give you one if you want it." Having always been spontaneous, somewhat of a risk taker, and looking for adventure, my response was "Sure!"

The next week I found myself in a pink uniform, on a bus traveling to a nursing home in Winchester, Kentucky, and a proud member of the Associate Degree Nursing program, class of December 1977. I never looked back. I had no idea when I agreed to sign up that there were even two different programs and that I was going into the associate degree program. Having done so, I have a unique and inclusive perspective of the many pathways into nursing and what we all bring to the table in our quest to improve the health of our patients, communities, and the nation.

Tracy McManaman-Bridges, EdD, MSN, RNC-OB, C-EFM, CNE

Assistant Clinical Professor, Texas Woman's University

When I was young, I would have said that I became a nurse because I wanted "to help people," but probably like most nursing students, I had little sense of what nursing practice really entailed. Nursing involves so much more than what most people imagine! The profession has evolved rapidly since I entered it almost 30 years ago, and I foresee its continued exponential growth in the future.

Looking back, my personal belief is that God led me to become a nurse, and I continue to consider nursing a divine calling. Today, with a fuller sense of what the profession entails and requires, I would answer the question a bit differently: I became a nurse to serve and mentor new nurses to accomplish great improvements in patient care and the nursing profession.

Staci S. Reynolds, PhD, RN, ACNS-BC, CCRN, CNRN, SCRN, CPHQ

Associate Professor, Duke University School of Nursing

Editor in Chief, *Journal of Nursing Care Quality*

When I was in junior high and high school, I was very interested in biology. I enjoyed biology classes so much that I took extra ones to learn as much as I could. I was a member of the Science Academic Super Bowl team, a highly competitive extracurricular science event designed to encourage students to enhance their research and study skills by delving into topics at a depth that could not be covered in a high school classroom. Upon graduation, I knew that I wanted to pursue a course that would involve further studies in biology. Nursing seemed a very practical option, as it included additional science classes and would allow me to make a significant, caring impact on patients and families.

Nursing also appeared to be a flexible field in which I could experience different roles. My perceptions of nursing were right on all counts! I have served as a staff nurse in the neuroscience ICU, clinical nurse specialist in neuroscience and infection prevention, faculty member, teacher, and researcher. I have thoroughly enjoyed each of these roles and appreciate being able to acquire and use so many different skill sets.

Elizabeth Walters, DNP, C-PNP

Assistant Director of Operations, Advanced Practice Initiatives and Certification Outreach, American Nurses Association

I decided to become a nurse because I was inspired by nurses when I volunteered in the emergency department while completing an undergraduate degree. I completed my undergraduate nursing program and took a new graduate position in the neonatal intensive care unit. While working in the NICU, I became passionate about improving outcomes for patients and families. I was fortunate to complete many quality improvement projects focused on improving outcomes for the patients I worked with. I changed roles throughout my nursing career from leadership positions to infection prevention. While working in infection prevention, I realized I missed patient care and decided to pursue graduate education and got my DNP and became a pediatric nurse practitioner. As a PNP, I work in the specialty of adolescent medicine. I value all of my experiences in caring for children and their families and continue to work to improve patient outcomes at a local, national, and international level.

Jennifer E. Wilson, DNP, RN, CPN

Clinical Professor & Nursing Honors Coordinator, Texas Woman's University

I came to nursing in a roundabout way. I was majoring in biology and had no desire to work in a lab with petri dishes. A biology of cancer course that tied cellular biology to the human experience convinced me that I wanted a career focused on people, but I wasn't certain which path to take. Although I had little knowledge of the nurse's role, I knew that I could get a job as a nurse until I devised a career plan. As a new graduate, I worked in pediatric oncology, caring for children who were fighting for life every day. That experience changed my perspective on life, and I fell in love with nursing.

I determined to expand my nursing knowledge and scope of practice. While I earned an MSN, I worked at National Institutes of Health as a clinical research nurse in the pediatric branch of the National Cancer Institute. Given my background in biology, I was acutely aware of the numerous people, wealth of expertise, and decades of research and preliminary work involved in the development of novel agents. As a nurse within this complex research continuum, I had exactly the kind of career role I had always hoped to find. Rather than working with cells in Petri dishes, I had the privilege of administering those therapies to children, sharing pivotal moments with them, and helping them on their journey, wherever it might lead.

Erin Elizabeth Whitaker, MA, MSIS

Assistant Professor & Student Success Librarian for Information Literacy, University of Tennessee, Knoxville

I always assumed that I would become a teacher. My father, two grandmothers, and a favorite aunt were teachers, so it made sense to me that I should become one. In college, I majored in English and went on to earn an MA in English. I considered earning a PhD but soon realized that although I enjoyed working with college students, the path toward becoming an English professor was not one I wished to follow. I knew that I didn't want to grade other people's ideas and writing. I decided to redirect my energies. I chose a new path based on the one basic thing of which I was certain: my love of books. I enrolled in an MSIS program. In library school, I came to the delightful realization that becoming an academic librarian would allow me to combine my love of books and enjoyment of teaching—without the need to grade! My teaching as a librarian differs somewhat from what professorial teaching would have entailed, and I love it. I help students every day to learn new ways of interacting with information.

Cindy G. Zellefrow, DNP MSEd RN CSN EBP-C

Assistant Clinical Professor, The Ohio State University College of Nursing

Director–Academic Core, Helene Fuld Health Trust National Institute for Evidence-Based Practice in Nursing and Healthcare

I've wanted to be a nurse since I was very little. My mom and two of my aunts were nurses, despite my tradition-minded, immigrant grandfather who insisted that his daughters would NEVER work with naked people. During World War II, my mother and her older sister went behind his back and signed a binding contract to join the Army Nurse Corps in return for a nursing education. These women were strong, smart, committed, and wonderfully adventuresome! Growing up, I loved hearing stories of their travels, adventures, and exciting work experiences. I wanted to be just like them, and I soon learned that determination was part of that goal. Initially, I found the foundational science courses in my BSN program so challenging that I changed my major to elementary education for one semester, but I quickly realized that I was a nurse at heart. I jumped back into the nursing program with new resolve and never looked back. I've been blessed to enjoy a career that has allowed me to transition from critical care to school nursing to nursing education. Like the women I so admired, I've traveled the world and worked with incredible people. The paycheck has been good, but the "paycheck of the heart" is priceless!

FSC
www.fsc.org
MIX
Papier | Fördert gute Waldnutzung
FSC® C083411

Zeitfracht Medien GmbH
Ferdinand-Jühlke-Straße 7
99095 Erfurt, Deutschland
produktsicherheit@kolibri360.de